Techniques of Stuttering Therapy

Richard Ham

The Florida State University, Tallahassee

Prentice-Hall, Inc., Englewood Cliffs, New Jersey 07632

Library of Congress Cataloging in Publication Data

HAM, RICHARD [date]
  Techniques of stuttering therapy.

  Bibliography: p.
  Includes index.
  1. Stuttering—Treatment. 2. Speech therapy.
  I. Title. [DNLM: 1. Speech Therapy—methods.
  2. Stuttering—therapy. WM 475 H196t]
  RC424.H23   1986   616.8'55406   85-9379
  ISBN 0-13-901844-1

Editorial/production supervision: *Edith Riker*
Cover design: *Wanda Lubelska*
Manufacturing buyer: *Barbara Kittle*

Printed in the United States of America

10 9 8 7 6 5 4 3 2

ISBN   0-13-901844-1   01

Prentice-Hall International (UK) Limited, *London*
Prentice-Hall of Australia Pty. Limited, *Sydney*
Prentice-Hall Canada Inc., *Toronto*
Prentice-Hall Hispanoamericana, S.A., *Mexico*
Prentice-Hall of India Private Limited, *New Delhi*
Prentice-Hall of Japan, Inc., *Tokyo*
Prentice-Hall of Southeast Asia Pte. Ltd., *Singapore*
Editora Prentice-Hall do Brasil, Ltda., *Rio de Janeiro*
Whitehall Books Limited, *Wellington, New Zealand*

CONTENTS

Preface and Dedication

This book was written to explain some of the many techniques that clinicians use in stuttering therapy. The orientation is toward specific skills and steps involved in various procedures rather than on overall programs or plans of therapy. It is an effort to fill a space between the ever-growing edifice of theory and research and the fluctuating patterns of different therapy programs. I hope that the clinician will use this book as a resource of methods and procedures, acquiring the same skills and the same experiences as do the clients.

This volume is a recognition of the clinician who has had the greatest and most enduring effect on me—**Charles Van Riper**. Stuttering therapy owes more to Van Riper than to any other clinician in our history. He has molded generations of clinicians, either to emulate his patterns or deliberately to contradict them. In our first meeting in 1952, he earnestly advised me to be skeptical of anything he said or wrote. In our second meeting, in 1952, we wound up in a barn where the "Wizard of Kalamazoo" was mending a harness. My time with him as a student, and the subsequent years of friendship and guidance, influenced my professional life. Superb teacher, demanding supervisor, amazing raconteur, and self-critical observer—he has enriched our profession and the lives of countless stutterers.

1

Considerations in Stuttering Therapy

INTRODUCTION

The background of stuttering therapy is ancient. Stuttering has plagued humanity for centuries, and undoubtedly therapy for stuttering has plagued us for almost the same length of time. Estimates of stuttering prevalence vary from 0.7 percent (Young, 1975b) to 2.1 percent (Porfert & Rosenfield, 1978) or to 5.5 percent in high school populations (Gillespie & Cooper, 1973). Socioeconomic factors relate to stuttering prevalence, and cultural standards contribute to the definition. In preparing to write this book I went through over 2,000 references and found more than half of them relevant to my topic of therapy procedures. In spite of this (or perhaps because of it) we have not arrived at an accepted definition or description of stuttering, a single theory to explain causation or rationalize therapy, or even consistent agreement in many replications of similar studies. In particular, we have not developed a therapy program, or subprogram techniques, universally acceptable throughout the profession. We need to consider carefully, and then reconsider, what we know about stuttering. The generalizations and conclusions already in place should be reviewed (Williams, 1982).

With all the confusions or disagreements just mentioned, it is not surprising that there are many different techniques for working with stuttering. Moreover, any particular technique typically has a variety of applications. As you read the literature on therapy there is a bewildering jargon of names and acronyms—desensitization, legato, GILCU, chewing, cancellation, pullouts, DAF, airflow, syllable-timed, shadowing, MIDVAS, prep sets, metronome, EMG, contingency, ventriloquism, elongation, and so on. All refer to techniques or to programs of therapy. Some of them are quite similar, but many are incompatible. Later in this chapter I will discuss some of the controversies in stuttering therapy. At the moment it is enough to say that clinicians today can make use of a variety of techniques—if they are aware of them and if they understand how to use them.

Use of this book is intended to be varied and is aimed at a wide audience. As you will see in the next section there is cause for concern about the training of clinicians in stuttering therapy. There also is evidence to indicate that many clinicians approach stuttering therapy with apprehension and avoidance. Blood and Seider (1981) surveyed more than a thousand stutterers, mostly in school settings. Their research indicated that 68 percent of the stutterers had one or more communicative disorders in addition to stuttering. Of this group, only 6 percent were receiving therapy only for stuttering. Where the subgroups had more than one concomitant in addition to stuttering, 76 percent to 92 percent were receiving *no* therapy for their stuttering. Granted, there can be wise decisions to work with the other problem first or to work with more than one problem at a time, but the extremely high percentages cited also suggest that many clinicians avoid working with stuttering when they can. (More will be said of this attitude later.) We thus seem to have limitations in the education and practicum training of students and some concern by professional clinicians over the best way to deal with stuttering.

This book is intended for students at the undergraduate and graduate levels of training. It can be used with instructor guidance, as an overview of some of the many techniques. On the other hand, it can be used for in-depth study and acquisition of selected techniques. Students often are apprehensive about applying methods because they may not have understood them completely. Step-by-step procedures are provided for the instructor to use (or modify) in class or in practice and for the student to refer to when needed. Professional clinicians, another target audience, perform therapy daily, often numbering stutterers among their clients. The chapters are intended to supply procedural information about techniques not acquired during training or techniques that have gained new variations. Teachers also can make use of the book. As a student, I was trained in "the one" approach to therapy and had to acquire other methods on my own in order to teach following students effectively. To a general audience, this book may be needed as an update resource on methodologies. As a supervisor, I am familiar with the clinician who announces dolefully that a certain method has not worked and expects me to provide a new technique immediately. I am writing, therefore, to three general audiences—student, instructor, practicing clinician. The purposes for each audience may differ, but my intent is to provide information for all three groups.

It is assumed that you will use this book for stuttering therapy, but many of the techniques can be, and are, used with almost any of the communicative disorders. I assume that the reader has been exposed to a basic foundation of information about stuttering or that such information is being acquired from other sources at the same time. If the reader requires additional information, a list of suggested sources is provided at the end of this chapter.

In studying techniques, the reader must be sure to learn the technique before a client does and be able to perform each step or level of progress at a level of competence. The practitioner should be able to use a technique in any setting and at any level of difficulty required. Some of the techniques will feel silly in artificial practice, and a few of them may provoke anxiety or fear in the practitioner. I have used the techniques in the book as class or clinic assignments and know that reactions sometimes occur. However, I never have received any feedback to suggest that time was wasted. Even when students disagreed with a technique and said they never would use it, they still profited from understanding the procedure and how it was applied.

Concerns about clinical preparation stimulated my original interest in writing this text. In thirty years of supervision and teaching, the supply of stutterers for practical experience has been a constant problem. Contact on the undergraduate level is, at best, minimal. Over the years, in a graduate seminar on stuttering, I have queried several hundred graduate student clinicians from all over the country about their undergraduate preparation. About 10 percent to 15 percent reported having had one-on-one experience with one stutterer in therapy; 40 percent to 60 percent never had had direct therapy; all but a fraction had never carried a stutterer from enrollment to dismissal. For most of them, therapy techniques had been discussed generally in class, and in some instances, therapy had been observed for brief periods. Leith (1971) surveyed fifty graduate programs in twenty-eight states, each program averaging thirty graduate students. The programs enrolled an average of fifteen stutterers for therapy. However, dividing stutterers into subgroups accentuated the problem in that the clinician-to-client ratios were 8:1 for preadolescent stutterers, 11:1 for adolescents, 4:1 for young adults, and 14:1 for adults. In many programs, meeting practicum requirements almost mandates rotation of clinicians around the same client and stimulates the student clinician to work quickly rather than thoughtfully. It is small wonder that many stutterers with concomitant problems receive therapy for the nonstuttering disorder once clinicians have graduated.

The actual training students can receive also is open to question. Volz et al. (1978) found that undergraduate students in training used few verbal responses helpful to client-clinician relationships. Crane and Cooper (1983) reported that supervisors rated only 51 percent of 135 MA graduate clinicians as dually effective in technical and interpersonal skills. Costello (1980) stated her opinion that therapy training in stuttering is no better than mediocre and undoubtedly contributes significantly to clinicians' fear of stutterers. Rudolf et al. (1983) supported the suspicion of stuttering fear and avoidance by clinicians. They relate these fears to lack of feelings of self-efficacy or competence on the part of the clinicians. They do not maintain that confidence and ability are the same but suggest that feelings of self-efficacy are important to good therapy. Wingate (1971a), a prolific contributor to and thoughtful critic of stuttering therapy, suggested that the "stuttering" label may engender anxiety in clinicians, that they are insecure about the adequacy of therapy techniques, and that the imagined dangers of damaging the client cause exaggerated concern. Van Riper (1974c), a major formulator of therapy procedures, also criticized inadequate training and experience of stuttering clinicians.

Academic courses in stuttering have an awesome amount of information to survey. In a ten-to-sixteen week course, the instructor must try to cover definition, description, theories of causation and maintenance, development, evaluation, philosophies or schools of therapy, prevention, parent counseling, current research, and therapy techniques. If a class met five days per week and gave equal attention to all topics, each topic, including therapy techniques, could be covered in only five to eight hours (with no time out for tests). That does not consider demands of other viable topics or the division of therapy into several age-group orientations. In many cases, the result is an "overview" course, where everything is sampled slightly, or a delimited course, where the instructor selects a preferred number of topics and omits the other considerations. Ryan (1979, pp. 168-69) expressed strong objections to the current status of stuttering therapy:

> These clinicians also often avoid working with people who stutter because they do not feel adequate because they have not been taught effective procedures. This problem has been produced by our authorities (clinician-researchers) who were so intent on "research" or "writing" or "theory building" that they neglected to clarify, describe, teach, and disseminate their procedures.

Ryan was expressing his preference for a particular approach to therapy, but his statement applies in general to stuttering therapy.

Introductory texts, appropriately, provide a very broad overview of stuttering therapy (Hixon et al., 1980; Perkins, 1978; Shames & Wiig, 1982; Van Riper, 1978.) However, texts devoted to stuttering alone tend to be similarly broad in their coverage. Wingate (1976), Van Riper (1973, 1982), Conture (1982), and others have excellent specialty texts in stuttering and therapy. These books contribute greatly to our understanding of the nature and treatment of stuttering. However, there is the implicit assumption in them that basic steps toward acquisition of skills will be taught by someone else or that experience with clients is readily available. Difficulties in both areas have been pointed out already. Some sources, such as Shames & Florance (1980) or Mowrer (1979), are very specific in describing therapy techniques and in giving step-by-step procedures. As opposed to the generalism cited earlier, these sources tend to tell the clinician exactly what to use, what to do, how to do it, when to act, and how to deal with failures or aberrant responses. The program can be used with a minimum of guidance. However, such sources tend to project only one program or technique. The basics underlying the program or technique may not be explained, making innovation difficult. If a stutterer happens not to fit the approach, the clinician faces frustration and the client faces failure of therapy.

The clinician working with stutterers may feel the need to invest heavily in an extensive library of therapy resources. Even then, many of the procedures are not described in print at a basic teaching level. Add this to the previous comments about training, and we have too many clinicians who have been prepared in overview, theory, and eclectic descriptions of therapy, or (even worse) we have clinicians who have been exposed to evangelical, one-approach systems of therapy. This latter, monotheistic approach consigns all other methods to the condemned category of heresy and leaves the clinician with a rigid therapy to which stutterers must adapt. As noted earlier, the clinician probably has had very little contact with stutterers during education and training, probably has never carried a client through a complete program, and is unsure about various techniques. As a result, clinicians tend to enter therapy careers with one of the following mind-sets toward stuttering:

1. Experience is the best teacher, and somehow the clinician and the client will survive while the former learns what to do and how to do it.
2. The one-and-only-way method learned in school will be used for all clients, regardless of age, severity, environment, or other factors.
3. Don't work with stutterers! Enroll other problems and avoid the uncertainty and anxiety.

The foregoing may be too distinct in its characterizations, but it does at least reflect some of the problems in clinician preparation, and the reasons for this book.

Another reason reflects a personal bias, and I believe other persons have the same bias. I believe clinicians should be able to duplicate the client's disorder, understand his or her feelings, and be able to perform any task that therapy requires of the client. There are obvious exceptions to this belief, but I feel a clinician should be able to duplicate most misarticulated sounds, reproduce an inflection pattern, simulate alaryngeal speech, and so on. In stuttering, the clinician should be able to duplicate a particular stuttering spasm, use controlled speech under DAF, use syllable-timed speech, practice airflow mechanics, and demonstrate other techniques. Sheehan (1970b, p. 283) expressed this view vigorously when he said,

> The Achilles heel of most normal speaking therapists who try to work with stutterers is simply they are not willing to do what they ask the stutterer to do and what is necessary for both to do.

Research has indicated that communication professionals have negative stereotyped images of stutterers, and these preconceptions seem to accentuate with experience, with little regard for the severity of the stuttering (E. M. Silverman, 1982; Turnbaugh et al., 1981; Woods & Williams, 1976). On the other hand, lay persons do *not* seem to stereotype stutterers, and our fictional literature appears to avoid stuttering stereotypes and presents stutterers' reactions in realistic fashion (Trotter & Silverman, 1976). There is ground for belief that our presumptions about stutterers may be more accurate *when they stutter*, and that some persons certainly will fit the presumptive pattern. In particular, normal-speaking persons who have "faked" stuttering report many of the feelings included in the usual stuttering stereotype (Woods, 1977).

The reluctance of clinicians to participate in therapy and the maintenance of inappropriate stereotypes can be a problem. Added to the limitations in education and training already cited, the approach to therapy becomes full of pitfalls. Overall, therapy has shifted from administration to participation, and students need more exposure to self-management (Lay, 1982) as part of learning self-management techniques. They need to understand better the importance of breaking learning into appropriately smaller steps, or subgoals. This can be achieved efficiently if the clinician learns how *to do* the techniques, rather than how to describe them for the client to perform. Clients are concerned about the therapy they receive and the competence of delivery. Research indicates that their perception of a clinician's technical skills, closely followed by her or his empathy, are the two most important factors in therapy (Haynes & Oratio, 1978). Client relationships, overall, will vary with the stages of therapy (Cooper & Cooper, 1969), but the continuing need of the client is to perceive competence on the part of the clinician. Doing, rather than just administering, is a valuable contribution to competence and feelings of self-efficacy.

HISTORY IN STUTTERING THERAPY

Eldridge and Rank (1968) state that our earliest known references to stuttering date back to about 2000 B.C. during the Middle Egyptian dynasty. Greek and Roman references have been found. Many of them blamed malfunction of the tongue for the halts and distortions of production. In the eighteenth century, Mendelssohn recommended slow rate, Erasmus Darwin proposed a system of easy attacks on articulated sounds, and a number of authorities championed various rhythm techniques. Arnot, in the nineteenth century, advocated using a continuous "e" sound between each word, and Hagerman suggested producing a continued "n" before each syllable (Klingbeil, 1939). For a period of time, intervention included surgery, popularized by the great German surgeon, Dieffenbach, and many European surgeons busily transected muscles, removed wedges of lingual tissue, and severed nerves. The popularity of these techniques in a preanesthesia and preantisepsis era waned rapidly, as the postoperative results failed to justify the pain and danger of the procedures. The metronome's apparent predecessor (muthonome) was used a century ago, and many patented devices were developed, even to the extent of clamping silver tubes inside the mouth, metal plates across the palate, and adjustable spring screws in leather collars that fit around the neck and put pressure on the larynx (Eldridge & Rank, 1968). Katz (1977) and Rieber (1977) describe a number of unusual devices used in the past, including one designed to keep the airway open even when the teeth were clenched and the tongue pressed against the roof of the mouth.

Over an extended time, the treatment of stuttering has been varied. Methods have included holding pebbles in the mouth, blistering or deadening applications to the tongue, clenching teeth, speaking on inhalation, talking out of one side of the mouth, alternating hot and cold baths, sticking fingers in a light socket, eating raw oysters, and traveling to religious shrines (Gottlober, 1953). One can agree that Van Riper (1971, p. 996) was restrained when he observed that stutterers have undergone ". . . an almost incredible variety of treatments. . . ."

Cycles

Cycles in stuttering therapy have been shown by different approaches in therapy throughout history. European developments early in the twentieth century formalized many approaches to communicative disorders. Gutzmann (father and son) had great influence in Germany, and Froeschels established important programs in Austria in about 1909 (Eldridge & Rank, 1968). Many approaches to stuttering were elocutionary, with "secret" methods abounding. In the mainstream, the psychiatric and the neurological variably concurred and conflicted with each other. At the University of Iowa, under Carl Seashore, a disciplinary program from psychology was developed for a doctoral program in communicative disorders. Persons such as Travis (1978), Bryngelson (1935), and West (1942) exemplified neurogenic approaches to stuttering. Boome and Richardson (1931) condemned syllable-tapping as a quack remedy, said practicing breathing or speech production was useless, and recommended relaxation under psychological principles; Bluemel (1957, p. 27) argued for emotional causation and appropriate therapy. In 1960 he still condemned rhythm, syllable-timing, and other fluency techniques as ". . . the secret remedy of quacks."

Van Riper graduated from the Iowa program and was in the neurological camp. However, his practice rapidly evolved into an eclectic symptomatic psychotherapy, and nearly fifty years later, he was still speculating on the continuing debate over stuttering (Van Riper, 1973). His chapter in Eisenson's first *Symposium* (1958) is a fascinating diary of twenty years of experimentation in stuttering therapy. In stuttering, Van Riper probably has contributed more techniques and revisions of past procedures than any other person in our short history. Also from the Iowa program, and equally provocative, was Wendell Johnson (1955). After World War II, his concept of semantogenic or diagnosogenic aspects of stuttering was schismatic. Neurogenesis, for all practical purposes, disappeared. His concepts had significant impact on therapy (or nontherapy) with children and on many of our approaches. Part of many clinicians' reluctance to work with preadolescent stutterers can be traced to teachers who were trained in the Johnsonian point of view and taught their students accordingly.

Recent Developments

Recent developments in therapy, and I refer to the past twenty years, have reflected a number of changes. The rejection of neurogenic causation did not appear to have a significant impact on mainstream therapy, excepting certain practices such as forcing unilaterality. As we will see, certain procedures such as DAF (delayed auditory feedback) appeared, but therapy otherwise tended to range from a continuum of purely symptomatic to purely psychotherapeutic, with many clinicians practicing in the mid-range area. Despite the firm belief of many professionals that a stutterer was no different from a person who did not stutter, the pendulum moved slowly back to considerations of organicity. Canter (1971) identified three stuttering subgroups and argued that diagnosis should function differentially. Overstake (1979) postulated a neurological basis and formulated therapy that included strong segments on relaxation, stabilization of vegetative breathing, and correction of faulty speech-breathing patterns. Zimmerman (1980c) made significant contributions to the resurgence of neurogenesis and will be referred to in the following section. Almost at the same time (1960–1980) there was a rapid emergence of clinical researchers allied with Skinnerian or other learning schools, who applied principles of behavioral modification and operant conditioning to therapy.

More will be said in the following section concerning so-called operant therapy. From the point of view that stuttering is a learned reaction and should respond to the presumed laws of learning, clinical researchers began to experiment with fluency promotion and stuttering suppression, rather than with symptom modification or emotional adjustment. The specific techniques were generally not new. Typically, they went back to the eighteenth, nineteenth, and early twentieth centuries and included such techniques as slow rate, prolongation, respiratory modification, masking noise, rhythm sequences, and so on. However, there was innovation in treating stuttering as a contingency reinforced behavior subject to adaptation, extinction, punishment and reward, and replacement with competing responses. In the past twenty years (approximately) there has been an explosion of "new" techniques that previously had been discarded or rejected. The last statement is not intended to be judgmental. It is factual. For decades, any clinician who used any technique or device to *prevent* stuttering, rather than to control it or deal with it, ran a very high risk of being called a quack or a charlatan. Today, however, nearly all these rejected techniques are in use, and many of them will be discussed in subsequent chapters.

CONTROVERSIES IN STUTTERING THERAPY

In general, stuttering never has lacked for controversy. In previous pages I have referred to various differences of opinion. Several of the sources cited at the end of this chapter, particularly Wingate (1976), Bloodstein (1975a), and Van Riper (1973, 1982) provide broad reviews of many of the controversies that have existed and still exist. However, I do not wish to consider many of these controversies, and I will restrict my coverage to those that relate more to therapy procedures.

Theory in stuttering has been and continues to be a source of controversy. The three references cited in the preceding paragraph provide much information about it, or one can refer to Hahn's book (1943) summarizing then current theories and therapies—and find many of them still present today. Wolf and Wolf (1959) theorized a neurogenic feedback disruption and suggested that therapy ultimately will involve an engineer-surgeon team to reconnect nerve tissue into proper feedback patterns. Wingate (1966) strongly attacked the operant programs based on learning theory, arguing that the results of adaptation research in stuttering are not in accord with learning theory. Wertheim (1974) criticized learning and personal construct theories and favored the bioadaptive theory for therapy approaches. Quinn (1971) more or less criticized everybody, suggesting that disciplines were more interested in supporting their theoretical constructs than in making applications to therapy. Fransella (1970) has been an articulate proponent of personal construct theory. She has applied this to therapy to a degree often lacking in other theories (1972, 1974a, 1974b, 1974c, 1975). Zimmerman (1980a, 1980b, 1980c) has presented neurogenic research and also suggested that theory and therapy should be compatible, that therapy should represent the theory, and theory should explain the therapy. Revolutionary concepts! It is quite safe to say that most theory, past and present, has been marked and is marked by its irrelevance to theoretical constructs. As Wingate (1976, p. 5) stated, ". . . most therapy methods have been developed on essentially empirical or pragmatic grounds. Many therapy methods exist independent of any particular theory."

As you can see from this small sampling, we still labor under a multi-theory load. Also, the techniques we use are often used by differing theoreticians. That may not be inappropriate, but it also may be a function of the philosophy "use what works, and we'll justify it later." There have been suggestions that we should forget about theory and just concentrate on developing therapy techniques that are effective. This is an understandable response to continued frustration, but it avoids the professional responsibility to serve our clients best by understanding and explaining their disorder and providing a therapy that fits the explanation. Although the rest of this book concentrates on therapy techniques with minimal reference to theory, I do not imply or suggest that we abandon pursuit of the elusive theory. I cannot settle the issue of single theory, multicausality, or no-model approaches to stuttering. I hope that I can aid the applications of therapy, whatever the theoretical orientation.

Symptom Modification and Fluency Reinforcement

Symptom modification and fluency reinforcement is one of our currently active controversies. Much heat has been generated, with some light shed. Until applications of learning theory mentioned earlier developed strong therapy programs, most therapy revolved around one of the following concepts: learn to control it or learn to live with it. Such approaches are represented by clinicians such as Adler (1966), Sheehan & Martyn (1970), and Van Riper (1973). The methods have been labeled variously as *symptom therapy, symptomatic psychotherapy*, stutter fluently therapy, and other terms. This does not imply that clinicians working in that continuum are a homogeneous group with theoretic and procedural unity. However, in various ways, they aim therapy at the stuttering itself and/or the emotional dimensions of the stutterers.

The other side of the major controversy is represented by clinicians such as Ryan (1974), Schwartz (1976), and Shames and Egolf (1976). The therapy has been labeled variously *speak fluently therapy, fluency reinforcement, symptom suppression*, and other terms. As in the preceding paragraph, there are many variations within this group also. The therapy goal is fluency. Stuttering is regarded as a learned response that can be extinguished by learning principles and replaced with fluency. To varying degrees, according to different practitioners, attitudes and fears, stuttering mannerisms, spasm types, avoidance behaviors, and so on receive less (or no) direct attention since it is assumed that the acquisition of fluency will render moot any need for direct work on these aspects. Strong feelings exist on both sides. Sheehan (1970, p. 272) attacks fluency reinforcement, saying,

> Techniques employing masking noise or delayed auditory feedback or "time out" postponement devices, or experimental manipulation of punishment contingencies, all have their forbears—the not very illustrious genealogy of the quacks.

He continued to accuse the operant therapy group of trying to dress up past quackery with the disguise of modern experimental psychology. An equally strong criticism, in the opposite direction, was directed by Ryan (1979, p. 137):

> It is too bad that our profession was so influenced by authority figures who stuttered, and convinced us there was no hope for the stutterer and tacitly held themselves up as models of what we could and should expect the results of therapy to be. In their effort to point out the "awful truth" about stuttering, they kept us from seeking ways to find a cure.

As you can see, both sides have their bombardiers. In general, many practitioners blend goals and methodologies from both sides. Some "stutter fluently" clinicians are very close to fluency reinforcement and use many of their approaches. On the other side, some "symptom suppression" clinicians pay close attention to attitude, relaxation, symptom management, and other modification parameters.

The problem in the disagreement generally is not the issue of operant conditioning therapy. Any therapy, ipso facto, is behavioral modification. Any behavioral modification procedures can be identified as operants and broken into progressive steps. Data recording and results analysis can be applied to any therapy mode. The so-called traditional therapies of symptom modification or emotional adjustment have been woefully remiss in subdividing therapy steps and applying data collection principles. Fransella (1970) has demonstrated that a psychotherapeutic approach, for instance, can adapt to a data matrix and be effective. Other clinicians have recorded examples of similar rigor. Such differences in practice are quite amenable to change. However, the basic differences in the two approaches lie in the goals of and assumptions about therapy, and the degree to which the believer expresses a separation philosophy. Following, I have attempted to delineate the two points of view and compare them. Extremes of position are set deliberately, and I emphasize again that many clinicians, of either persuasion, will exemplify elements from both points of view. In each comparison, fluency points are presented first, followed by symptom points in italics:

1. Goal is to have stutter-free speech by establishing and supporting fluency. *Goal is to develop ability to control stuttering and turn it into acceptable dysfluency.*
2. Elimination of struggle and mannerisms is not necessary since fluency itself eliminates them. *Stuttering spasms are to be eliminated/reduced by eliminating/reducing struggle and mannerisms.*
3. Secondary mannerisms will disappear as fluency is established. *Direct work is required to eliminate secondary mannerisms.*
4. Fears and attitude problems will disappear when fluency replaces stuttering. *Fears and malattitudes must be faced and dealt with on a direct basis.*
5. "Stutterer" labels should disappear from client's concepts. *Client must admit he or she is a stutterer, accept it, and learn to live with it.*
6. Fluency will remove any need to develop tolerance for stuttering. *Client must learn to stutter without avoidance or behavioral collapse.*
7. Client needs to establish good speech habits, find a basal fluency, and expand it. *Client must learn and experiment with various dysfluency control techniques.*
8. Information about stuttering is not needed; understanding and use of fluency are needed. *Careful analysis of stuttering patterns and behavior, plus general information about stuttering, is important.*
9. Success is fluency, and fluency generally is defined as one or fewer dysfluencies for every two minutes of talking time. *Success is the capability to control dysfluencies in any situation and to behave appropriately in communication situations.*

It should be noted that I deliberately took the extreme position on both sides, and there certainly are many clinicians who would find themselves falling on both sides of this list.

The separation between symptom and fluency therapies is not mended by the statement just made. As you consider the techniques in this book, the goals you seek will have some effect on which techniques you use, and great effect on how you use them. I was trained in the original symptom techniques and initially rejected those who strayed from the righteous pathways. Experience and learning persuaded me that there were times when fluency reinforcement therapy would be more appropriate than symptom therapy. However, I find instances where fluency reinforcement, per se, does not meet the speech or personal needs of the client. Times occur when a mix of the two approaches is useful to me.

Other Controversies

Other controversies in therapy have a more variable relationship to the techniques in this book. Gregory (1978) has covered a number of the controversies in some detail and from multiple points of view. There also is a basic controversy that revolves around most of our research. Wingate

(1962) points out that the bulk of our research in children's speech characteristics, in the significance of stress, and in critical evaluation of speech either is equivocal or contradictory. St. Onge (1963) cites the theory disarray and the research conflicts and suggests that we start over again. Schissel et al. (1978) criticize most of our research on judging or evaluating articulation (and, indirectly, all judgment studies) because of inadequate information provided about judges, their competence, and other factors. Sommers et al. (1979) reviewed a decade of stuttering research (181 articles) and found that many of the procedural faults identified in the past are still operative. Adams (1976) criticizes the design and conduct of research because there are so many circular definitions of hypotheses, lack of specificity in defining stuttering, research based on invalid assumptions about stuttering, and other faults. In short, we have a controversy over the adequacy of the research on which our techniques and theories supposedly are based. Small wonder that therapy so often is pragmatic!

The significance of the stutterer's pretreatment attitude is controversial and will be dealt with later in this book. Guitar (1976) claims high significance for the relation between attitude and outcome of therapy, whereas Ingham (1979) questions his research. Ryan (1979) emphasizes that operant therapy programs do produce attitude changes, as measured by verbal comments. Cooper (1977) feels that whether or not to attend to the feelings and attitudes of stutterers may be our most important controversy. He expresses concern that operant orientations may foster many clinicians who are actually technicians lacking in interpersonal skills. Sheehan (1980) also points out that human beings are not as simplistic as operant models are. Similar arguments develop over the role of the clinician as a psychotherapist. Some advocate avoidance and rejection of the role, and others argue that the question is one of degree only.

Therapy with children has been controversial for decades. As indicated earlier, for some period of time our philosophy often was to avoid therapy with children because of the dangers of labeling and exacerbating the problem. Many clinicians, for various reasons, still avoid children's therapy. Other clinicians have made a point of developing programs directed specifically at children (Luper & Mulder, 1964; Shames & Florance, 1980; Shine, 1980). This book will not deal with children's therapy as a specific topic. However, many of the techniques are directly applicable, or adaptable, to children.

Transfer, maintenance, relapse, and criteria for measuring the foregoing currently are actively debated. The Banff Conference (Boberg, 1980b) devoted its entire agenda to transfer and maintenance. The high relapse rate of dismissed clients (estimates range from 50 percent to 70 + percent) has made this a stormy issue. Coincident with this problem is the question of what is called "success" in therapy. Fluency reinforcement advocates criticize what they see as the endorsement of pathological speech behavior by symptom clinicians, and the latter attack the fluency clinicians for allowing X percent dysfluency to be reached before speech becomes "stuttering," and also to call speech fluent when it may be at extremely slow rates with elongated, timed, or other fluency device patterns.

A ticking bomb lies in the controversy over stuttering subgroups. For many years, authorities have acknowledged that all stutterers are not alike. However, in more recent years, a growing number of persons have called for categorization of stutterers into subgroups. Myers and Wall (1982) suggested a multiple-factor model in stuttering, with similar applications in evaluation and therapy, whereas St. Onge (1963) suggested that we needed to divide stutterers into perhaps three distinct syndromes, with gray areas and subgroups. Bayly (1965) strongly criticized the single-factor attitude, and many other researchers are proposing subgroup divisions. The potential confusion is great because many clinician researchers will subdivide on observed behavior; others will subdivide on history; others will be multicausal; and some surely will point out that this subdivision parallels non-stuttering persons, proving that stutterers are no different from non-stutterers.

Other controversies include debate over the spontaneous recovery rate of stutterers (Cooper, 1972; Sheehan & Martyn, 1970), which is pegged at about 80 percent. This has created concern over the inappropriate enrollment of some children in therapy and the possibility that many "cures" may only be spontaneous recovery (Fritzell, 1976). However, Young (1975b) has disputed the 80 percent figure, saying it must be lower. Arguments also exist over group versus individual therapy (or a mixture), the differential evaluation of dysfluency and stuttering in young and school-aged children (early intervention), what we should evaluate when we evaluate stuttering, and the extent to which clinicians should be involved in environmental therapy. We also have disagreements over the extent to which clinicians should use covert or overt methods to monitor stutterers, as an ethical and a pragmatic issue.

There are other controversies that could be cited, and more are sure to develop. The main points, however, are these:

1. The student clinician, or professional, should be aware of controversies. All too often we learn from single sources and are slow to realize other points of view.
2. In presenting techniques I generally ignore controversies. However, readers should be aware of the current controversies as they approach the procedures presented in the following chapters.

CRITERIA FOR EVALUATING TECHNIQUES

General applicability of techniques in therapy actually is another controversy. Particular methods have been praised or condemned according to their natures and the philosophies of the critics. Unfortunately, some look at the source of a procedure rather than examining the method itself. In the same vein, certain techniques that have a sound basis in theory will be objected to because of some of the implementation procedures (which could be changed easily). Before looking at criteria to evaluate particular techniques, certain generalities might be considered:

1. People often do not practice techniques the way they were taught. This can be due to planned variations, but frequently it is due to incomplete instruction and inadequate listening.
2. Techniques are evolutionary, partly because of the practices just mentioned. However, deliberate experimentation and revision also alter techniques and their uses. Techniques evolve, and clinicians should move with them.
3. One technique or one method or one program cannot cover all dysfluency possibilities. There always will be exceptions, and simply slowing and prolonging a program's steps (Webster, 1979) will not always solve the problem. Techniques and programs require flexible application and the readiness to shift to other approaches.
4. In applying any technique, you must remember that efficacy is a compound of technical skill, knowledge, and interpersonal adequacy. No technique is adequate on its own.
5. All techniques are composed of sections or steps, whether they are explained that way or not. A frequent cause of failure is to explain a procedural goal and then ask the client to "go do it." Too many clinicians move too quickly in procedures and then feel frustrated when the client fails to perform. The client did *not* fail, and neither did the technique; the clinician failed. Step sequences are important. If they are not clear, figure them out.
6. When you read research studies on techniques, be cautious in your acceptance of results. Question the subjects used, the persons applying the procedure, the degree to which measurement interferes with the procedure, and any changes made in the procedure. Some research studies are evaluations of therapy in place, but others are limited tests of specific techniques, used without relationship to clinical settings. Shames (1976) notes that we should not confuse laboratory and clinical control capacities.
7. Finally, as a general principle, you should understand that techniques only produce responses; clinicians change behavior. The interpersonal skills, self-confidence, and ability of the clinician are the most significant qualities. Some clinician researchers now argue that the clinician's relevance has been reduced significantly by the development of operant programs that anticipate therapy variations. This theme has been heard before and will repeat in the future. It is not, and never will be, a valid approach to the facilitation of behavioral growth and change in reasoning, social, interactive organisms.

Criteria in evaluation of techniques are necessary. We too often tend to learn through the authority system. We are taught particular techniques in a classroom, observe specific methods in therapy by others, or are told by supervisors to follow certain procedures. In this section I will present several approaches to evaluative criteria. Remember that evaluation of techniques, based on clear criteria, is a functional step in the analysis and description of the technique.

Sheehan (1975) presented a list of criteria for technique evaluation. One must remember that he was an approach-avoidance theorist and therapist. He rejected fluency reinforcement, symptom modification, instrument intervention, and other procedures if they did not involve acceptance of the role of stutterer, acceptance of stuttering, and resolution of speech conflicts. I have revised his list from question form to declaratory form. Accordingly, a stuttering therapy technique should

1. Lead to approach, not avoidance, behavior.
2. Be true to the self of the stutterer and not create a false role of fluency.
3. Allow for future fear and fluency failure and provide means for dealing with both.
4. Call for expressive behavior and not for (stuttering) behavior suppression.
5. Provide for eventual speech behavior freedom and not for dependence on the technique.
6. Not call for "control" of something that is not there.
7. Act to produce fluency by changes in attitude and behavior, not through a spread of artificially induced fluency.
8. Produce results that are lasting and minimally subject to adaptation, stress, or other long-term factors.
9. Create eventual independence of the client from the clinician.
10. Be related systematically to a comprehensive theory of stuttering, and supported by scientific evidence.

As a list of criteria, there are few objections to most of the items, barring a certain theory bias, but the criteria are not sufficiently inclusive. Messbarger (1982) developed a series of criteria to apply in evaluating techniques for use in public schools. With PL 94-142 mandating certain procedures, and school requirements exerting other influences, she asked whether the technique

1. Lends itself to measurement for record keeping and reports.
2. Allows for differences in clients' chronological and mental ages.
3. Is cost-effective in terms of initial and operational costs.
4. Will function under school scheduling and time restraints.
5. Is adaptable to space and facility constraints.
6. Lends itself to transfer outside the therapy room.
7. Provides for parental awareness, involvement, and counseling.
8. Provides for maintenance and follow-up over an extended time period.
9. Has skill requirements reasonably within range of clinicians' abilities.
10. Provides for eventual client independence of the clinician.

The items were developed by an experienced public school clinician and lean heavily toward the practicalities of daily therapy. Many of the in-practice professionals I have talked with express levels of irritation with "laboratory clinicians" and package program developers who seem to miss some of the constraints of their jobs. Shames and Egolf (1976) provided an abbreviated, but relevant, list of criteria. They are associated with learning theory contexts, but their criteria are applicable generally:

1. Is the technique related to a theoretical point of view, with a base of research data? Absence of this indicates trial-and-error function.
2. Does the theory itself lead to therapy strategies and specific methodologies, or just describe another position on the nature of stuttering?
3. Does the therapy change the stuttering and/or its associated behaviors? A "happy stutterer" approach is not therapy *for* stuttering.
4. Is it possible to evaluate therapy and its results? Is there evidence and supporting data to recommend it?
5. Can the therapy program, and activities, be revised and modified in a systematic, orderly fashion?
6. Does the therapy cover emotional and social contexts, concerning what goes on outside the therapy room?

Borrowing from some of the previous lists, and adding items, I have prepared the following list of criteria. It is not complete for every use of a technique. In the general comparison of techniques you might find it useful; you could provide a 1 to 5 score value for each item and see how considered techniques compare on this basis:

1. Is procedure explained clearly, with steps indicated, methods described, and (if appropriate) examples provided?
2. How easily can the typical clinician learn this technique?
3. How easily can the typical client learn this technique?
4. Can you evaluate progress by steps rather than only by final outcome?
5. Does the explanation indicate common problems of acquisition, errors likely to occur, and typically appropriate remedies?
6. Is there a clear goal in itself, or does it prepare for a following technique?
7. Is the technique rational in terms of a theory of stuttering?
8. Is the cost justifiable in terms of your budget, frequency of use, anticipated life span, and so on? Is the operating cost justifiable?
9. Can you vary aspects or applications of the technique as needed?
10. Are there special limitations on the use of the technique?
11. Can the client reasonably understand what the technique is doing?
12. What is the probable reaction of the client to the technique?
13. Can you measure the results of the technique for charting and data?
14. Are the effects of the technique amenable to transfer (generalization)?
15. Is the technique contributory to ultimate maintenance where the client assumes responsibility for his or her own performance?

Some techniques will be too molecular or transitory for application of all fifteen questions. Even if you use none of the lists specifically, every clinician should develop an inquiring, even sceptical, attitude when considering therapy techniques.

STRUCTURE AND USE OF THE BOOK

Previous sections of this chapter have reviewed aspects of stuttering history, theory, controversies about therapy, and criteria for evaluating techniques. It is evident that much of our therapy is based on trial-and-error pragmatism or on artificially structured simulations of laboratory conditions. We know *so much* and understand *so little* about stuttering and its remediation that almost any approach can acquire the label of "therapy" and be used. We even have a therapy text entitled *Stuttering Solved* (Schwartz, 1976), but very few of us believe it. Indeed, most clinicians feel sympathetic to Bluemel's title, *The Riddle of Stuttering* (1957). Against this background I have tried to structure subsequent chapters about techniques in stuttering therapy.

Objectives of this book are limited to a number of specific items, followed by the objectives that are not embodied in it. Of course, planned objectives do not always match actual use, and individuals using this book may add to its objectives by their own needs and applications. With this reservation, the objectives can be summarized as follows:

1. Provide exposure to a range of therapy techniques and procedures used with stutterers, covering different philosophies, cutting across age lines, and encompassing group as well as individual applications.
2. Describe each technique in general terms, provide known background about origin and history, review research conducted with it, and consider various uses.
3. Detail the step-by-step procedures involved in learning or teaching the technique so clinicians can acquire the skills at progressive levels of competence.
4. Identify where appropriate the preliminary skills needed and the criteria for adequacy in using a method.
5. Structure practice assignments for the clinician to use in learning techniques, to apply them in situations, and to evaluate efforts.
6. Recommend a sample of model assignments for use in therapy or to serve as ideas for planning activities.

As you can see, the objectives are specific and limited. Not all of them will be met completely in every chapter, and this will be more a reflection of the technique itself. A number of possible objectives, typical to many books on stuttering, have not been proposed.

Objectives not considered are those particularly apart from specific techniques. Some exclusions were by choice, and others were unavoidable. Following I have listed the planned omissions. The accidental exclusions are not listed, since I don't know about them yet.

1. All possible techniques were not covered. The original design for the book was twenty-two chapters, but space limitations pared that down. Some techniques are so overlapping or redundant that I chose not to repeat them. Other techniques require expensive instrumentation or special facilities or specialist (e.g., medical) involvement or have other limiting factors. Some also may have been missed.

2. No overall plans of therapy are presented, although general outlines may be attached to detailed techniques. At times, as in the Curlee and Perkins use of DAF (1969), the overall program steps are outlined, but specifics are limited to the particular techniques discussed.

3. There is no espousal of symptom modification versus fluency reinforcement. I use and teach both approaches. By years of experience I lean to a more frequent use of symptom techniques, but I wish a plague on both houses of the nihilistic purists in either camp, hoping they would abandon rhetoric in favor of communication. Techniques can be used for different purposes, and different clients need different methods.

4. No technique is covered completely in all its variant forms. Basic methods and certain variations will be suggested. In general, it is assumed you will develop the variations you need.

5. To emphasize the previous point—descriptions provided are not "the way" to perform a particular technique. There is no one-and-only way to perform any procedure.

6. Generally, the extremely important area of psychodynamics of the therapeutic relationship is not dealt with. It is mentioned fairly often, but no special section is devoted to it. Nevertheless, your most important abilities are in the areas of insight, accurate empathy, genuineness, manipulation, and relationship. Without these capacities, the clinician is only a technician.

7. Theories of stuttering generally are ignored.

8. Information about the general topic of stuttering is omitted most of the time. Many other texts cover this area far more adequately.

9. Research, per se, about stuttering is not reviewed. However, quite a few research studies will be cited as they relate to a particular area of stuttering and/or to specific techniques. It would be simpler in those sections to save space by saying, "Research has shown that . . ." and then follow that with many citations. At times this is done. However, in many areas I have elected to present many of the studies, pro and con, and let the readers be guided to their own conclusions about what the research actually does show.

10. Controversies cited earlier will not be discussed further except where they are germane to particular techniques.

Arrangement of the book is such that the instructor or individual reader can follow any sequence desired or select from among the chapters. The next two chapters seem logically to concern techniques of evaluation, self-analysis in speech, and use of assignments. Following these is a detailed chapter on pseudostuttering in therapy and how the clinician can learn to fake stuttering. The next chapter considers relaxation and desensitization procedures, followed by a discussion of DAF techniques and their uses. Although there has been a move away from DAF (Ingham, 1984), in our overemphasis on rate control therapies, DAF still is accorded a separate chapter because of the extensive research associated with it and the many ways in which it can be used for therapy. Three chapters, in sequence, separately consider cancellation, pullouts, and preparatory sets. These techniques go beyond symptom control and their specific use and have applications to other methods, such as prolongation, easy onset, airflow, rate control, and others. As methods that involve prespasm, in-spasm, and postspasm applications, they are accorded separate chapters. A chapter is devoted to laryngeal function in stuttering and breathing-airflow approaches to therapy. After that, a series of techniques, including masking, rhythm, role play, and other methods, concludes the coverage possible in this book.

Use of the book has been commented on already. If an academic class is involved, the instructor may want to precede technique by study of some of the areas omitted from this book, to provide foundation or background. After this chapter, the reader might progress logically to the evaluation chapter following and then move to Chapter 3 on description, self-analysis, and assignments. These two chapters more or less prepare the reader for the pseudostuttering and learning-to-stutter activities of Chapter 4, and I would suggest it come next. After Chapter 4, sequence pretty much depends on the desires of the instructor or the needs of the reader. Within any chapter, you may want to vary your depth of coverage, and flexibility is encouraged.

In each chapter, it is suggested that you read the first part first. Definitions, general descriptions, and known history about techniques will be provided. Controversies will be noted. Research studies relevant to the methods will be cited. Following this, most chapters will include discussion of background to learn a technique. Where appropriate, suggestions are provided for clinicians' learning and client-teaching methods. Most chapters will end with detailed sequences for the clinician to use in learning the techniques (they also can be used with the client), followed by practice assignments for clients.

The reader may quarrel with my use of the term *spasm* instead of other terms—blocks, dysfluencies, stutterings, and so on. I have elected the older term deliberately because of its neurological connotations. *Block* I prefer to use as a type of stuttering spasm. *Stuttering moment* and similar terms are too long and clumsy for my preference; besides they suggest to me the *overall* events of stuttering—physical struggle, general behavior, and personal feelings before, during, and after the spasm.

The reader should be warned concerning time commitments. I have used all the assignment sequences, or similar ones, in my classes. I was surprised frequently, at first, at how long it took students to complete the assignments and how much work they felt was involved. Student psychology aside, I had forgotten that most of the material was strange, unfamiliar, and sometimes anxiety-provoking for the students. Things I had practiced for thirty years they were experiencing for the first time. You may wish to shorten practice sequences, trim individual subassignments, eliminate certain requests for written reports, and so on. All such adjustments are the prerogatives of the instructors or individual readers.

I strongly recommend the use of practice partners. Desensitization in using some techniques will be facilitated by a partner. Practice, criticism, and observation of another person learning the same skills will help you learn. There are advantages if your partner is a professional major, but tolerant others also can be used. Partners must learn to be objectively critical with each other—praising when warranted but responding honestly to poor performance. Therapy has to include negative as well as positive feedback, and practice in such balanced behavior is important.

The use of a three-inch, three-ring notebook, with divider tabs to correspond to the sections of this book can develop into a therapy resource reference, to be added to as classes, workshops, articles, and photocopies generate more information. You might want to add new sections to the notebook in areas not covered here (for example, use of tranquilizers, counseling, and play therapy). Such a growth file would help keep you up to date and, just as important, remind you of where information can be located. You may prefer file folders or some other physical arrangement instead of a notebook. To those who use this book, I would welcome as much feedback as you care to supply in terms of omissions, expansions, variations, and other ideas that relate to therapy.

SOURCES FOR ADDED INFORMATION

The following sources are a sampling of material available in areas of therapy, theory, overview, counseling, children, and so on in stuttering. It goes beyond the scope of this book and may lead you to additional areas of information in which you are interested.

ANDREWS, G., CRAIG, A., FEYER, A.M., HODDINOTT, S., HOWIE, P., & NEILSON, M. (1983). Stuttering: A review of research findings and theories circa 1982. *Journal of Speech and Hearing Disorders,* 48:226-46. An excellent, brief summary of research to the time cited. Their conclusions are debatable at times, and the invited commentaries following the article are very useful.

BLOODSTEIN, O. (1975). *A Handbook on Stuttering.* Chicago: National Easter Seal Society for Crippled Children and Adults. A very good overview book on definition, description, theory, therapy.

CHAPMAN, M. E. (1966). *Self-Inventory, Group Therapy for Those Who Stutter.* Minneapolis: Burgess Publishing. Group therapy for adolescents. Somewhat dated, but has many good ideas for therapy.

CONTURE, E. G. (1982). *Stuttering.* Englewood Cliffs, N.J.: Prentice-Hall. Brief overview, with particularly strong emphasis on dynamics of therapy.

FALCK, F. J. (1969). *Stuttering: Learned and Unlearned.* Springfield, Ill.: Charles C Thomas. Excellent overview of a variety of techniques and theory and research concerns.

GREGORY, H. H. (1979). *Controversies About Stuttering Therapy.* Baltimore: University Park Press. Series of chapters of noted clinicians, about controversial topics in stuttering therapy.

INGHAM, R. K. (1984). *Stuttering and Behavior Therapy.* San Diego, Calif.: College Hill Press. An excellent overview book on current therapies for stuttering and the state of our knowledge and practice in stuttering.

RYAN, B. P. (1975). *Programmed Therapy for Stuttering in Children and Adults*. Springfield, Ill.: Charles C Thomas. Excellent overview of behavior modification approaches to therapy.

SHAMES, G. H., & FLORANCE, C. L. (1980). *Stutter-Free Speech, a Goal for Therapy*. Columbus, Ohio: Charles E. Merrill. Very specific procedures in DAF rate control and fluency therapy.

SHEEHAN, J. G. (1970). *Stuttering Research and Therapy*. New York: Harper & Row. Very good summaries of many research areas of stuttering. Therapy from an approach-avoidance frame of reference.

SPEECH FOUNDATION OF AMERICA. M. FRASER (DIR.). Memphis, Tenn. This is a series of monograph publications on many different areas of stuttering. The title list should be checked periodically.

VAN RIPER, C. (1973). *The Treatment of Stuttering*. Englewood Cliffs, N.J.: Prentice-Hall. A strong symptom therapy orientation, but probably the best therapy overview book in print.

VAN RIPER, C. (1982). *The Nature of Stuttering*. Englewood Cliffs, N.J.: Prentice-Hall. Very good review of theories, development, and description of stuttering.

WALL, M. J., & MYERS, F. L. (1984). *Clinical Management of Childhood Stuttering*. Baltimore: University Park Press. Child-directed. Limited review of therapy in general, but has excellent final chapter on therapy approaches for children.

WINGATE, M. E. (1976). *Stuttering Theory and Treatment*. New York: Irvington Publishers, John Wiley. Overview, particularly strong on synthesis of research and information. Challenges many notions about stuttering, and has excellent review of therapy techniques.

2

Evaluation of Stuttering

CONSIDERATIONS ABOUT EVALUATION

Children

Evaluation of children will not be covered to the degree that is possible. It is a topic that could take at least several chapters. At the time I was a student, stuttering was divided into primary and secondary levels, children being placed in the first category. By definition, primary stutterers exhibited easy, effortless repetitions, usually of whole words and phrases, with little or no awareness or struggle. Secondary stutterers were marked by awareness, tension, rhythm breaks, struggle, and avoidance behaviors. When it became difficult to maintain this dichotomy, transitional stuttering was added; it was supposed to occur typically in preadolescence.

Many years ago, Van Riper (1954) described four stages in stuttering development. Bloodstein (1960) evaluated over 400 stutterers, ages two to sixteen, and found many contradictions to the neat stages and separations in the first paragraph. He noted awareness, tension and struggle, acute emotional reactions, substitutions, consistency, and other advanced symptoms occurring in children younger than five. Some children matched the earlier definitions, but any combination of factors seemed possible. Later he described (1975b) four stages of development which reflect the variable possibilities mentioned. Children *tend* to follow a track of easy repetition, low awareness, avoidance, on up to growing reaction and struggle in adolescence, and then into adult levels of stuttering. However, any degree of awareness, emotional reaction, struggle, mannerisms, and avoidances can happen at any particular age.

Metraux (1950) evaluated fluency patterns in over 200 children, at six-month intervals, starting at eighteen months. Repetitions are noted in the first two groups with "developmental stuttering" appearing at thirty months and again a year later. Wall and Myers (1982) provide an excellent review of fluency research, noting that about 35 percent of stuttering children also exhibit language delay. In addition, Murphy and Fitzsimmons (1960) suggest looking for tics, nail biting, eye contact avoidance, or other anxiety indicators. They also recommend evaluation of willingness to speak, length of responses, defense modes (denial, withdrawal, fantasy, and so on), self-attitudes, and reactions to groups.

Much has been written concerning the parents of stuttering children. Of the many studies, some have reported parents to be more submissive, with the fathers particularly less well adjusted (LaFollette, 1956) and mothers showing greater covert rejection of the children (Kinstler, 1961), reductions in parent-child positive interactions (Egolf et al., 1972), higher levels of negative verbal comments (Kasprisin-Burrelli et al., 1972), and poorer attitudes toward and less accurate knowledge about stuttering (Crowe & Cooper, 1977). Many other studies could be cited, but Bloodstein (1969) compresses information nicely in noting that parents of stutterers seem more competitive and perfectionistic, tend to set unrealistically high goals for their children, and tend to dominate them. Mothers may be less socially stable and not successful in creating or maintaining a well-balanced home environment. The general consensus seems to be that parents are not clinically neurotic or psychotic, but they tend to foster an environment not favorable to stress-prone speech development. Data do not allow us to neatly label parents as a cause of stuttering but suggest they be evaluated as part of the identification and pretherapy process.

As we will see later on, there is a development toward dividing stutterers into subgroups. Bloodstein's four stages suggest this developmentally. Another source (Riley & Riley, 1979) evaluated nearly 200 children and factored them into four groups on the bases of auditory skills, fine motor coordination, linguistic output, and other variables. They suggest that speech dysfluencies be regarded as abnormal if repeated syllables show airflow disruptions, rate variations, or vowel substitutions during production. Other criteria include tension surges during repetitions or prolongations, the presence of phonatory arrests, or the development of articulatory postures in consonant production. Also, reactions of frustration, avoidance, or escape are negative indicators. Webster (1974) feels that we easily can distinguish stuttering and nonstuttering, but that is not the same as evaluating the syndrome—even if the assumption is true. Van Riper (1982, p. 25) summarized an earlier formulation of factors differentiating stuttering and normal dysfluency. He stipulated the tentative nature of many of the items. The list carries twenty-six factors under seven categories. Some of the items (for example, more than two repetitions per unit, more than 2 percent occurrence, insertion of the schwa vowel, phonatory arrest, inappropriate articulatory postures) are familiar in evaluation. Other items (monotone, poor eye contact, fast rate, tension) are less helpful in that they often can occur for a number of reasons unrelated to stuttering. Nevertheless, the list can be helpful in directing attention to various considerations. Curlee (1980) provided a succinct series of differentiating factors between stuttering and normal dysfluency. He listed signs of visible struggle, noticeable emotions and/or avoidances associated with stuttering, and self-criticism about speech. Other factors identified were

1. Marked variations in frequency and severity of stuttering as speech situations vary.
2. Part-word repetitions of two or more repetitions per unit on 2 percent or more of the words spoken.
3. Prolongations of greater than two seconds' duration on 2 percent or more of the word spoken.
4. Noticeable increases in loudness, elevations in pitch, or abrupt terminations in behaviors in the two preceding items.
5. Involuntary stoppages or hesitations that last longer than two seconds during otherwise continuous speech.

Recent research (Yairi & Lewis, 1984) focused on evaluating as soon as possible children labeled as stutterers by their parents. These children, twenty-four to thirty-six months of age, were evaluated no later than sixty days after initial parental diagnosis. The ten children were matched with a fluent control group for speech analysis. Results indicated all typical dysfluencies were present in the nonstuttering children in fairly equal amounts. However, the stuttering children showed a disproportionate increase in part-word repetitions and in disrhythmic phonations. Findings disagreed with Bloodstein's (1960) emphasis on whole-word repetitions and with Adams' (1977) criterion of three, rather than two, repetitions of a speech unit that is repeated (to differentiate between stuttering and normal dysfluency).

The preceding paragraphs touch lightly on questions about stuttering in children. The questions of genetics, environment, parental relations, fluency versus dysfluency, subgroups, early intervention, and spontaneous recovery are only some of the additional possible areas of discussion. However, in the orientation of this book, attention will focus on procedures involved in the evaluation of established dysfluency rather than on differential evaluation of early fluency disruption.

Reasons for Evaluation

Reasons for evaluation might seem obvious at first. We evaluate to identify, to describe characteristics, to assess severity, and to define behavioral variables: identify, describe, assess, define. Those seem clear. However, what are we evaluating? Stuttering, as a label, covers a diverse collection of behaviors with conflicting explanations (Gottinger, 1981). We have significant problems in defining stuttering, and we need greater precision in describing it and the behaviors associated with it (Hood, 1974a). At one time I was taught that stuttering was an anticipatory, apprehensive, hypertonic, avoidance reaction. With some qualifications this is a functional definition of stuttering. It also defines how many people feel about a visit to the dentist, preparing one's income tax, attending certain social events, or studying for an academic test. At the opposite end of the verbosity spectrum is Wingate's definition (1964, p. 498) encompassing some 150 words in six complex sentences. Van Riper's definition proposes interruption of the forward flow of speech by motoric disruption or by the speaker's reactions to the interruption itself (1982, p. 15).

The obverse problem (since it is more important) is that we also have no acceptable definition of fluency. As will be shown later, fluency often is defined negatively in terms of the absence of dysfluencies. We therefore face evaluating a problem we cannot define, in terms of its departure from a fluency state we cannot define either. However, most clinicians feel they can distinguish between the two most of the time on a practical basis. Perkins (1980, p. 469) has provided three terse reasons for evaluation:

1. To describe the nature and severity of the problem.
2. To determine a prognosis.
3. To provide direction of the appropriate treatment.

We could rework definitions for years and still not improve on Perkins' rationale. From the previous section, I would add this: to determine if a problem exists. In general, our reasons are to explore the problem in its various characteristics and severities so that remedial efforts are possible. On the basis of our knowledge about the problem and its possessor, we want to give some estimate of prognosis. Finally, in avoidance of one-approach therapy systems, evaluation should generate information that will allow us to select the most appropriate model(s) of therapy and suggest adaptations in them.

What to Evaluate

What is to be evaluated brings up the residual diathesis, or the remaining "unknown" after any diagnosis. We never can find everything out about a problem. One clinic I trained in conducted its stuttering evaluation for about twenty-five hours over a period of five days. Many clinics average about three hours. Others fall between, and some take even less time. In some situations, the clinician has about one hour and then must fit any continuing evaluation into ongoing therapy. I have no time prescription, but suggest the following areas should be encompassed:

1. The current fluency of the client. Stuttering behavior aside, describe the nonstuttered speed. Include language, response length, rate, rhythm, stress, pitch, respiration, phonation, articulation, and other elements. Compare the client, nonstuttering, to other persons.
2. The current dysfluency of the client. Describe the speech productions and associated behaviors. Bear in mind that repeated observations are needed to plumb the variety of dysfluency behaviors.
3. The history of speech and language development and stuttering development.
4. Factors that affect the stuttering and speaking behavior. This extends from the specifics of phonemes, positions, and stress points up to broad aspects of situations, people, or any other variations.
5. The attitude of the client toward stuttering and toward speech and the adequacy of his or her general adjustment.
6. The environment in which the client lives, works, studies, and socializes. What are the limitations, enhancements, and opportunities?
7. What other factors need to be considered? This is to make you stop and ask yourself, "Is there something else I need to know?"

Reliability

Reliability of evaluation is important to every clinician. When we make a judgment or read a report, we want assurance that the information is reliable. We try to improve reliability by repeated measurements and cross-testing procedures, but we know that our sampling process extracts only a tiny fragment of the client's speech behavior. The testing situation is a biasing factor in itself, and we may see a change in the stutterer's speech between the time of evaluation and the initiation of therapy (Andrews & Harvey, 1981). In compensation, clinicians have tried covert evaluations, where the stutterer is unaware of any evaluation or attention. Some research indicates that covert and overt measurements produce no significant difference in dysfluency frequency (Andrews & Craig, 1982), whereas other studies report significant differences between covert and overt measures (Howie et al., 1982; Ingham, 1975b).

What can we do to increase or at least maintain the reliability of evaluations? One step is to refer to the previous section and know exactly what it is we want to find out. A second step is to take the time needed to complete the assessment procedures, without inappropriate economies. Immediately I must add a warning against taking refuge in evaluation in order to avoid the uncertain fears of therapy. Spend the time when it is needed, but don't waste it. A third safeguard is to use, but not be limited to, standardized testing instruments. A form that yields total speech time, stuttered moments, percentage stuttering, and so on is *not* an evaluation of speech or of stuttering. It is a useful, very limited, data-base counting procedure, and behavior is not data. Testing forms are valuable, but they are adjuncts to observation and skill. Observation and information are the key steps in evaluation. With them travel understanding, accurate empathy, synthesis, interpretation, and planning.

The personal knowledge of the clinician rests on prior learning and experience. I have discussed earlier the problems of gaining experience with stutterers. Time will compensate for these lacks. However, a number of diagnostic techniques can be practiced on yourself or fellow students. Many procedures or forms can be applied to nonstutterers. Tape recordings (audio or video) can be useful. Experiencing pseudostuttering, self-analysis, and other practice assignments in this book will be of assistance. Do all that you can to gain these experiences and areas of knowledge, for there truly is no substitute for the clinician in an evaluation.

PREPARATION FOR EVALUATION

Evaluating Fluency

Practice in the evaluation of fluency is important in preparing for evaluation of stutterers. In undergraduate and graduate classes I assign projects in monitoring fluency of self and others. Postproject critiques frequently comment that listening for how speech is produced is hard, tiring, distracting, and at times frustrating. When I first started the assignments I was surprised that students complained about not knowing what to listen for. I needed to give a better grounding in normal nonfluency before considering stuttering. One of the steps, therefore, in evaluating stuttering is the evaluation of fluency. When you have information and awareness about fluency and its variations, you will be better prepared for your stutterers. Remember, a stutterer typically will be "fluent" 70 percent to 95 percent of the time, and you need to evaluate all aspects of speech, not just stuttering.

Evaluation of stuttering is enhanced if the behavior is audible or visible (Martin 1965), if recorded examples are time-expanded (O'Keefe & Kroll, 1980), if various error-producing factors are controlled (Young, 1975a), and if adequate samples are taken. Young and Prather (1962) suggested that very short (twenty seconds) speech samples are comparable to the total production. However, other clinicians (Sheehan, 1969) disagree with this opinion as one moves away from simplistic, counting analysis. Specific training for judging fluency and dysfluency does not seem to be significant (Hoops & Wilkinson, 1973; Schaef & Matthews, 1954) although some research suggests experience and training do affect judgments (Manning & Jamieson, 1974). Listeners apparently can be affected by the fact that they are listening for "stuttering," so that more normal nonfluencies are rated as stuttering than if the judges are told to listen for normal nonfluencies (Williams & Kent, 1958). Curlee (1981) reported that setting up firm criteria (of dysfluency) did not make judgments more reliable. On the basis of time-lapse, Cullinan and Prather (1968) reported that a three-month interval between reratings did not materially reduce reliability of stuttering judgments (but did on fluency judgments; apparently we have a consistent internal definition of stuttering). Perhaps our disagreements stem more from the gray areas separating stuttering, fluency, and normal nonfluency (Hulit, 1978).

Equipment

Equipment and material needed for evaluation is a potentially endless problem. It would be very useful to have a video recording unit, electromyograph, frequency/intensity analyzer, sound spectrograph, pneuompolygraph, and many other specialty items. All of them contribute to an evaluation and provide baseline data for measuring therapy changes. However, many clinics and most clinicians do not have such an armamentarium. In most instances it must be substituted for by the observation and knowledge referred to previously. To that should be added an emphasis on the need to organize and record information, analyze it, and transfer resulting outcomes to a report form. I earlier noted criticism that too much stuttering therapy is done without data to support progress or even maintenance measurement. Some clinicians have turned data accumulation into an onerous chore that reduces the client to a laboratory specimen responding to a digital counter, but such excesses by a few insecure clinicians are no justification for failure to elicit and record adequate information.

As noted, many instruments can be used, and you should use what you have. In general terms, you will be served very well by an audio tape or cassette recorder, a stopwatch, and a digital counter. Several recorders would be useful—a laboratory quality unit for analysis of acoustic parameters, a standard table-top unit for use in the clinic, and a miniature unit that can be carried out of the clinic. Pragmatically, a single portable cassette (AC/DC) unit can serve most purposes. Recorders are so common that a client or clinician could carry a unit in one hand while performing outside the clinic (you might want to cover clear plastic "doors" or signal lights that would indicate the unit is operating). The stopwatch can be obtained very cheaply, although I recommend the slide-bar (or electronic) control type to avoid the constant stop-start clicking noises of older types. Digital counters come in all sorts: mechanical or electrical, single or multiple dials, table or rack or wrist models, and with or without various accessories. You can use the simplest type (pencil and paper), but a unit that can count at least three separate phenomena is very useful. These items, supplemented by your observation, can provide valuable data in the evaluation.

Particular tests and forms cannot all be surveyed here. A variety of them will be presented. Many clinics develop their own forms and adapt tests to particular needs. Just as I have recommended a minimal amount of equipment, I will suggest very few specific tests or forms for acquisition, although a number will be described or at least cited.

Procedures

Procedures in evaluation vary as much as the materials used, and it also would be inappropriate to stipulate one procedural structure. However, certain sequencing can be recommended. Many clients approach evaluation with tension and fear, or at least anxiety, which can result in an atypical speech performance. It helps if you can observe the client talk with other people while he or she is waiting for you. Younger clients may be with parents or other family members. Some clinics set up situations with special waiting areas. The speech still tends to be subject to any perceived stress but temporarily avoids the immediate influence of the stranger, the clinician.

Second, it helps to audio record everything you can, listening and watching as you do. Students sometimes turn off their monitoring behavior except when they are administering a formal test or procedure. Every word the client utters, every aspect of the behavior, should be part of the evaluation—even in the last minutes of the postevaluation counseling session. Keep and file an adequate sample of the recorded material for future reference and comparison.

Formal testing for dysfluencies, speech behaviors, adaptation, speech rate, and other factors should be performed thoroughly. I suggest that formal adaptation testing be placed near the end of the schedule. This is done in hopes of having the stutterer start out nearer to his or her mean average level of stuttering and, hence, give a more accurate adaptation profile. Throughout various tasks, periodically ask the client to report her or his own stuttering behavior, feelings, comprehension, or other factors. You will want to know the client's self-awareness and information capacity, regardless of the anticipated therapy mode.

Adaptation measures aside, it often is useful to repeat several tasks (not identically) from earlier in the session and then compare results of the two performances. Several times, play back a recorded segment of the client's stuttering and ask the client to describe or evaluate it. This provides another check on awareness, information, and tolerance. Observe emotions and behaviors when you do this. Ask the client to compare the overall level of stuttering in the session with the usual level. If other family or friends have been involved, query them similarly.

Finally, other areas of evaluation completed, probe the client to discover the desired or anticipated outcome of therapy. You will want to secure the following information whenever appropriate:

1. Why did the client come for help? Was it a planned decision, a desperate effort, a routine effort to reassure self of no relief, a forced compliance, or for other reasons?
2. What is his or her understanding of therapy? The client may be totally uninformed, an experienced veteran of several past remedial efforts, or aware of one of the miracle cure articles in popular publications.
3. What is the client's therapy goal? There can be a strong halo effect here, and the clinician can be misled. Probe into very general "to talk better" types of answers.
4. What time and effort will the client invest, and can he or she conform to your time schedule? Again, be alert for stock answers. Some clients will be willing to work for as long as it takes, but others believe that anything from six lessons to six weeks should be the maximum. Popular publications have had many accounts of two-day, five-day, or whatever programs. Gauge your client's motivation and available time.

EVALUATION OF FLUENCY

As noted earlier, we are in trouble when we try to evaluate fluency. Most of the time we define negatively by stipulating the absence of certain dysfluencies (Adams, 1982b). To complicate this confusion, there is disagreement over whether the fluent (nonstuttered) speech of stutterers can be differentiated from the fluent speech of nonstutterers. Few and Lingwall (1972) found no consistent difference. Wendahl and Cole (1961) found that listeners could distinguish between the two, but Young (1964) replicated their study and obtained opposite results. Many research studies support the thesis of difference at finer levels of movement, breathing patterns, acoustic parameters, and so on, but whether these fine differences are perceptible to listeners is open to argument. Until we accumulate data by stutter types, severity, concomitant problems, and other factors, it probably is wise to assume that some stutterers have fluency that perceptibly is different from the speech of nonstutterers.

Total Talking Time (TTT)

Duration and amount of speech can be measured in fairly straightforward fashion. Duration refers to the amount of time a person speaks from onset of the first phoneme to final termination. It is called *total speaking time* (TST), *total talking time* (TTT), and other labels. Since several labels use *s* to refer to stuttering or to syllables, I will use TTT in this book. Simply measuring the onset-to-termination time does not provide a universal TTT value. In a recent study I had sixty normally speaking students read a passage aloud. Their TTT values ranged from twenty-two to thirty-six seconds, a difference of almost 40 percent in talking time. Speech production rate and pause time will significantly affect TTT, as will delays from stuttering. Measuring the length of time to read a passage is simple, but be sure to look at the production behavior. Measuring talking time for spontaneous speech is meaningless except as a comparison to typical responses or longitudinal measurements of the same client.

The amount of speech measures how often the person engages in speech communication and the amount of time spent talking in a particular situation. This measure of behavior can be gained by keeping a record of speaking situations encountered and the time the record keeper (only) talked. Such form was developed at the University of Iowa (Johnson et al., 1963) and was called the Speaking-Time Log. Users are to keep a record from the time they awake in the morning until they sleep at night. Every situation, even a "Hello!" in passing is to be noted. For each notation users are to estimate their talking time (not of the other participants) in seconds. At first, users tend to overestimate. The Iowa study reported that college students spent an average of forty-five minutes per day in actual talking time. I have developed a revised version of the summary form (see the charts at the end of this chapter) where shorter time intervals are estimated, not measured, and situations are grouped into categories. Students report that the activity is distracting, timing is difficult, and remembering is a problem—but the results are very interesting.

In addition to actual talking time, the summary will provide information about who the person talks to, what types of situations are met, and other data. This information can be very useful in a stutterer's self-analysis and in establishing situation hierarchies for desensitization, transfer, and maintenance activity. By omissions it can help identify situations that are avoided or are not presently part of the person's behavioral pattern.

Rate

Measurement of rate is a high priority in fluency or stuttering. We know that listeners tend to correlate fluency and rate. We also know that the primary effect of many fluency reinforcement techniques is to retard rate, and a number of symptom modification techniques have a similar effect. Rate can be measured by recording a speech sample, obtaining the TTT value, counting the number of words read, and dividing to get a word-per-minute (wpm) rate, so that a 250-word passage, read in 100 seconds, would yield 250, divided by 100 and multiplied by 60, for a wpm rate of 150.

$$\text{wpm} = \frac{\text{number of words spoken}}{\text{TTT in seconds}} \times 60$$

Research at the University of Iowa reported a median wpm rate of about 176 in reading, 120 to 130 for telling a story, and 136 to 147 for discussing a future vocation (lower figures are male; higher figures are female). Johnson et al. (1963) recommend three steps in measuring rate, recording as the client

1. Talks for three minutes about a past, present, or future job or vocation. Allow preplanning time, and ask leading questions if needed. Job task.
2. Reads a 300-word passage aloud. Instruct only to "Read aloud as you normally do." Reading task.
3. Tells a story about card 10 of the TAT (Thematic Apperception Test). Any picture suitable to the age level can be used. Ask the client to tell a story about what is happening, what preceded the current situation seen, and what will happen in the future. Elicit about three minutes of production. Allow a minute or so of planning, and ask questions if needed. TAT task.

You also can devise your own rate sampling by eliciting three minutes of reading, three minutes of monologue about self-interests, and three minutes of storytelling or improvisation. Count only complete words, or words intended to be complete. Subtract any participation on your part from the time record. (An assignment in rate calculation is found at the end of this chapter.)

Rate measurements are affected by intervening factors, mainly pauses, although intruded stuttering can significantly slow the rate (Perkins, 1975). This is particularly true at fairly low levels of word output (Martin & Haroldson, 1979), where unfamiliarity with the topic, anxiety over one's impression, or other factors may intervene. Overall wpm rate can be misleading since we can vary considerably in our individual phrase and sentence productions. Research has indicated a much better correlation between listener perceptions and mean sentence rate than with wpm rates (Kelly & Steer, 1949). However, counting every word in every sentence and calculating the rate for each sentence can be quite tedious. Fortunately, Kelly and Steer noted a positive correlation between wpm and sentence rates so, at least for clinical use, the former is quite appropriate. Another variable to consider is whether or not words are the most appropriate unit of measure. A number of clinicians prefer to use syllables per minute (spm) as a measure of rate. This can be affected by the educational or cultural level of the speaker. Andrews and Ingham (1971), with the precaution just noted, suggest a measure of 1.5 syllables per word:

$$spm = \frac{\text{number of words spoken} \times 1.5}{\text{TTT in seconds}}$$

If in doubt, select ten distributed sentences from spontaneous discourse, and count the syllables. The number of syllables divided by the number of words will yield an average syllables-per-word measure for use.

Other Aspects

Rhythm, inflection, and stress—prosody elements—are an important part of fluency. As will be seen in the section on stuttering evaluation, some feel prosody elements are critical to the loci of stuttering. Evaluation of these elements cannot be stated easily in formulas or criterion measures. However, the clinician should use elicited speech samples to check for

1. Broken, exaggerated, or inappropriate rhythm patterns. Stuttering will break rhythm, but fluent utterances may show patterns that are atypical.
2. Constricted, exaggerated, or stereotyped inflection patterns.
3. Stress that is inappropriate for the word or syllable or stress that is over-emphasized or lacking.

Other aspects of fluency need to be considered. Vocal loudness and variability should be noted, and pitch level and variation also should be checked. Both acoustic parameters are closely related to rhythm, inflection, and stress. They form a collection of clues that are less dramatic, less noticeable than tonic or clonic stuttering spasms. However, fluency is the bedrock on which therapy must build. If we modify a symptom, toward what end do we modify it? If we reinforce fluency, exactly what is it that we are trying to reinforce? Just to modify a symptom or suppress dysfluency— neither are valid goals for therapy. Fluency is a composite of rate, rhythm, inflection, stress, and many other factors. An evaluation should include a description and assessment of fluency skills, and not just concentrate on the moments of nonfluency.

EVALUATION OF STUTTERING

Identification

Identification of stuttering as a dysfluency appears to be feasible. Even naive judges can make reliable discriminations between stuttered and normal dysfluencies. However, describing the dysfluencies and rating their severity is more complex. Van Riper (1937) evaluated 50 stutterers and found that tonic (continuous muscle tension) or clonic (intermittent muscle tension) spasms were the only universals. Bar (1940) measured 500 moments of stuttering and identified twenty-five different phenomena, with nine of them occurring 25 percent or more of the time. Stutterers will have a commonality of symptoms but show variations within their range. This variability should warn us to be discriminating in assessing stuttering and not to regard stuttering as a functional unit (Sakata & Adams, 1972). Part of the uniformity question probably relates to the factor that much of our information base about stuttering phenomena stems from university clinics, where severity levels often are low. Soderberg (1962b) surveyed the populations used in four studies, finding that they were typically "mild" in severity, and Sheehan (1974) reported that a sample of twenty stutterers averaged less than two seconds in spasm duration. To move from such a base and assume that increased severity is simply a matter of "more of the same" is incorrect (Yairi, 1972). High dysfluency stutterers showed a reduction in revisions and phrase repetitions and increased proportions of part-word repetitions (most significant), whole-word repetitions, disrhythmic phonation, and tense pauses. McClelland and Cooper (1978) suggested that male stutterers have more complex stuttering patterns than females.

Differences between reading and spontaneous discourse dysfluencies were established classically by Johnson (1961a). These data were reexamined by Young (1980), who reported that the difference was due largely to reading reductions in whole-word repetitions and interjections, and the difference is reduced further as severity increases. Nevertheless, Prins and Lohr (1972) found reading and self-formulated speech to be one of six combined factors significant in evaluating stuttering. Wohl (1970) proposed five classifications of stuttering (festinating,[1] phonatory blocking, articulatory blocking, ataxic, and psychiatric). These observations warrant the point made by Hood (1974b)—that what we observe a stutterer doing is a dynamic moment that is partly the result of behaviors preceding it. We could add, it also is affected by the anticipation of subsequent consequences.

Stuttering can be divided into the muscular spasm states associated with production and the behaviors associated with the speaker's efforts to overcome, control or avoid the spasms. The muscular spasms basically are tonic (where the tension state is continuous) or clonic (where the tension state is regularly or irregularly interrupted). Brestovici (1976) adds clonotonic and tonoclonic spasms where both types mix, with one predominating. The clonic spasms are observed in repetitions, the most commonly identified stuttering behavior. Repetitions can be on phrases, words or word groups, syllables or syllable groups, phonemes, or articulatory postures preliminary to the phoneme production. Sheehan (1974), in evaluating twenty stutterers, observes that 83 percent of the repetitions were on phonemes and syllables and only 5 percent on phrases. Repetitions may be slow or fast, few or many, easy or forced, sequential or broken into clusters, and may or may not be accompanied by other dysfluency productions (interjections, loudness or pitch variations, and so on) and physical behaviors. The reverse of the clonic spasm is the tonic spasm, or block.

The nomenclature or semantic problem complicates description. Some clinicians use *block* to mean any dysfluency, and others use it to indicate a complete stoppage in speech effort. I use the latter referent and apply *spasm* to the physical occurrence of stuttering. This can be criticized on purely neuromotor grounds, but it separates the other terms. By *block* I

[1]Involuntary rapid rate, typically increasing as the production continues.

mean a tonic spasm where the vocal folds and/or articulatory structures block the release of air so that the speaker temporarily is mute (can be a thoracic fixation also). As in repetitive spasms, blocks may be variable in severity, duration, physical struggle, and associated behaviors. As just indicated, blocks will occur at points of articulatory constriction—lips, linguaalveolar, linguavelar, and glottal areas. If complete, a block will be soundless, but it may intermittently be interrupted by vocalization and/or articulatory moments (clonotonic).

Prolongation is a tonic form of spasm, but constriction of the aperture points in the vocal tract is not complete, so sound or air is released. However, the speaker cannot transit into the next vocal fold adjustment or vocal tract modification so there is fixation at one particular moment of production, without termination or transition. Some clinicians feel that prolongations are vowel-oriented, occurring on vowels or in an effort to reach a following vowel, but this is arguable. Prolongations, as in other spasm types, can vary in tension, struggle, continuity, and associated behaviors. Sheehan (1974), in his sample of stutterers, noted that prolongations averaged slightly less than one second. In my own experience I have found prolongations to be of briefer duration than blocks or repetitions, in most stutterers. However, I have observed fifteen-to-twenty second prolongations in a number of stutterers. Often the production is cut short and the person tries again.

Repetition, prolongation, and blocks account for the basics of the physical act of stuttering. Over the years I have seen four stutterers who showed no overt symptomatology and no observable tension. They sat quietly for a few, or many, seconds and then said the word in normal fashion (yet they reported all the classic fears, avoidances, and so on). More typically we find gray areas where the spasm types merge and/or mix. By merge, I mean the stutterer has, for example, repetitions that involve prolonged productions. By mixed, I mean the stutterer displays the separate behaviors in the same production sequence:

Merged: whaaaa-whaaaaa-whaaaa-what?
Mixed: whaaaa-wh-wh-wh-what?

Of course, you can merge and mix in the same utterance. As a rule of thumb, increasing severity will result in more varied, complex spasm patterns.

Associated Behaviors

Associated behaviors complicate the basic stuttering, contribute to perceptions of severity, and provide indications of attitude and adjustment of the stutterers as far as speaking is concerned. It is possible to divide associated behaviors into covert and overt patterns, where one type attempts to hide from or avoid stuttering, and the other (overt) type, to struggle with and overcome stuttering. Some divide the behaviors into secondary mannerisms and avoidance behaviors. The nomenclature is not particularly important. I prefer to divide the behaviors into three categories:

> *Struggle behaviors* are the physical behaviors that are an integral part of the stuttering spasm, no matter how distal. They always occur, when they occur, during the spasm and either are a reflection of overflow neuromuscular effort and/or an habituated effort to break the spasm and complete an utterance.
>
> *Avoidance behaviors* focus on a particular spasm and seek to eliminate the possibility that stuttering will occur on a specific utterance. They usually are habituated and reflect growing awareness of stuttering and fear of it.
>
> *Antiexpectancy behaviors* do not focus on a particular spasm but seek to eliminate or reduce the probability that any stuttering, on any utterance, will occur. They may or may not be habituated. They can be specific to speech behavior only or general to the overall adjustment pattern of the person.

Spasm types and associated behaviors will be discussed again in the chapter on self-analysis. However, for evaluation, they should be delineated further at this point.

Struggle behaviors, as defined, are an almost indivisible part of a stuttering spasm. The more proximal they are, the closer the association. Lip, jaw, and tongue struggles are maximally proximal, whereas actions such as leg flexion or fist-clenching are distal. In between will lie head postures, facial grimaces, eye movements or fixations, and neck and shoulder involvement. They are overt patterns and indicate nonsurrender by the speaker. Some will be grotesque or ridiculous. I have seen a stutterer "wrinkle" his lips seventy to eighty times without stopping, another protrude her tongue until she (literally) could touch her chin, and another blink his eyes so rapidly he could not see. In many instances, struggle reactions are overflow. They are progressively habituated avoidance or antiexpectancy behaviors that no longer function as intended. The girl (aged twelve) with the tongue protrusion started by licking her lips just prior to a feared utterance. For awhile it seemed to help, and she used it consistently. Later, she had to increase the licking motion to achieve the same effect. By the time I saw her, the action was no longer effective and had become involuntary. The same can be true for other struggles and mannerisms. Struggle also may include interjected sounds, words, pitch shifts, or alterations in loudness. These also may be habituated avoidance efforts, or overflow phenomena. A particular frustration for clinicians is when techniques from previous, failed therapy have become incorporated into the struggle pattern. This exacerbates the stuttering and undermines the credibility and perceived efficacy of subsequent therapy.

Avoidance behavior was defined as keying to anticipated stuttering on a specific utterance. It may include any body area or aspect of the speech sequence—respiration, phonation, articulation. It can be categorized in a variety of ways, as follows:

Postponement is any device used to delay the effort to initiate phonation and/or form articulatory contact for the production of a feared word. It can be silent hesitation, perhaps masked as a pause for thought. It can be an interjected sound, word, or phrase: *uh, er, but, what, well now,* and so on. It is temporally separated from initiation of the feared word and is intended to allow for relaxation and control to occur before utterance. Postponements can be very sophisticated and logical or very blatant. I always will remember "Aw, heck . . . aw, heck . . . aw, heck. . . . Four score and seven years ago. . . ."

Starters are any device used to initiate the feared utterance in hopes of avoiding stuttering. Starters can be almost anything used as a postponement and can be mixed:

> Postponement: "My name is uh . . . uh . . . uh . . . Richard."
> Starter: "My name is . . . uhRichard."
> Mixed: "My name is uh . . . uh . . . uhRichard."

Starters can be physical movements such as head jerks, jaw movements, or leg kicks. A few times I have seen very sophisticated use of gestures timed to coincide with the initiation of a word. As noted earlier, starters can become habituated and integrated into the involuntary aspect of the spasm.

Retrials combine elements of postponement and starters. There is a cessation of effort to utter a particular word (usually stuttering has occurred) and a new effort is made. The retrial may just be a simple starting over on the word, or it may back up and resay several previous words. It may also include other devices:

> "My name is Ri . . . [stutter and pause] . . . Richard."
> "My name is Ri . . . [stutter and back up] . . . my name is. . . ."
> "My name is Ri . . . uh [postponement] . . . call me [substitution] . . . uhRichard [starter]."

Release devices are difficult to separate from struggle phenomena and often have become habituated components of the spasm. They are not retrials but are added to the ongoing spasm in an effort to break out. As before, they can include limb jerks, flexions or extensions, interjected sounds, gusty exhalations, appropriate or inappropriate gestures, shifts in pitch or loudness, or other methods. If successful, they break the closed-loop cycle of neuromuscular fixation and oscillation and allow continuation. I have seen one stutterer who used starter and release gestures so effectively that no one knew he stuttered. When we persuaded and coerced him to immobilize his upper limbs, he stuttered severely. In his study of fifty stutterers, Van Riper (1937) reported that 84 percent to 98 percent admitted using postponements, starters, and releases, and up to 85 percent reported habituation of these efforts.

Substitution simply refers to the replacement of the feared word with a synonym—*large* for *big*, *hi* for *hello*, and so on. Stutterers have reported using nicknames to replace feared proper names. Acquiring a large vocabulary of synonyms is quite feasible, although hard; of the 600,000+ words in our language, less than one-half of 1 percent account for 85 percent of our utterances. A few stutterers substitute to an extreme, and like our gesture artist, are almost undetectible unless they confess. Of course, there are some words that defy substitution.

Circumlocution can operate alone or as a backup to other avoidance behaviors. In its simplest form, a circumlocution is the replacement of one feared word with a phrase or phrases that convey the same content or action. It also can replace more than a single word:

Straight: "My office is in Lindley Hall."
Circumlocution: "My office is in the building on Court Street, across from the library."
Straight: "May I have a bottle of Myer's Shampoo?"
Circumlocution: "May I have a bottle of shampoo, the one in the red box with the blue lettering?"

Omission also can be an avoidance device. I do not refer to mutism or speech avoidance (see later) but to the deliberate omission of, usually, one word. This can be done in a way that the message is not compromised, and context fills in for the listener. It also can be delivered in the "It's on the tip of my tongue . . ." style, and the auditor fills in the word or completes the sentence. There is no substitution or circumlocution, just a gap in ongoing speech.

The various avoidance behaviors can appear in a great variety of combinations, frequencies, and intensities. It is necessary to observe the stutterer over time in a variety of situations to develop a clear picture of the pattern and nature of avoidance behaviors. By now you probably have observed that many of the behaviors are common to nonstutterers. You probably engage in most of them yourself. Inevitably, then, the question arises as to when to assume that a stutterer's associated behaviors are related to stuttering and when they are the ordinary behaviors we all function with. Most of the time it will not be difficult to decide. As you come to know the person better, it will be easier. Otherwise, it is easiest to assume that any such behavior is associated with stuttering.

Anticipatory behavior involves actions or attitudes intended to reduce the probability that stuttering, in general, will occur. It subdivides into two categories, speech behavior and social behavior. Speech behavior can involve any aspects of the acoustic parameters or prosody elements: speaking in higher or lower pitches, at louder or softer levels of loudness, with faster or slower rates. Efforts to control or stereotype rhythm, change or omit stress, breathe frequently, engage in physical distractions, have tic-like behaviors, and so on may occur. Rhythmic timing movements are not uncommon. These are deliberately performed and are under conscious control, even when they become more or less automatic. Eye contact may be omitted or fixated. Occasionally, past therapy techniques intended for symptom modification or fluency reinforcement are misused. Social behaviors can range from aggression to constant humor (another form of aggression) to overly submissive, placatory modes. The stutterer may reduce expectancy by avoiding situations or remaining silent when speech is invited or encouraged. "If I don't talk, I don't stutter" is absolutely safe behavior.

Severity

Evaluation of severity rests on several perceived or measured factors. Frequency, how often stuttering occurs, is used most often to indicate severity and correlates well with listeners' judgments (Dalton & Hardcastle, 1977). Earlier, Prins (1972) reported five factors significant in severity: duration of stuttering, frequency of stuttering, slow or labored rate, presence of lip tremors, and the number of different anatomical parts involved in a stuttering occurrence. Lewis and Sherman (1951) described the first widely accepted scale for measuring severity, and a year later, Sherman reported that it could be used reliably by judges (Sherman, 1952).

Berry and Silverman (1972) determined that the Sherman scale was ordinal, not interval, and suggested eliminating the "Very Mild" and "Mild" categories to form a seven-point scale that was more interval in nature. Van Riper (1982) criticized the scale because of the grouping of the variables and the implied suggestion that the variables are highly correlated. He revised or replaced the scale with the structure in Table 2-1. Van Riper suggested using this scale in initial evaluations and then reapplying it periodically during therapy and charting results to determine amount and areas of progress.

Next to the Lewis-Sherman scale, the Riley Stuttering Severity Instrument (SSI) (Riley, 1972) is one of the most popular scales. It is based on three parameters: frequency of repetition and prolongation of sounds and syllables, estimated duration of the longest spasms, and severity of observable associated struggle behavior. It omits or partially covers Van Riper's

TABLE 2-1 Profile of Stuttering Severity

SEVERITY	PERCENT STUTTERING	TENSION-STRUGGLE	SECONDS OF SPASM	PERCENT POSTPONEMENT-AVOIDANCE
1	Under 1	None	Under 1	None
2	1–2	Rare	About ½	Under 5
3	3–5	Mild	About 1	5–10
4	6–8	Severe	About 2	11–20
5	9–12	Very severe	About 3	21–31
6	13–25	Overflow to eyes, limbs	About 4	31–70
7	25+	Overflow to trunk	5+	70+

From C. Van Riper, *The Nature of Stuttering*, 1982, p. 201.

postponement-avoidance and tension-struggle areas and similarly misses some of the Lewis-Sherman points. The SSI is arranged to be used with almost any age group. It has a high correlation with the Lewis-Sherman, and its reliability is favorable. I teach it to undergraduate students but find it too limited for graduate clinicians except as a preliminary step in evaluation. It is commercially available and is useful as a quick measure of severity.

In evaluating severity, it is necessary to evaluate speech in a variety of situations and degrees of complexity. Simply having the stutterer read aloud or sampling speech during an interview will not be sufficient. A very comprehensive sequencing of evaluation situations was presented by Shames (1976). He suggests you record and observe the following:

1. Vary audience size from one, to two, to three, up to seven persons. Spend at least five minutes with each size factor.
2. Secure from the client the names of three people with whom the most stuttering occurs and three people providing the least stuttering. Contact these persons and arrange for short sessions with the stutterer.
3. Secure from the client an identification of his or her three easiest and three hardest speech situations. Arrange for the client to enter these situations.
4. Arrange for various interruptions while you and the client are talking.
5. Vary length of client's utterance with five yes-or-no questions, five two-word responses, progressive lengths of sentence completion, a standard interview, and a free conversation where you check utterance length against stuttering.
6. Vary topics in terms of familiarity, sensitivity, and so on.
7. Request client to describe and re-create various situations that were happy, sad, angry, relaxed, anxious, and fearful.
8. Observe actual short interactions with family, friends, strangers, and so on. Apply measures of verbal interaction.
9. Vary linguistic structure—answering questions, giving directions, explaining concept, justifying opinion, correcting clinician, confirming, disagreeing, and so on.
10. Vary time pressure by controlling duration of stimulus and the time allowed for response.

The foregoing would provide a thorough range of situations and influencing factors. Unfortunately, few clinicians will have the time or resources available to encompass such an ambitious schedule. This does not criticize but simply recognizes the pragmatics of many professional situations. It is to be hoped that one will go beyond the limitations of the SSI and further than the three Iowa situations (job, reading, and TAT tasks).

Descriptive accounts of stuttering are involved in the component parts of most scales. One approach by Johnson et al. (1963) established twenty-six categories of stuttering behavior and provided a rating sampling procedure to describe the stuttering behaviors. I have taken their idea and developed a reporting chart that can be used in a series of situations where the stutterer can be seen and heard. The situation should be recorded to aid memory and later comparisons. The rating scale values are:

0 = behavior did not occur
1 = behavior occurred rarely, on up to 10 percent of spasms
2 = behavior occurred periodically, on up to 50 percent of spasms
3 = behavior occurred frequently, on more than 50 percent of the spasms

The percentages are guidelines and not precisely computed divider points. Overall, you would count the number of stuttering spasms recorded in a situation and also enter the frequency of the behaviors listed (see Chart 2-1). Blanks are provided for additional behaviors to be noted. In self-analysis you could designate different types of situations in advance, give the form to the client, and have him or her estimate the frequency of the various behaviors. You can compare the client's estimates to your own observations.

Hood (1974b) presents a very thorough descriptive assessment in which verbal output, stuttering frequency, and stuttering types are mea-

CHART 2-1

MEASURE	SITUATIONS (identify)			
Number of stutterings				
1. Part-word repetitions				
2. Whole-word repetitions				
3. Other repetitions				
4. Prolongations				
5. Block (stoppage)				
6. Silent postponement				
7. Oral postponement				
8. Starter				
9. Retrial				
10. Release				
11. Failure to complete word				
12. Heavy exhalation before utterance				
13. Air wastage during speech				

14. Improper respiration				
15. Speaking on inhalation				
16. Lip distortion				
17. Tongue distortion				
18. Mouth/jaw distortion				
19. Nasal dilation/wrinkling				
20. Eye contact loss				
21. Head movements				
22. Torso movement				
23. Arm/hand/finger movement				
24. Leg/foot movement				
25. Thoracic fixation				
26. Neck tension				
27. Interjected sounds				
28.				
29.				
30.				

sured. With this information, ten different ratios can be calculated, such as spm, fluency disruptions per syllable, avoidance-escape behaviors per disruption types, and so on. The measures are taken on reading, spontaneous speech, and picture description. The resulting measures and ratios yield fifteen data points per speech mode, or forty-five in all. The time consumption and skill requirement are significant, but the yield is high.

As you can see, the evaluation of stuttering is complex, and there are many different approaches to it. I have omitted quite a few. There are enough research studies, enough tests and forms, and sufficient different approaches to evaluation that an entire volume could be dedicated to the subject. You will need to use what is appropriate for you, from the preceding and following sections and your own experiences.

Currently certain data measures are popularly used to provide baseline data for pretherapy, progress, and maintenance checks. Some of them have been covered already but may usefully be repeated:

1. Words per minute (wpm) = meaningful words spoken, divided by total talking time in seconds, and the result multiplied by 60.

2. Syllables per minute (spm) = meaningful words spoken, multiplied by 1.5.[2] Divide by total talking time in seconds; multiply by 60.
3. Stuttered words per minute (SW/M) = number of stuttered words divided by total talking time in seconds, multiplied by 60.
4. Stuttered syllables per minute (SS/M) = number of syllables on which stuttering occurred, divided by total talking time in seconds, and the result multiplied by 60.
5. Percentage of stuttered words (%SW) = total number of stuttered words divided by the total number of words spoken. The result in multiplied by 100 and the percent sign is attached.
6. Percentage of stuttered syllables (%SS) = the total of stuttered syllables (actual count) divided by the total of syllables spoken (see 2). The result is multiplied by 100 and the percent sign is attached.

ADAPTATION AND CONSISTENCY IN STUTTERING

Adaptation

Adaptation is a learning concept which states that if unreinforced behavior is stimulated repeatedly, its frequency of occurrence will progressively reduce, theoretically to zero (extinction). This has been demonstrated in the laboratory many times. Johnson et al. (1963) claim that Johnson and Knott (1937) first reported and named the stuttering adaptation pattern. Their subjects repeated readings of the same passage from 2 to 123 times. The standard today is 5 consecutive readings with brief pauses between each reading. Shulman (1955) reported a number of factors related to adaptation:

1. Increasing the number of auditors on each successive reading did not prevent adaptation, but it was greater and faster if the auditor factor remained constant. Siegel (1964) increased and decreased audience size.
2. The delay between successive readings of the same passage, up to twenty-four hours, did not significantly affect adaptation, but adaptation was greater when the separation interval was fifteen minutes or less.
3. Length of reading passage (up to 500 words) did not significantly affect adaptation, although the percentage was higher on longer passages.
4. Adaptation correlated negatively with stuttering frequency on the first reading; that is, the higher the stuttering percentage on the first reading, the greater the adaptation on the successive readings.

Before providing additional information about adaptation, it may help to discuss the procedures for measuring it:

1. Provide the client with a (preferably) standardized reading passage and instruct her or him to read it over silently for familiarization.

[2]See earlier cautionary note. Some clinicians will prefer an actual count of syllables rather than the approximation.

2. Have the client read the passage aloud ". . . as you ordinarily would . . ." while you follow a copy of the passage. For each stuttering, mark the number 1 over the appropriate word. Treat each occurrence of stuttering as a single event, even if there is retrial, mannerisms, and other complex behaviors. Circle omitted words and write in interjected words.

3. Do not respond critically to the stutterings. After the first reading, thank the stutterer (do not praise) and direct him or her to read it aloud a second time. Follow on your copy and mark each stuttered word with a 2. Repeat this for readings 3, 4, and 5.

Be sure to tape-record the consecutive readings. Some clinicians mark all nonfluencies, of any type, and others mark only those they identify as stuttering. As you gain experience, you will find you can mark your copy with personal abbreviations concerning type and severity of spasms and indications of types of associated behaviors. Time the total reading duration for each reading (then or from the tape), and use the data for wpm or spm scores (reading rate typically increases over consecutive readings).

When the client has completed five consecutive readings, enter the information for each reading on the first three lines of the chart (see Chart 2-2). In counting total words used, reduce the total by any omitted words and increase by any interjected whole words that are new to the text. Do not add repeated words or retrials to your count. You can calculate wpm or spm (line 4) if you wish, using the formula provided earlier. Next, calculate the percentage of stuttered words (%SW) by the formula given earlier; we

CHART 2-2

Measurement	Reading Number				
	R1	R2	R3	R4	R5
1. Total words read					
2. Reading time in seconds					
3. Total stuttered words					
4. Words per minute/ syllables per minute					
5. Percentage stuttered words					
6. Adaptation % between R1 and each following reading					
7. Words stuttered on in R1 also stuttered on in the particular R_1					
8. Consistency % between R1 and each following reading					

will use this figure for each of the five readings, later, in consistency evaluation. Adaptation percentages (line 6) can be calculated between any two readings by this formula:

$$\frac{\text{stuttered words on prior reading minus stuttered words on following reading}}{\text{stuttered words on prior reading}}$$

Multiply the result by 100 and attach the percentage sign. If a client stutters 30 times on R1 and 20 times on R2,

$$\frac{30-20}{30} = \frac{10}{30} = 0.33 \times 100 = 33\%$$

If the client then stuttered 18, 9, and 7 times, respectively, on readings 3, 4, and 5, the calculations of

$$\frac{30-18}{30}, \quad \frac{30-9}{30}, \quad \text{and} \quad \frac{30-7}{30},$$

each multiplied by 100, would yield adaptation percentages of 40 percent, 70 percent, and 77 percent, respectively. Simply stated, from R1 to R5, the stutterer shows a 77 percent reduction (adaptation) in stuttering. Remember that these are adaptations compared to the first reading, R1. Adaptation from R4 to R5,

$$\frac{9-7}{9} \times 100 = 22\%$$

You might want to inspect all adaptation combinations (ten are possible on five readings), but most analyses are as presented.

You can calculate adaptation on anything you wish to count—total time, wpm or spm rates (usually negative adaptation), severity ratings, particular spasm types, and so on. There has been a great deal of research on adaptation. It has been measured in many ways—compared to spontaneous speech (Newman, 1954), in successive readings of different material, by prolonged reading, and so on. Bruce and Adams (1978) had one group read aloud five times and a second group read aloud on R1 and R5 but read in a whisper on R2, R3, and R4. The lowest adaptation percentage of the whisper reading was greater than the highest adaptation percentage of the all-aloud readings; that is, there was much less stuttering on the whisper reading. However, the aloud R5 reading of the whisper group returned to a stuttering frequency greater than that of R2, R3, R4, or R5 of the all-aloud group. Other studies approached many variables. Soderberg

(1969a) compared adaptation between stutterers and superior and inferior normal speakers. They read consecutively on the same passages, and they read consecutively where the passage was changed each reading. All three groups showed insignificant adaptation on the changing material. On repeated material, the stutterers and inferior speakers reduced all types of errors. The superior speakers had a negative time adaptation but no particular adaptation on the errors they made.

Adaptation measures by a simple comparison to R1 has been criticized (Quarrington, 1959) because the method is too subject to a high initial frequency of stuttering. F. H. Silverman (1970) noted that although stutterers adapt more than nonstutterers, the difference is due to the high R1 figure for stutterers rather than to a higher adaptation rate per se. Tate et al. (1961) reviewed four methods of measuring adaptation, finding various deficiencies in all of them. The least satisfactory one was the straight percentage method. Despite this, today the straight percentage method still is the most commonly used formula for clinical purposes.

There is a question of what to do with adaptation scores once we obtain them. Johnson et al. (1963) very cautiously suggested that negative adaptation (more stuttering on consecutive readings) may indicate a person with significant fears and anxieties, who is very vulnerable. Minimal adaptation could be as just suggested, or the stutterer may have "adapted" in advance. Over the years I have been told that negative adaptation indicates the fearful and unstable stutterer, no adaptation indicates the resistant type or perhaps a clutterer, and a very high adaptation rate suggests a stutterer who may "take refuge in fluency" under the pressure of therapy. Oddly enough, I have seen stutterers match each of these interpretations. However, I also have seen stutterers whose outcomes were at variance with those suggestions. Lanyon (1965) failed to find a usable correlation between adaptation (weighted percentage) and improvement in therapy. Prins (1970) also failed to find a useful prediction factor in adaptation.

Despite these discouraging words, there are several values in obtaining adaptation scores. Frequency levels suggest a stutterer's response to possible stress situations, and subsequent reductions suggest the flexibility of his or her responses. Also, you have an opportunity in reading to observe cyclic patterns of stuttering, changes in severity, phonetic changes in the same spasm types, and personal reactions of the client. Shames (1953) suggested its use in symptom modification therapy, possibly relating to Bloodstein's (1975b) hypothesis that the adaptation effect is due to rehearsal and short-term memory storage of motor patterns for a particular complex of speech productions. Finally, many persons cited adaptation and its presumed equivalent, laboratory extinction, as support for the concept that stuttering is learned behavior, and therefore, adaptation is "unlearning." In an excellent summary, Wingate (1976) disputes this concept and notes that results of adaptation study conflict with aspects of the learning theory models.

Consistency

Consistency of stuttering has preoccupied clinicians for generations. It is the degree to which words stuttered on in a prior performance are stuttered on again in a repeat performance. It also has a more general application, where we simply observe for commonalities; for example, does the stutterer more frequently have difficulty with certain words, certain sounds, certain sentence positions? Measurement of the first consistency type is made by the consecutive readings described previously. Johnson and Knott (1937) reported consistency effects of 65 percent to 75 percent. Many others duplicated their study. Hendel and Bloodstein (1973) found an average consistency of 48 percent, with a range of 24 percent to 78 percent. However, they also reported that different stutterers reading the same passage showed an average congruity factor of only 18 percent. Congruity denotes different stutterers stuttering on the same words. Hamre and Wingate (1973) simulated a speaking task and found a consistency measure of only 36 percent. As you can see, there is a consistency factor, and some stutterers will be very high, but we have poor agreement on the average amount. The classic method for determining consistency is the use of the system described earlier for measuring adaptation. Since you have marked stuttered words with numbers to indicate which reading they occurred on, you can return to Chart 2-2 on page 45 and enter data there on line 7. In R2, count the words stuttered that also were stuttered on in R1, and enter this figure under R2. Then count the stuttered words in R3 that also were stuttered on in R1, and enter that figure under R3. Repeat this step for R4 and R5. To obtain stuttering consistency compared to R1,[3]

$$\frac{\text{R2 stuttered words also stuttered on in R1}}{\text{total stuttered words in R1}} \times 100$$

Then repeat with R3, R4, and R5 in order to obtain the consistency measures for those readings.

Johnson et al. (1963) suggest that the value of the consistency measurement can be approximated by dividing the consistency percentage for the following (second of the pair) by the %SW of the previous reading. For example, if consistency from R1 to R5 was 40 percent and the R1 %SW was 20 percent,

$$\frac{40}{20} = 2$$

---

[3]You can make different comparisons, for example, R2 to R3 or R3 to R5, but research (Rosso & Adams, 1969) suggests that stutterings in R1 are more likely to be stuttered on in successive readings.

The authors suggest that any value above 1 represents repeated stuttering not attributed to chance as the value increases. Unfortunately, the stability of this value is affected by severity (frequency) of stuttering in the first reading:

MEASURES	STUTTERER A	STUTTERER B
Consistency % from R2	35%	35%
%SW from R1	40%	10%
Consistency ÷ %SW	0.88	3.50

As you can see, two stutterers with identical consistency percentages have two markedly different value scores, one well above chance and the more severe one falling into the range of chance consistency effect. This is unfortunate, since research indicates that severity of stuttering relates positively to consistency scores (Hamre & Wingate, 1973). The simple percentage method has been criticized as being unstable in evaluating consistency (Cullinan, 1963). Over a three-day period of readings, the simple percentage correlation was only 0.62, with a very high standard error. Three other methods were applied, with correlations ranging from 0.92 to 0.96 and a standard error that was 80 percent to 90 percent lower than that of the simple percentage method. Unfortunately, these methods are considerably more complex to use, and the simple percentage method is still used generally.

Consistency involves a number of considerations; what, basically, contributes to consistency? This will be discussed further on but requires some comment now. The so-called loci of stuttering have been studied intensively since Brown's time (1938) or earlier. He noted more stutterings on the first three words (in decreasing order) of a sentence or paragraph, and he reported the significance of stressed syllables and stuttering. Brown (1937) also reported a grammatical ranking in consistency and that information value of words affected stuttering. Trotter (1956) found that stuttering correlated with word position in the sentence, word length (above five letters), and the initial consonants. Word length has been correlated with stuttering in many studies (F.H. Silverman, 1972; Danzger & Halpern, 1973), and also longer sentences seem to increase stuttering (Tornick & Bloodstein, 1976). However, a number of studies suggest that the information value of a word, rather than length, is critical to stuttering (Soderberg, 1967, 1971; Kaasin & Bjerkan, 1982); but Peterson (1969) disagreed, and Lanyon (1968) reported that spontaneous speech, unlike reading, showed the highest correlation between stuttering and words with low information value. Researchers have found that severity affects loci (Ronson, 1976), that eliminating previously stuttered words reduces stuttering, that rearranging sentence structure is even more effective (Brutten & Gray, 1961), that stuttering does (Trotter, 1956) or does not (Soderberg, 1962a) relate to phoneme type, that expectation influences stuttering (Knott et al. 1937), that knowing what word comes next reduces stuttering (Schlesinger et al. 1965), and so on. Wingate (1979b) feels that linguistic stress is the essential feature in grammatical class and sentence position for stuttering. He suggests that we are neglecting prosody and stress and should consider them (1979a).

The foregoing discussion may have confused you concerning loci of stuttering and consistency. It is obvious that most of the research done in these interrelated areas cannot be applied to stutterers in general. Age, severity, mode of speech, environmental conditions, experimenter variables, and so on will have affected outcomes and limited applicability. However, for clinical purposes the following observations can be offered:

1. To varying degrees, stutterers will show consistency in their stuttering, the consistency generally increasing as the severity of stuttering increases.
2. Consistency of stuttering relates to a complex of factors that can include word position, length, familiarity, grammatical class, transition value, information content, initial phoneme, stuttering expectation, mode of speech, difficulty of material, linguistic stress, prosody, and others.

In evaluation, use the research variables as clues to examine consistency measurements, looking for various factors. I urge against setting up a firm standard for defining consistency against which to measure every stutterer.

Prediction

Prediction is useful in therapy. Stutterers displaying high consistency values provide for prediction of stuttering. Whether prediction explains expectation, or vice versa, is arguable. Suffice it to say that higher consistency allows the clinician to plan therapy, as needed, to emphasize or to avoid factors that favor stuttering. As noted before, you can also look for consistency in spasm type, form, rate, and so on, situations that consistently result in stuttering and associated behaviors. Shames and Egolf (1976 p. 50) have suggested that consistency of loci ". . . may well be the only form that differentiates stutterers from nonstutterers." In therapy, consistency measures can have many values.

Attitude and Adjustment

Evaluation of attitude and adjustment has been the source of frequent debate. We have been through stages of strong neurosis theory and they still exist. Bender (1939) said flatly that stuttering was closely associated with personality maladjustment. Other clinicians insist that the stuttering population distributes itself in an adjustment pattern similar to nonstutterers, and some clinicians are eclectic. At this point I will not consider cause and adjustment but discuss the client at the time of evaluation. Many studies have approached this aspect. Duncan (1949) reported that stutterers had an unsatisfactory home life and poor parental relations. Walnut (1954) found them to be slightly paranoid and depressive but not different overall from nonstutterers except in reactions to speech and speaking situations. Most other studies tend to follow lines similar to those cited—some find differences, and some find a fairly normal distribution. Woods (1977) summarized the stereotype stutterer from various studies. Stutterers are expected to be quiet, reticent, hesitant, guarded, avoiding, introverted, passive, and self-derogatory. Also, they are assumed to be anxious, tense, nervous, afraid, less friendly, and more sensitive. Interestingly, Woods states that when stutterers and nonstutterers carried out pseudostuttering (faking) assignments, their reports expressed many of the feelings just listed.

Clinicians have questioned the significance of considering attitude and adjustment because of conflicting research and/or because the therapy that induces fluency is supposed to eliminate emotional concerns (Ryan, 1979). Others provide extensive considerations of fears, anxieties, frustrations, hostilities, guilt, and other attitude and adjustment factors (Van Riper, 1982). In between, there is space and need to consider the attitude stutterers have toward speech and speaking situations. Early efforts to evaluate attitude were variable in terms of reliability. Ammons and Johnson (1944) published an attitude scale, which although of uneven reliability, was a standard test of attitude for many years. This scale provided forty-five statements with which the person agreed or disagreed, on a scale basis. Statements such as "A stutterer should not become a teacher" or "People should feel sorry for a stutterer" were rated on the level of agreement scale. Although temporally and socially dated in certain areas, the scale can provide some information in evaluation. The halo effect is strong, and clients should be counseled concerning objectivity when taking the scale. It also can be used with nonstutterers.

A related measure of attitude is the Stutterer's Self-Ratings of Reactions to Speech Situations (Shumak, 1955). This scale lists forty situations involving speech. Each situation is rated four times: degree of avoidance by the stutterer, attitude toward the situation, amount of stuttering in each, and frequency with which each situation is met. Using ninety-five adult stutterers, Shumak found moderate positive correlations between stuttering frequency and situation avoidance and stuttering frequency and attitude toward situations. She obtained a better (0.84) correlation between attitude and avoidance. An adapted form of instructions and the original scale (see Chart 2-3) are presented:

> For each of the 40 situations, use the four ratings that most accurately describe you most of the time. If there is a situation you have not met, try and think of a similar situation you do meet, and answer as best you can; but inform the examiner about these items. Answer all 40 items in one column; then fold a piece of paper to cover your answers, and answer the next column. Each time, cover your previous answers until you have responded to all four columns. The four rating groups are:

AVOIDANCE

1. I never try to avoid this situation and have no desire to avoid it.
2. I don't try to avoid this situation, but sometimes I would like to.
3. Usually I do not try to avoid this situation, but sometimes I do.
4. Usually I try to avoid this situation.
5. I avoid this situation every time I possibly can.

REACTION

1. I definitely enjoy speaking in this situation.
2. I would rather speak in this situation than not speak.
3. It's hard to say whether I'd rather speak in this situation or not.
4. I would rather not speak in this situation.
5. I very much dislike speaking in this situation.

STUTTERING

1. I don't stutter at all (or very rarely) in this situation.
2. I stutter mildly (for me) in this situation.
3. I stutter with average severity (for me) in this situation.
4. I stutter more than the average (for me) in this situation.
5. I stutter severely (for me) in this situation.

FREQUENCY

1. I meet this very often, two or three times a day, or more, on the average.
2. I meet this at least once a day with rare exceptions (Sunday perhaps).
3. I meet this from three to five times a week on the average.
4. I usually meet this once a week and, occasionally, twice a week.
5. I rarely meet this, certainly not as often as once a week.

CHART 2-3 *Stutterer's Self-Ratings of Reactions to Speech Situations (Shumak, 1955)*

SITUATIONS	RATINGS			
	Avoidance	Reaction	Stuttering	Frequency
1. Ordering in a restaurant				
2. Introducing myself, face to face				
3. Telephoning to ask a price				
4. Buying a plane, train, or bus ticket				
5. Short class recitation (10 words or less)				
6. Telephoning for a taxi				
7. Introducing one person to another				
8. Buying something from a store clerk				
9. Conversation with a good friend				
10. Talking with a teacher after class or in office				
11. Long-distance telephone call to someone I know				
12. Conversation with father				
13. Asking girl for a date or talking to a man who asks me for a date				
14. Making a short speech (1 or 2 minutes) in a familiar class				
15. Giving my name over the telephone				
16. Conversation with my mother				

CHART 2-3   *(Cont.)*

SITUATIONS	RATINGS			
	Avoidance	Reaction	Stuttering	Frequency
17. Asking a secretary if I can see [the] employer				
18. Going to a house and asking for someone				
19. Making a speech to an unfamiliar audience				
20. Participating in committee meetings				
21. Asking an instructor questions in class				
22. Saying hello to a friend going by				
23. Asking for a job				
24. Telling a person a message from someone else				
25. Telling a funny story with one stranger in a crowd				
26. Parlor games requiring speech				
27. Reading aloud to friends				
28. Participating in a bull session				
29. Dinner conversation with strangers				
30. Talking with my barber or beauty operator				
31. Telephoning for an appointment or to arrange a meeting with someone				

32. Answering roll call in class				
33. Asking at a desk for a book or a card to be filled out				
34. Talking with someone I don't know well while waiting for a bus or class				
35. Talking with other players during a playground game				
36. Taking leave of a hostess				
37. Conversation with a friend while walking along the street				
38. Buying stamps at the post office				
39. Giving directions or information to a stranger				
40. Taking leave of a girl (boy) after a date				
Add each column and divide by the number of items answered to obtain the average score				

Shumak reported a series of response patterns which are summarized as follows:

Interpretation of Scores on Stutterer's Self-Rating of Reactions to Stuttering

MODE OF RESPONSE	MEAN	SD	25TH %TILE	50TH %TILE	75TH %TILE	RANGE OF SCORES
Avoidance	2.31	.66	1.82	2.20	2.80	1.02-4.00
Reaction	2.57	.62	2.10	2.56	2.80	1.41-3.97
Stuttering	2.54	.60	2.08	2.53	2.98	1.20-3.02
Frequency	3.80	.45	3.48	3.88	4.11	2.30-4.72

The overall score averages may or may not be meaningful to you. However, observation of the individual situations and the client's responses may be very useful (this will be referred to again in the chapter on self-analysis). You also can add situations unique to age, sex, vocation, social status, hobbies, and so forth of the client. This will preclude comparisons with norms but might provide very useful information.

Lanyon (1967) developed a paper-and-pencil measure of stuttering behaviors and attitudes, finding a clear separation between stutterers and nonstutterers. Brutten (1973) presented a speech situation checklist and noted it was important to screen out stutterers who have significant fears not associated with speech or the act of speaking. F. H. Silverman (1980) provided a form to evaluate therapy results, which could be revised for diagnostic use. He makes the valid point that what is important to the clinician may not be important to the client.

Erickson (1969) reported on a form assessing communication attitudes of stutterers, called the S-scale. A total of thirty-nine items are designated as "true" or "false" by the respondent. There was wide variation in responses, but stuttering groups averaged 25.65 and nonstutterers 13.24, with 95 percent of the stutterers falling above the median of the nonstutterers. I administered the full form to twenty-nine college juniors in a stuttering class and obtained a mean score of 14.6 and a median of 13, based on a range of 4 to 24 points. Andrews and Cutler (1974) deleted fifteen items from the S-scale that were not suitable for repeated administration, deriving a twenty-four-item scale that is more valid and reliable. The retained items and their scorable answers (*) are listed in Chart 2-4.

Guitar and Bass (1978) used the modified Erickson Scale (S24) and found a significant relationship (S24 score of 9 or below) between stutterers' scale scores and their long-term response to therapy. This study was criticized strongly (Ingham, 1979), but Guitar's response (1979) supported his original findings. E. M. Silverman (1980) used the modified form of the S-scale with women who stuttered, finding that they averaged about 66 percent (about 16), whereas nonstuttering women averaged about 24 percent (about 6), and male stutterers averaged about 78 percent (about 19). A recent study (Ulliana & Ingham, 1984) has raised questions about the prognostic values of S24 as it related to overall speech attitudes, but this doubt does not change the test's usefulness in evaluating stuttering and progress in therapy.

Whether you wish to administer projective tests or other measures of psychological adjustment is a matter that concerns your philosophy, your time, and your expertise. Concerning attitudes toward speech, speaking situations, and self-concept as a speaker, there seems ample justification to assess the stutterer. I would suggest an evaluation of attitudes toward stuttering specifically as assessment of reactions to speech situations, similar to Shumak's and the S-scale or its equivalent. Whether you decide to cate-

CHART 2-4

Answer the following by circling "T" if a statement is generally true for you, or circle "F" if the statement is generally false for you. If the situation is unfamiliar or rare, judge it on an "If it was familiar . . ." basis.

1.	T	F*	I usually feel that I am making a favorable impression when I talk.
2.	T	F*	I find it easy to talk with almost anyone.
3.	T	F*	I find it very easy to look at my audience while talking to a group.
4.	T*	F	A person who is my teacher or my boss is hard to talk to.
5.	T*	F	Even the idea of giving a talk in public makes me afraid.
6.	T*	F	Some words are harder than others for me to say.
7.	T	F*	I forget all about myself shortly after I begin to give a speech.
8.	T	F*	I am a good mixer.
9.	T*	F	People sometimes seem uncomfortable when I am talking to them.
10.	T*	F	I dislike introducing one person to another.
11.	T	F*	I often ask questions in group discussions.
12.	T	F*	I find it easy to keep control of my voice when speaking.
13.	T	F*	I do not mind speaking before a group.
14.	T*	F	I do not talk well enough to do the kind of work I'd really like to do.
15.	T	F*	My speaking voice is rather pleasant and easy to listen to.
16.	T*	F	I am sometimes embarrassed by the way I talk.
17.	T	F*	I face most speaking situations with complete confidence.
18.	T*	F	There are few people I can talk with easily.
19.	T	F*	I talk better than I write.
20.	T*	F	I often feel nervous while talking.
21.	T*	F	I often find it hard to talk when I meet new people.
22.	T	F*	I feel pretty confident about my speaking ability.
23.	T*	F	I wish I could say things as clearly as others do.
24.	T*	F	Even though I knew the right answer I have often failed to give it because I was afraid to speak out.

gorize your client with a psychological label is not important; but you should have a basic understanding of his or her attitudes, feelings, and coping behaviors as a communicating person.

OTHER FACTORS IN EVALUATION

How much territory you can cover in evaluation is open-ended and has been discussed earlier. The research studies are very fertile. Strother and Kriegman (1944) suggested rhythmokinesis[4] differences between stut-

---

[4]Ability to move feet, fingers, lips, tongue, and other body parts so as to imitate stimulated or modeled rhythm patterns.

terers and nonstutterers. Wingate (1967, 1971b) reported stutterer inferiority on phonetic manipulation and translation tasks. Reaction time on voicing and whispering vowels was reported as being prolonged for stutterers (Venkatagiri, 1981), and close scrutiny of interarticulation positions was recommended by Zimmerman (1980b). Auditory processing studies reported that stutterers are significantly slower in oral responses to auditory stimuli (McFarlane & Prins, 1978), that stutterers had lower central auditory function scores (Wynne & Boehmler, 1982), and that stutterers were inferior on Illinois Test of Psycholinguistic Abilities (ITPA) auditory processing (Riley, 1980). Liebetrau and Daly (1981) divided stutterers into organic and functional groups; the organic group was reported to be poorer in auditory processing and perceptual abilities. Shearer (1966), among others, commented on the significance of stapedius middle ear muscle contractions in stuttering, and Brutten and Janssen (1979) reported that stutterers show more eye fixations and more forward and regressive eye movements in reading. In two reports (1966, 1970), Neaves summarized the factors related to over 150 stutterers, in age groups from eight to twelve years and thirteen to seventeen years, and their success in therapy. Success was defined as 0 percent to 4 percent stuttered words (4 percent or less SW), and failure as 5 percent or more stuttered words. The following factors were studied:

1. Age—surprisingly, more (60 percent) of the successes were in the thirteen-to-seventeen-year-old group than in the eight-to-twelve-year-old group (44 percent).
2. Motor ability—58 percent of the success group was normal; only 22 percent of the failure group was normal.
3. Lateral dominance—61 percent of the success group displayed clear lateral dominance, compared to only 43 percent of the failure group.
4. Intelligence—the success group was significantly (.01) higher on both verbal and performance scale measures.
5. Adjustment—the successes in the eight-to-twelve-year-old group tended to be assertive and self-reliant, compared to the nonsuccessful group; the successes in the older group tended to be expressive, self-sufficient, and more relaxed, whereas those in the failure group tended to be more depressed, threat-sensitive and withdrawn, more excitable, and more tense.
6. Speech history—the failure group had significantly (.01) more abnormalities of speech development.
7. Age of onset—the success group significantly (.01) more often had onsets later than those in the failure group.
8. Familial history—the failure group had a significantly (.01) higher incidence of family history of stuttering.
9. Social class—the higher the social class, the better the chance for success (.05 level).
10–13. Birth history, traumatic experiences, number in family and ordinal position, and occurrence of significant illnesses were not related to the outcome of the therapy.

If a stutterer was negative on only one of the thirteen items, the possibility for success in therapy was 80 percent. The probability dropped to 50 percent if two factors were negative, to 10 percent for three negative factors, and only to 5 percent if four of the factors were negative.

Many clinicians evaluate respiration, more so than in the recent past. Some give it preeminence in the diagnostic scheme and recommend use of instruments such as the pneumotachograph to generate a paper printout of breathing and diaphragm movements (Brankel, 1961). Rather than discuss respiration to any degree here, I will cover it in the chapter on airflow techniques. In general terms, you will want to assess both vegetative (quiet, nonspeech) breathing and deep breathing for speech and normal activity. Details and procedures will be indicated in Chapter 10.

The anamnesis, or case history, is a basic information source in the evaluation, often mailed in advance to the client, to be returned before or at the time of evaluation. Case histories come in many forms, with considerable variation in length. In addition to the usual history about birth and development, health, education, and so on, you will want to secure additional information about stuttering. The following topics can be refined into individual questions or used as a guide for a narrative interview:

1. Familial stuttering—in the immediate family and several generations back. Try to elicit descriptions, reactions, and treatment information. Porfert and Rosenfield (1978) found positive family histories in all categories of stuttering, but Kidd et al. (1980) found no relation between severity of the stuttering and family history.
2. Onset of stuttering—age first noticed, events or conditions at the time, how noticed and by whom, initial characteristics, reactions of auditors and of the client.
3. Early stuttering history—thorough description of early developmental stages, fluctuations, remissions, awareness and reactions of the client over time, environmental responses, related events.
4. Ongoing stuttering history—continued development of stuttering, symptom changes, awareness and behavior, environmental responses, therapy efforts (naive and professional), fluctuations or remissions, apparent effects on functions.
5. Current stuttering—complete description of current stuttering, in detail, to describe
   a. Physical characteristics of spasms in terms of types, forms, and severities.
   b. Associated behaviors or mannerisms and variations in them.
   c. Self-concept and social behavior with regard to stuttering and speech.
6. Attitude—does the client regard him- or herself as a helpless victim or as a fighter? What is the client's motivation to therapy? Does the client use stuttering as a crutch or alibi? Is the pattern of the covert or overt type? What is the attitude toward speaking in general? And what is the level of social adequacy?
7. Knowledge—what does the client know about stuttering in general, and about stuttering therapy in particular?

8. Goals—a careful exploration of the client's goals. Refer back to the level of knowledge. Check for superficial objectivity. How would fluency change the client's behavior? What time and effort are perceived as necessary for therapy? Does the client want to be a passive recipient, an active participant, or a critical evaluator of therapy activities?

The foregoing could be expanded for different clients. However, it will be useful as a start on a basic history addition for stuttering evaluation.

Laterality, at one time, was regarded as highly significant, a linking to the lateral dominance of the cerebral hemispheres. Bryngelson and Rutherford (1937) reported a high level of ambidexterity among stutterers, as well as a large number who had been forced to shift from sinistral (left) to dextral (right) handedness. However, Records et al. (1977) indicated that stutterers did not differ significantly in terms of their peripheral lateral dominance. Van Riper (1982) reviewed the lateral dominance question, generally concluding that it has minimal value in diagnosis. However, he noted a number of studies that suggest that stutterers, or some of them, have a shift in central (cerebral) laterality. He also discussed sixteen dichotic (competing auditory messages presented simultaneously, one to each ear) listening studies and found reason to support a difference between stutterers, or subgroups of them, and nonstutterers. Many tests of laterality are available. In general, I suggest that the usual diagnostic observation of overall motor coordination and laterality should determine whether more extensive testing is needed.

The differentiation between stuttering and cluttering can complicate a diagnosis. Superficially, the two seem similar, but the clutterer typically presents a much broader picture of deficit in speech and language. Perkins (1978) and others refer to it as a symptom of a central language imbalance. Darley (1964) describes the clutterer as talking with an irregular rate, slighting or omitting consonants, and displaying syllable elisions. There will be occasional repetitions and revisions, slips of the tongue, and self-interruptions. In reading, clutterers will tend to ignore punctuation as they read in a rush, neglect phrasing, omit and insert syllables and words, transpose words, and breathe at inappropriate points. General comparisons are as follows:

1. The stutterer usually is aware of every nonfluent event, whereas the clutterer rushes along without awareness.
2. If the stutterer concentrates on her or his speech, it usually becomes more nonfluent, whereas self-attention of the clutterer typically improves fluency.
3. Compared to reading or directed speech, stutterers often are better in spontaneous speech, and clutterers generally are worse.
4. Stutterers usually are more nonfluent with strangers, and clutterers are better.
5. Brief verbalizations are more difficult for stutterers to control and easier for clutterers.
6. Structured retrials usually do not improve in stuttering but do in cluttering.

This list is general and not complete. Also, there will be stutterer-clutterers (or vice versa) to complicate evaluations.

Examination of the peripheral speech mechanism is part of any complete evaluation and should be done in stuttering. As part of the procedure, check for tactile and kinesthetic awareness:

1. Use a sterile tongue depressor or cotton swab and have the client's eyes closed. Touch various parts of the lips, tongue, and palatal vault (do not elicit a gag reflex) and have the client locate in terms of structure touched, right-left-middle and front-back-middle.
2. With client's eyes closed, direct him or her to place the jaws, lips, and tongue in various positions. Observe the accuracy. Repeat the directions while the client looks in a mirror and performs.

You also may wish to check diadochokinesis and rhythmokinesis. For the former, Johnson et al. (1963) suggest that rapid production of [tʌ] can be used, with a below average speed being less than three productions per second, and above average speed being more than 5.5 productions per second.[5] Rhythmokinesis is very subjective, and you want only to determine basic skills. Be sure you don't wind up testing auditory memory span. On the basis of clinical experience, I suggest the following rhythms, using [pʌ], [tʌ], and [kʌ]. Notice the stress marks:

1. pʌ—pʌ—pʌpʌpʌ
2. pʌ'pʌ—pʌ'pʌ—pʌpʌpʌ
3. pʌ'pʌpʌ—pʌpʌ—pʌpʌ'
4. pʌ—pʌpʌpʌ'—pʌpʌ' (Shave and a haircut, two bits!)

Using these examples, you can devise your own patterns. You may want to combine the syllables in various ways and culminate in the old favorite [pʌtʌkʌ].

Autobiography

The autobiography has its ups and downs in stuttering. If you are planning fluency therapy you may not use it, whereas it is often used for counseling and symptom modification. I have found it useful for several reasons: for the information you obtain, for the degree of insight and knowledge the stutterer displays, for the attitude and motivation shown by the client in terms of what is produced, and as a preliminary step in self-analysis. I will discuss the autobiography in the self-analysis chapter, but a basic outline follows:

Respond to the questions below as best you can, and say as much as you wish. Use a separate sheet for each area, even if your answer is short; we may add to

---

[5]Use a recorder with at least two speeds. Record at the faster speed and play back at the slower while you count. Remember to adjust the time span.

it later. Remember, your answers are confidential and will be used only as we have discussed the evaluation information.

1. Provide a summary of what you can remember about the onset of stuttering. When, where, how, and what was it like? How did you feel? What did you do? How did others respond?
2. After onset, how did your stuttering progress? What changes occurred and when? How did your speech attitudes change? What help did you receive, and how did various people respond to you?
3. Describe your speech now; be as exact and informative as you can. How does speech affect what you do or don't do?
4. If you did not stutter, what things would change—what plans or goals would change?
5. What people have had the most influence, positive or negative, on your speech?
6. Describe three occasions you regard as the most difficult or embarrassing, because of your speech.
7. Discuss what you hope to achieve in therapy, what you think therapy will be, and how long you think it will take you to achieve your therapy goals.

The list can be reduced or expanded. At times I have used the first three items only and then added more questions as therapy progressed.

Counseling

Counseling the stutterer is an important part of evaluation and subsequent therapy. The client should receive your information and recommendations so that your competence is enhanced and her or his uncertainties reduced. Provide a statement covering the relative severity, speech situation behavior, and attitude. Recommend the therapy approach you intend to follow and secure the client's commitment to the therapy process. Invite and encourage questions, taking the time to make the client feel that questions are welcome. Periodically ask the client to summarize or interpret what you have said; misunderstanding or mistaken emphasis is common and you want the client to perceive what you think you are saying. Whatever your therapy plan, don't mislead the client about time. If a two-year maintenance program is part of the plan, be sure that is explained initially and not later in therapy. Varying with the types of therapy planned, I like to send the client away with an assignment of some type. It may be a paper-and-pencil scale to take, an autobiography, a preliminary list of fear hierarchies, or other tasks. Finally, the business aspects of schedules, rooms, fees, parking, releases, and so on should be completed.

PRACTICE ASSIGNMENTS IN EVALUATION

Projects in this chapter are difficult to structure since I cannot provide stutterers or audio or video tapes or ask you to simulate stuttering (at this point). Also, a number of the procedures need real stutterers to be at all useful. Some of the procedures mentioned earlier are indicated, rather than specifically described, and those would not be appropriate for practice assignments. In class your instructor may stipulate certain procedure projects or add procedures she or he recommends. The projects can be done in any sequence, with omissions or additions and reporting requirements as needed. As suggested in Chapter 1, I recommend that you secure a partner for some of the assignments. In several instances I have suggested that you get an audio or video tape of certain performances or that you observe a stutterer; your own situation will establish the availability of such responses.

1. Write or type the following form on a sheet of paper. Separate each category line by an inch or more of space. Fill in the data from the activities that follow.

Nonfluency in Fluent Speech

	SITUATIONS			
NONFLUENCIES	1	2	3	4
Interjections				
Phrase or word repetitions				
Syllable or sound repetitions				
Inappropriate pauses				
Misarticulations and mispronounciations				
Omissions				
Prolongations				

a. Monitor a program on radio or television in which talkers do not use a script, prompter, or memorized lines. Accumulate three minutes of talking time on one talker, counting each dysfluency and putting a mark by the appropriate line in the first column (label your column). For this and other assignments, ignore behaviors that seem to be deliberate, for example, a long pause for thought or a deliberate repetition for emphasis. Otherwise, if in doubt, call it a nonfluency.

b. Repeat the assignment with a different person and different program. Label the second column and enter your results.

c. Use a book, magazine, or newspaper and have your partner read aloud for three minutes. If possible, tape-record the reading. Mark each nonfluency in the third column. Play back the recording and check your scoring.

d. Call a friend, tape-recording the conversation (your side only). Talk until you think you have accumulated at least five minutes of talking. Later, play back the tape, skipping approximately the first minute of talking time (your talking). Then listen to the next three minutes of your talking time, marking nonfluencies in the fourth column.

2. Listen to three different speakers (teachers, preachers, public speakers, and so on) who are talking to groups. For each, count the total nonfluencies (not by type) during about three minutes of talking time. Write a short paragraph on each speaker—describe the situation, report the number of nonfluencies, and describe their predominant pattern.

3. Throughout an entire day, rate every spontaneous speaker you hear long enough (at least one minute) to apply one of the following criteria:
    a. Unusually fluent—no perceptible nonfluencies.
    b. Fluent—rare, mild nonfluencies.
    c. Average fluency—occasional mild or moderate nonfluencies.
    d. Nonfluent—frequent nonfluencies.
    e. Very nonfluent—frequent, noticeable, and distracting nonfluencies. How many persons fell into each category? How did they differ?

4. Take the different nonfluency categories in 1 and collect twenty speakers (spontaneous) who talk long enough for you to identify their predominant nonfluency type(s). Report each person's sex, the estimated age, the situation, and the nonfluency type(s) most predominant.

5. On a separate sheet of paper or on a file card, prepare the following format:

Speaking Time Summary

SITUATION	NUMBER MET	TIME (IN SECONDS, THAT YOU TALKED IN EACH SITUATION)
Social greetings		
Social conversation		
Telephone—social		
Telephone—business		
Classroom—social		
Classroom—academic		
Business		
Mealtime		
Job—social		
Job—work		
Other:		

From the time you wake up until you go to sleep, count and estimate your talking time (in seconds) for every situation:

a. Count all social greetings as three seconds.

   b. Carry the report form with you. Each hour, or nearly so, fill in the Number Met and Time blanks for the previous hour.

   c. Tape-record several telephone calls. Estimate your time as usual. Then play the tape and actually time yourself to check the accuracy of your estimates. Tape only your side of the conversation.

   d. Add up the times and events and report. Indicate if this was a typical day for you. What did you find out?

6. Use a cassette recorder and any paragraph from a printed source.

   a. Read the paragraph aloud while recording. Make sure the recording lasts at least one minute. Following the procedures in this chapter, calculate your wpm rate. Multiply the total number of words by 1.5 and calculate your spm rate. Now count the actual syllables read, divide by the number of words, and see how close you come to 1.5.

   b. Record yourself talking for the same length of time you read in 6.a. Talk about any topic, such as a book or movie. On playback (make sure your time here matches the reading time in 6.a), count the words spoken and calculate your wpm rate. How did it differ from your wpm rate for reading?

7. Listen to a recording of a stutterer reading or talking for at least one minute. On a separate sheet of paper, copy the following information categories and provide the information needed:

   a. Total talking time, in seconds   ————————

   b. Total words spoken   ————————

   c. wpm rate   ————————

   d. spm rate   ————————

   e. Total words stuttered   ————————

   f. SW/M   ————————

   g. %SW   ————————

8. Listen again to the tape used in 7. On a separate sheet of paper, copy these information categories and provide the information needed:

Repetitions	————	Prolongations	————	Blocks	————
Postponements	————	Starters	————	Retrials	————
Releases	————	Average duration of spasms	———— sec.		

9. Observe a stutterer, live or on video tape, until you have accumulated approximately three minutes of talking time. On a separate sheet of paper, copy the stuttering behaviors on Chart 2-1 and mark the occurrence of each behavior, adding any that are not on the list. Also, answer the following questions:

   a. On the average, how long did spasms last?

   b. What was the SW/M score?

   c. Using the severity references on page 42, what severity rating would you apply?

10. Select any paragraph or reading passage of 300 to 500 words and have your partner record it five consecutive times, reading in his or her normal fashion. Make a copy of the paragraph, leaving several spaces between each word and

about one-half inch between each line. As your partner reads, mark each nonfluency with 1, 2, 3, 4, or 5, depending on the reading. If you are cursed with a very fluent partner, have her or him deliberately insert errors of the types identified in the first footnote below. Play the recordings back for analysis. On a separate sheet of paper, copy the following categories and provide the information needed:

Adaptation and Consistency

CATEGORY	R1	R2	R3	R4	R5
Total words spoken					
Total talking time, in seconds					
Number of nonfluencies[a]					
Words per minute					
% of nonfluent words					
Time adaptation[b]					
Nonfluency adaptation[c]					
Nonfluencies in R1 also present in Ri					
Consistency % between R1 and each following reading[d]					

[a] Interjections, repetitions, prolongations, inappropriate pauses, omissions, misarticulations, mispronounciations, and other errors.

[b] $\dfrac{\text{Time (sec.) R1} - \text{time (sec.) R2}}{\text{Time (sec.) R1}} \times 100$. Repeat for R3, R4, and R5.

[c] $\dfrac{\text{Nonfluencies in R1} - \text{nonfluencies in R2}}{\text{Nonfluencies in R1}} \times 100$. Repeat for R3, R4, and R5.

[d] $\dfrac{\text{R2 nonfluencies also nonfluent in R1}}{\text{total nonfluencies in R1}} \times 100$. Repeat with R3, R4, and R5.

11. On a separate page, copy the following form. Number the lines 1 to 40 and use the self-rating section on page 52 (don't copy each of the 40 items). Use the rating scale on page 55 and fill out the form. Note that "Fluency" replaces the "Stuttering" column, and substitute criteria for that column are

1. I am very fluent in this situation.
2. I am usually fluent, but may produce a few nonfluencies.
3. This is about my average fluency level.
4. I will be more nonfluent than usual in this situation.
5. I am liable to be very nonfluent in this situation.

Compare your results to those of your partner.

SITUATION	AVOIDANCE	REACTION	FLUENCY	FREQUENCY
1.				
2.				
etc.				
40.				

12. On a separate page, number 1 through 24, one line per number. Take the revised S-scale on page 57 and score it according to the instructions. How did you compare to the norms? Compare your score to those of others in your class.

13. Use a stopwatch or timepiece that shows seconds and a cassette recorder. You and your partner are to take turns producing a five-second series of [pʌ], [tʌ], and [kʌ]. Move as rapidly as you can, recording the productions (use a slower speed, if possible, on playback). Divide each set of productions by five to obtain the per second average. What was your rate? How did it compare to your partner's?

14. Write a brief autobiography covering the following areas:
    a. Your early speech development—when did you start to talk? What was your progress? Problems?
    b. What have been your hardest and easiest academic subjects in school, and why?
    c. How did you learn about this profession, and why did you enter it?
    d. What persons have been most influential (positively or negatively) in your life?
    e. What are your professional and personal goals?
    Compare your autobiography with that of your partner. Ask her or him appropriate questions to clarify the statements, or secure more information. What did you learn about using autobiographies?

3

Self-Analysis Techniques

BACKGROUND TO SELF-ANALYSIS

The analysis of stuttering and speech behavior by the client has a long history. Review of the literature discloses a number of references (Berry & Eisenson, 1945; Bryngelson et al. 1944; Chapman, 1959) that stress the application of self-analysis procedures. For many it was regarded as a standard, or required, procedure for the stutterer to be able to analyze his or her own stuttering in terms of its varying symptoms, and to recognize and understand feelings associated with speech and stuttering (Van Riper, 1958). In a direct address to the stutterer, Johnson (1961b) advocated intense self-study of stuttering by deliberately repeating stutterings over and over to study every aspect of the spasm. In some instances, the application of behavior therapy reduced or even eliminated analysis procedures in therapy (following the diagnostic evaluation). Some behavioral practitioners argued that concentrating on the abnormal behaviors (see Chapter 1) was, at best, inefficient, and at worst, a reinforcement of pathological behavior. Many clinicians find this view to be an "if-loaded" presumption based on a shaky theoretical foundation. Cooper (1971a) described a therapy procedure combining behavior control and traditional therapy for stuttering, with stress on identification, examination, and confrontation. Ryan (1978) noted for his behaviorist stance described an operant program in which spasm counting and description were taught contingently, preliminary to moving into a mixture of symptom modification and fluency reinforcement. However, Ladoucer et al. (1982) reported that systematic awareness training did not affect the outcome of a therapy program based on two ninety-minute regulated-breathing training sessions (Azrin & Nunn, 1974). Opposite this report, Ingham (1982) had stutterers practice monitoring stuttering and speech rate, structuring it into self-managed, performance-contingent maintenance schedules. Covert and overt checking systems were used, and he felt the results strongly supported the use of even this very limited self-analysis procedure.

Rationale

A rationale for self-analysis goes beyond the extremely limited, laboratory-type count data just described. Counting and classifying (while important) bear the same resemblance to self-analysis that inhalation-only does to speech. Both are requisite capacities but are not the whole process. There are many other overt features of stuttering that require analysis, and as Naylor (1953) pointed out, the audible-visible signs of stuttering ignore the "inner disturbance" that makes the stutterers' evaluations unique. For these reasons, the following definition of, or goal statement for, stuttering self-analysis is offered:

> Self-analysis encompasses the awareness of each stuttering occurrence when it happens; cognizance of the type, severity, and physical location(s) of the stuttering; description of the struggle, overflow, and associated behavior patterns; understanding of attitudes concerning stuttering in particular and speech in general; and a perception of the environmental reactions to moments of stuttering, as they occur. Further, to varying degrees, self-analysis encompasses the characteristics of nonstuttered speech of the stutterer and of other speakers. These elements of self-analysis should be available as part of the stutterer's own knowledge and be functional during any situation in which he or she participates.

On the basis of the foregoing definition, a rationale can be structured.

Simply understanding a significant aspect of one's behavior can be a worthwhile justification in itself. However, I do not believe that simply knowing oneself is an acceptable therapy goal. Knowledge generally has its greatest value when it facilitates the change of existing behaviors and/or the development of new behaviors. Its value is to the clinician as well as the client, and possible benefits are these:

1. Addition to or correction of diagnostic information.
2. Guidance in the selection of the major therapy mode(s) to be used.
3. Suggestions for adaptations in sequence, content, and time schedule of the steps comprising the therapy mode(s).
4. Assistance in applying and interpreting specific procedures.

5. Awareness by the stutterer of her or his behaviors and the factors related to them.
6. Early desensitization to stuttering.
7. Greater awareness of self-fluency and nonfluencies of others.
8. A progressive development of self-structured monitoring, evaluation, planning, and management.
9. Facilitation of transfer and maintenance activities.

Although, as stated earlier, self-analysis has strong roots in symptomatic psychotherapy, I am not proposing it as a preliminary step to a program of symptom modification therapy. If I were planning a program of DAF rate control, regulated airflow, GILCU, relaxation, or other procedures covered in this book, I would want a thorough self-analysis program for the reasons already stated. Many clinicians would not apply such a program, or would apply it very selectively, to stutterers in the age range of eight to ten years or below. With appropriate awareness of the different, intermingled tracks of stuttering development (for example, Bloodstein, 1975a, discussed in Chapter 2), I would agree with those who reduce or avoid self-analysis. However, in most instances above the age range cited, failure to stress self-analysis is likely to result in unthinking symptom modification or induced symptom suppression. Both approaches serve the stutterer poorly.

Areas to Analyze

Areas requiring analysis have been covered more or less in the definition offered earlier and will be discussed in following sections. A brief summary follows. It should be stressed that clients will differ in the emphases needed for the various areas. These differences will vary according to prior knowledge of therapy, therapy experience, awareness capacity, attitude and tolerance, and orientation to therapy. The goals are these:

1. Awareness of stuttering when it occurs, each time.
2. Identification of spasm types, locations, and severities.
3. Description of tension levels, struggle, and overflow phenomena.
4. Descriptions of associated behaviors and mannerisms.
5. Awareness of antiexpectancy behaviors.
6. Evaluation of attitude, tolerance, fears, and so on, associated with stuttering and with speech in general.
7. Evaluation of client's own nonstuttered speech and the speech of others.
8. Awareness of the attitudes and responses of auditors during stuttering.

Each of these is an evaluatable complex of information and skills. Each can be broken into a number of subareas, and a subarea of particular significance to a client could be separated as a major component of analysis.

Scheduling

Scheduling and combination factors are important in self-analysis. As has been indicated previously, the time taken, sequence followed, and emphasis distribution can vary from client to client. One client may need to start with item 8 because of strong fears of and incorrect assumptions about auditors and the environment. Some clinicians prefer to start with item 7 to prove to the client that he or she is "fluent" most of the time. A few clients may need some demonstrated improvement in their speech before they can be motivated to work on self-analysis. At times the more production-performance aspects of the first four items are accomplished as a sequenced unit, and the remaining items are applied in progressive steps during stages of symptom or fluency work. It probably is most efficient to decide what area to start with, and let initial reactions determine your scheduling needs and times for the remaining areas.

The organization of this chapter will follow the eight items cited. In some sections, related considerations (for example, use of assignments) will be inserted. Since simply telling you, "Have the stutterer read aloud and count spasms" will not be very helpful, I will attempt to arrange each analysis section systematically. The area will be described, any relevant information provided, and special considerations mentioned. A series of activities will be suggested, as examples, in approximately progressive levels of difficulty. The reader should understand that these activities are exemplary, and are not the only method or a rigid sequence. Many factors, such as client's employment, client's type, locale of clinic, and personal considerations, can change opportunities and needs. Be flexible and inventive. At the end of this chapter will be some general assignments for you, followed by several examples of multiple assignments for clients.

THE CLINICIAN IN SELF-ANALYSIS

Stuttering Stereotype

The stuttering stereotype is a factor in therapy. For many years it was said that stutterers were like any other person except for the fact that they stuttered. Nevertheless, as noted before, many clinicians seem to fear stutterers. Wingate (1971a) comments on this, believing that stuttering is regarded as an enigma or mystery, that many of us really believe it is a psychological problem, that the therapy methods are of doubtful efficacy, and even the name or label has acquired potential for anxiety, so that we use euphemisms such as "dysfluency" or "the stuttering problem" rather than the word itself. Two excellent articles on stuttering stigma and stereotype come from Australia (Woods, 1976, 1977). The first article reports on the views of teachers, public school clinicians, college students, adult stutterers, parents of stutterers, and parents of nonstutterers. Generally, all the groups had a strong stereotype of the stutterer, including the stuttering group. They projected a stereotype of a submissive, tense, insecure person who was afraid to talk to people. In the second study, Woods performed a factor analysis to determine some of the dimensions of the stereotype. The Expansive-Restrictive (bipolar attributes) was the principal dimension, leading to stereotypes such as quiet, reticent, withdrawn, hesitant, guarding, avoiding, introverted, passive, and self-derogatory. Closely related to the prime dimension was the one of Composure-Anxiety, with stereotypes such as anxious, tense, nervous, and afraid. However, Woods noted a tendency for persons to feel that the stutterer, once you came to know him or her, would be a warm and considerate person. Turnbaugh et al. (1981) reinforces this view, stating that listeners tend to have an initial negative stereotype of stuttering, one that changes after contact. Clinicians need to be aware of these stereotypes and deal with them in therapy. The negativism extends to clinicians, regardless of experience, who tend to project negative personality traits to mild, moderate, or severe stutterers (Turnbaugh et al. 1979).

In short, we are dealing with a mythical figure—the stereotypical stutterer. The public believes it, we believe it, and even the stutterer believes it. Since we cannot easily change the public, we have to change ourselves and also provide the client with an opportunity for change.

Qualities Needed in Therapy

Anxiety on the part of the clinician is bad for therapy (Gregory, 1968). The characteristics of the clinician may tend to be rigidified also. One study (Crane & Cooper, 1983) evaluated 135 graduate-level, female clinicians at several different training centers. They were found to be a very similar group, resembling profiles of women engaged in nursing, home economics, and education. They consistently were higher on interpersonal than on technical skills, but the two were highly correlated. The women were normal in adjustment, tending to be passive and compliant. They also were "stereotypically feminine," that is, sensitive, energetic, anxious, creative, and highly imaginative.

The client is looking for a stereotypical clinician. In a study of 162 subjects covering a variety of ages and communicative disorders (Haynes & Oratio, 1978), it was found that qualities of directness-immediacy (don't waste time), technical skill, empathy-genuineness, and concreteness were all highly desired, the technical skill being most important. In other words, clients wanted a very competent, efficient, specific, caring clinician. Clinicians' frequent concerns about their own age, sex, race, or other demographic factors were not important on a group basis. Hood (1973) stressed the importance of relationship, acceptance of the client, and the ability to see the client's world as the client sees it. Volz et al. (1978) studied undergraduate clinicians who received sixteen hours of training in "helping skills" before therapy assignments were made. Subsequently, an evaluation of client-clinician sessions could find few verbal responses of the clinician that were regarded as helpful in developing the interpersonal relationship.

Feelings of competence, or self-efficacy, are important qualities for the clinician. One of the significant contributions to fear reduction and therapy avoidance (and self-efficacy) is practicing therapy with stutterers. Rudolf et al. (1983) used a self-efficacy rating scale with clinicians before they began assigned work with stutterers and with clinicians not scheduled. Subsequent retesting showed a significant increase in self-efficacy of clinicians scheduled with stutterers, whereas the nonexperienced group did not change significantly. Interestingly, the degree of fear of stuttering professed by the student clinicians had little relationship to the supervisors' evaluations of their work.

The clinical relationship, as we can see, is important to both persons in therapy. The client does not need (just) a machine or a computer to analyze responses. Human participation is vital. Cooper and Thompson (1971) found that self-observation by the client of audio-video recordings did not seem to improve perceptions of stuttering—unless the viewing was guided by the clinician and the observations discussed. The clinical relationship will vary as therapy varies and the interpersonal dynamics shift. One study of symptom modification therapy showed that client affect was lowest during the analysis phase, followed in rank sequence by the initial phase, introspection-testing, and ending with modification at the highest affect (Cooper & Cooper, 1969). In short, clients felt most positive about the clinician when they actually worked on the overt problem. This result emphasizes the importance of relationships during the self-analysis stage of therapy.

Other qualities needed in therapy relate more to the universals of remediation with any communicative disorder. I tend to stress several of them in teaching:

1. Knowledge—more than usual, the stutterer can be concerned whether the clinician is knowledgable about the disorder. Some will test to find out. It is impossible to learn everything about a disorder, but you might want to make frequent reference to the sources listed in Chapter 1.

2. Eye contact—people have a psychocultural response to look away from embarrassment, pain, or strong emotion. In therapy, you want to have good eye-face contact every time a stuttering occurs. The information gained is useful, and the stutterer should not feel that you are visually avoiding her or him. At times, clients and I have negotiated a penalty system if either of us catches the other looking away during a stuttering moment.

3. Accurate empathy—the capacity to understand another's feelings without becoming victim to them. Pseudostuttering by the clinician is part of this, but it extends further to the individual feelings of each client.

4. Data keeping—every session and every assignment should generate data that you write into a therapy record. I do not subscribe to the therapies that

measure wpm, SW/M and %SW on every utterance every time and/or make those the only measures taken. On the one hand, the clerical demands of counting are ridiculous and conflict with therapy needs. On the other hand, such data are too limited. Count data are useful and should be gathered regularly; but data on attitude, cooperation, feelings, verbal content, eye contact, alterations in degree, and so on are important, too. Don't fall into the mode of, "Well, he was better . . . worse . . . the same . . . this time" type of evaluation. Collect data and use it, but don't become a data robot.

5. Consistency—initially give the stutterer the support of consistency. Scheduling the same days, times, and rooms will help. Don't introduce an observer or an assistant unless it is a planned change in the therapy program. Abrupt additions or alterations in therapy should be minimized, unless done deliberately. The client wants to feel secure, and consistency is a great aid. I think the greatest basic fault in many training programs is the practice of rotating clinicians to gain experience. Some authorities disagree and downgrade the importance of the clinician. Ryan (1978) spoke of using seven different clinicians with no reduction in client's performance, and he criticized the unwillingness of clinicians to follow proper programmed formats. Ryan is correct—if the clinician's role is to turn on the machine, punch the digital counter, trip the timer, and say "wrong" or "good boy" according to preplanned criteria. For such automation, it doesn't matter too much who does it, but it is consistent.

6. One-system systems—any procedure, no matter how subjective or empirical, can be broken into learning steps and have measurable performances assigned to each step. Any procedure, no matter how mechanistic, can be enriched with interrelationships and personal application. Just as any one approach can be varied for different clients, totally different approaches also can be used. No one approach is going to meet the needs of a population of stutterers. Consider flexibility, adaptability, and change and always be curious about new-to-you techniques.

Motivation

Motivation of the client is part of the clinician's concern. There are obvious motivation problems with the person who is more or less forced into therapy by parents, teachers, employers, or spouses. Negativism or apathy that can result from coercion will have to be dealt with. However, motivation also is significant for the self-referred client. Too often there is an assumption that self-referral means self-motivation. A few clients enter therapy to reassure themselves that they are helpless victims and therapy will fail (justifying their own failures). Many clients are motivated but need extra support and demonstration to help them deal with anxieties about therapy. Most clients will need support to help carry them through the pedestrian levels of fluency or symptom therapy. Often, as therapy progresses, new problems in motivation arise as the stutterer takes over a self-management role and develops new anxieties in the transfer. Some clients will have motivation problems in advanced therapy as they realize they are losing their crutch, their alibi, their never-fail excuse for nonperformance or failure. At the end, motivation will make or break the maintenance program. Ultimately, motivation determines the outcome of therapy, and the clinician should deal with it in the very first meeting, in self-analysis, and in every session thereafter.

USE OF ASSIGNMENTS

Most teachers use assignments, and clinicians follow that pattern. Learning through practice, transfer of skills, and stability of maintenance are involved with assignments. Many of us are familiar with the client who speaks one way in therapy sessions and promptly reverts to the old speech pattern after leaving the room. Habituation of responses, automatizing of motor patterns, refinement of skills, and variation of responses depend on practice. These factors apply also to stuttering therapy, regardless of the control mode. Other factors also enter in when assignments are used, in that they

1. Increase tolerance for and desensitization to the stuttering or the symptom control or the fluency system being used. This enhances the client's feelings of self-efficacy while still under the control of the supporting clinician.
2. Develop self-management and direction by the client. Some assignments are designed for use in a therapy session with a clinical auditor present, but many are solo assignments for the stutterer. These progressively make the client responsible for his or her own actions and reduce dependency feelings of being "done to" by the clinician. This is particularly important in fluency induction modes of therapy.
3. Encourage the stutterer to practice and adopt patterns of self-monitoring, self-evaluation, and self-consequation, to provide the capacities that self-management requires. It is particularly significant in breaking clinician dependency. Some current programs foster dependency by scheduling frequent follow-up visits or cassette recording submissions (or "hot line" telephone numbers), and this is reprehensible when it substitutes for adequately teaching self-management. Clinicians should have follow-up procedures, and the client should feel encouraged to ask for assistance when needed, but umbilical programs impede normal behavioral maturation.
4. Change behavioral patterns, or at least, offer opportunities for change. Many stutterers have become habituated into a limited set of speech behaviors and reactions to different speech situations. Assignments provide opportunities to restructure old approach-avoidance patterns and add new behaviors previously stifled.
5. Provide practice in planning. Clients often express the feeling that not knowing what to do or how to arrange for doing it is a major part of their problem. Assignments that teach planning, step development, option programs, and so on turn the client into a quasi-clinician who is better prepared to cope with the unique problems that occur after dismissal from therapy.
6. Involve the environment of the stutterer. This is particularly important for young stutterers, but it can apply to any age. Assignments can involve parents, spouses, neighbors, coworkers, and employers. Assignments may result in attitude enhancements of the environment, along with better understanding of the client's struggles, vicarious participation in achievement, and better

acceptance of changes in the person they knew before therapy. The last point sometimes can be crucial since environmental others may be concerned or even nonaccepting of behavioral changes resulting from therapy.

Other values of assignments are possible, and there will be unique values for different clients.

Good Qualities

Qualities of a good assignment are important, and we should avoid frustrating, busy-work assignments. As I have said, most of us use assignments, but we don't discuss them very often. They are taken for granted. All too often, the clinician takes them for granted, too, and routinely gives the client items to take home and practice with little care and planning. One of the more visible proponents of assignments has been Van Riper. In 1958, he published an extensive list of various assignments for different aspects of a symptom modification program. Looking at them, one can see that it takes time and thought to plan good assignments. I found this out when I was first required to originate, for one client, five assignments per day over a period of sixteen weeks, a total of 400 assignments for one person to use. Later, I spent two years planning 10 assignments per week for fourteen weeks, for twenty-five stutterers. I did not devise 250 new assignments every week; many were variations on the same theme. However, I did have to consider each individual and not just give every person the same tasks. Van Riper (1978) recommended that assignments should be structured so that objective reporting is possible, there is enough stress to be useful, success is feasible but not guaranteed, and the clinician's approval or reward is involved. Using these tenets as a base, it is possible to structure a set of assignment criteria. In general, a good assignment should

1. Be relevant to therapy, and the relevance should be explained to the client. You may not disclose all your reasons for using a particular assignment, but the client should feel that it is valid, whether she or he likes it or not.
2. Utilize capacities already present or learned in therapy and, preferably, practiced under the clinician's supervision. You rarely want to initiate anything new in an assignment.
3. Be feasible, with failure a possibility but not very probable. Some stress is needed to avoid ennui and enhance success. Rarely, you may want to introduce a high-failure probability. If you do, or if you are concerned about possible failure, the assignment should include what-to-do provisions if failure is experienced.
4. Provide some options or levels of difficulty for the client to elect. I usually like to have more assignments than the client has to do and let him or her select. Within each assignment, I prefer three or more levels of difficulty for selection (see end of chapter for examples).
5. Require varying levels of monitoring, measurement, scoring, evaluation, and so on by the client. Practice on skills is not sufficient if the client does not learn judgment.

6. Require a report, preferably objective and written, from the client. Every assignment performed should be reported and the report responded to. If the project is important enough to be done, reported on, and responded to, the client typically will try harder to perform.
7. Be verifiable by the clinician. Absolute replication may not be possible, and you do not have time to check every assignment, but the client should feel that any assignment might be duplicated for follow-up checking.
8. Consider the attitude, motivation, fears, and so on of the client. This relates strongly to criterion 4, but goes beyond it to the individuality of each person. Stock assignments, without tailoring, are poor therapy.
9. Allow the client to explain his or her own evaluation of the assignment itself. This should affect future assignments and encourage self-management.
10. Provide for reward and/or approval from the clinician.

Problems

Problems with assignments will occur. Ordinary problems are the time assignments take to plan, how original you can be over and over again, and fitting them into the schedule. Some clients will be lazy or apathetic toward assignments, and you will have to deal with the problem of motivation. Some clients will sabotage assignments or lie about results. Most will do it occasionally. If you have verification procedures you will spot consistent defaulters easily. The solutions are more complex. Usually, the client is dishonest for one or more of the following reasons: apathy, fear, or contempt. Apathy has been commented on already. Fear may be your fault because you pushed too hard, or you were misled by the client's apparent in-session confidence. Either way, you will need to devote therapy time to attitude. A few clients sabotage or lie because of lack of respect for or confidence in the clinician. I have seen this particularly when clients were required to attend by other persons and when clinicians were rotated frequently for experience.

An occasional client will reject an assignment or a series. This need not create a crisis. Find out why the stutterer is doing this, and if possible, explain or encourage the person so that the assignment will be done. If this does not work, or if you find the objections valid, revise the assignment and learn from it. You should be willing to carry out the assignment yourself, while the client observes. You also can turn and request the client to devise an assignment that is acceptable and achieves the same goals, helping him or her to evaluate the assignment along the criteria mentioned earlier. Both of you will learn. Sometimes none of these responses works, and the client still rejects assignments. I have heard clients say, "Look, I'm paying good money for you to cure my stuttering, not for me to do it" and "I gotta come here, but I don't gotta do nothin'." Reactions to this can vary. On the basis of personal experience and philosophy, I first check myself to see if I have scheduled assignments for directly appropriate reasons or if I perhaps was guilty of some automatic planning. If the latter is the case, and I can find no special value in the assignment, I should save what face I can with the client, restructure the therapy sequence, and go on. However, if careful reflection affirms to me the value of assignments with this client, I will elect one of two options:

1. Advise the client of my decision, explain carefully why, and then assist a transfer to another clinician.
2. Advise the client of my decision; explain why as the start of a tangent program to explore his or her attitude; and ultimately, change it by degrees through negotiating a stress sequence that can be tolerated.

ANALYSIS OF THE STUTTERING SPASM

Awareness

Awareness of stuttering is the foundation for any mode of stuttering therapy. The stutterer needs to respond to moments of stuttering with awareness, not withdrawal. Some spasms may be very brief and, in running speech, be largely unnoticed. Beyond this, stutterers may engage in behaviors that reduce awareness. As with fluent speakers, stutterers will vary in terms of the adequacy of their naive monitoring processes.

Some speakers are externally oriented and pay little attention to their self-characteristics, whereas other speakers have an internal orientation and a precise awareness of nearly every facet of general production. Starting with awareness, we will want to move as rapidly as possible to more complex monitoring and evaluation. All advanced skills rest on this first level of awareness, and you should not move from it until your performance criteria are met. In the following paragraphs are examples of activities arranged in an approximate sequence of increasing difficulty for developing spasm awareness by the stutterer.

The stutterer is asked to read aloud and to speak spontaneously for brief periods. The time elapsed before the client is stopped will depend on the frequency of stuttering, perhaps as brief as fifteen seconds or as long as several minutes. After each time unit, the client is asked to indicate how many times she or he stuttered. Usually, you will not allow the client to stop during a spasm and report; this comes later. You want her or him to experience complete dysfluencies, not truncated ones. If the response is fairly accurate, the clinician confirms it with several more performances and then moves to the next phase. Accuracy is defined as 100 percent of severe, 90 percent of moderate, and 75 percent of mild spasms. When there are few spasms, ask the client to identify which words were stuttered on.

Check on the monitoring ability by bringing in one or more auditors while the performance is repeated. Have the stutterer make several telephone calls, and go on to two or three easy assignments while the client practices monitoring for stuttering. On the calls and assignments it would be appropriate for you to model first, faking spasms and reporting; ask the client to report first on you, and then you reinforce or correct the report. Give the stutterer a series of solo assignments, such as to count stutterings in every speech situation (or every easy speech situation) for a whole day.

When you are satisfied that the client is making progress in being aware of stuttering spasms, and while he or she works on more demanding levels of awareness, start work on expanding the awareness. Instead of simply responding to the existence of a spasm, he or she now is to identify it by type (repetition, prolongation, or block). As in the first level, start with short time units and low demands. If several spasms accumulate quickly, interrupt and call for a report. You aren't trying to test cumulative memory but to stress awareness of ongoing speech. One method is to provide reading material or ask questions, recording the exchange for analysis. After two or three spasms, stop and ask,

> How many times did you stutter?
> What words did you stutter on?
> What type(s) of spasms did you have?

After the client has answered the questions, play back the tape and verify the report. The playback also will be a modest desensitization. Any time you use playbacks of any type, or if you fake spasms for modeling, try to observe the client's reactions to stuttering by him- or herself or by others. As the client improves in reporting ability, increase the stress and complexity of the tasks, striving for continuous increases in objectivity and accuracy. Bring in other auditors, use the telephone, go out together, and use solo assignments.

Location

Location of the spasm is the next step. From simple awareness, to type awareness, you will now want to move to identifying where the spasms are localized. Many stutterers are aware only that they get "all tied up" and the word cannot be produced. At this point it usually helps if you provide information about where tension points are likely to be. With appropriate levels of terminology, teach the client about labial, lingual, velar, glottal, and thoracic points of tension. When you are satisfied that there is a basic grasp of essentials, inform the client about how stuttering tends to localize:

> Sometimes spasms get so covered up with other behaviors or devices that we forget where the trouble really is. We're going to look at the devices later, but right now we want to find out where you stutter when you stutter. Sometimes there will be a single tension area; sometimes several. Almost always, one area will be the primary spot. That's what we want to locate.

This is an excellent time to model simple pseudospasms for the client, illustrating various areas of tension. Instruct him or her to watch you closely, touch your throat during glottal tension fakes, and try to mime some of your fakes to get the feelings (more desensitization).

Select a point at which you ask the client to evaluate the nonfluencies of normal speakers. It usually seems to run better if the client first has had some practice in basic self-appraisal, sharpening monitoring skills. Use some of the material from Chapter 2 to devise assignments, if needed. If you have a local radio personality who does strange things to fluency, tape a segment to bring to a clinic session for practice. You can model "normal nonfluencies" for the client to detect. Give outside assignments and have the client bring back reports. Such fluency evaluations are good practice for self-analysis; they help turn the client more toward looking and listening to auditors rather than making assumptions about them; they are a desensitizing source; and usually they provide positive motivation when the stutterer becomes more aware of the frequent nonfluencies that occur in so-called fluent speech.

When the client is prepared, have her or him read, answer questions, or perform other simple tasks. After each spasm the client is to stop and tell you the type of spasm, the location(s), and the severity. Frequently ask him or her to imitate the spasm without actually trying to say the word. Have the client repetitively produce tension in the designated area(s) to increase familiarization with tactile and kinesthetic cues of tension. Imitate spasms for the client to duplicate, tape and play back, and so on. As before, bring in other auditors and work through situations with greater stress and complexity.

As part of locating the spasm, once the client has the basic ability, try to get her or him to stop as soon as stuttering is complete, but don't allow termination before the word is uttered completely. Stopping immediately after the spasm can be useful for other techniques, it promotes self-discipline, and it prevents the contingency reinforcement of the stuttering spasm. At first you may have to regress in complexity and stress to have success. You also will find out, if you haven't already, that people can differ sharply in self-awareness. Some persons, stuttering or fluent, are just not good monitors. Beyond that, some who can monitor adequately have difficulty in interrupting their own forward flow of speech. One practice method is to have the client read while you intermittently trigger a signal (light, tone, tap, bell) which requires the client to stop talking when the word being said is complete. Reading is a good starting point because you can look ahead to select (at first) words easier to stop after. Shift to monologue and dialogue, increase stress, and give solo assignments. You can, if needed, use a second signal that is more obvious if the client misses. For stopping after stuttering spasms, your criteria again are 100 percent, 90 percent, and 75 percent for severe, moderate, and mild spasms in the clinic. Outside the clinic, at this point in therapy, you should be fairly lenient in applying criteria and be flexible in criteria when practicing with a signal.

How long the awareness, spasm type, and location sequence takes is variable. I have had clients master all three steps, in the clinic, in one sixty-minute session, with outside practice developing as we shifted to other tasks in the clinic. On the other hand, very mild or covert or fearful stutterers may take a dozen sessions just to achieve basic skills. One thing almost sure to occur is a situational adaptation effect. As the client comes to know and respect you, becomes familiar with the clinic, and loses other anticipation fears, she or he typically will start to stutter less and less. Stuttering may even become too minimal for effective practice. You then will have to plan to introduce topics that generate more stuttering and make greater use of added auditors and outside situations (after in-clinic practice).

Struggle and Overflow

Struggle and overflow factors refer to what the stutterer does that is integral to the stuttering spasm and cannot be divorced from it. The girl who stuck out her tongue (Chapter 2) is an example of this. A series of glottal stops, loss of eye contact, head jerks or neck twists, leg flexions, and much more can be part of the struggle and overflow phenomena of stuttering behavior. The first step in this stage of stuttering self-analysis is to have the stutterer describe all such behavior she or he does as an information exercise. Probe and ask leading questions, but do not supply answers to the client. Find out the level of awareness and willingness to discuss the topic. You can provide examples and variations of them. Many clients will want to avoid an unpleasant subject with evasions or general answers. Pin them down and probe. Question degrees of severity according to affecting factors, variations in form, feelings, and other aspects of a spasm. If you find some behaviors are not mentioned, resist the impulse to name them, but go back to probing and asking cue questions for the client to find the answer or admit the behavior.

In this stage, a video recorder is immensely helpful. If you do not have one, a mirror can be substituted. Give the stutterer a list of words or sentences to be delivered one at a time while looking straight into the mirror. Eye contact with oneself is to be 100 percent, with no exceptions, while talking. You will prefer a mirror large enough to display the entire image of the speaker (for example, pier glass). I like to seat the stutterer four or five feet away from the mirror, with no masking furniture in front. She or he is to look at the list, recognize the word or sentence, look up at him- or herself, repeat what was on the paper, and then respond to my questions. I ask the client to describe what, how, and where about anything or about stuttering. As a part of awareness and tolerance, I may ask for demonstrations of behaviors we discussed, without accompanying speech, or I repeat the stimulus material and simulate a particular behavior on every word. This promotes both awareness and desensitization and is early practice of pseudostuttering. From reading, have the client progress to answering your questions or engaging in a monologue. Be sure stutterers maintain good eye contact with themselves, and stop them instantly every time it shifts. Position yourself so you are not in the mirror but can see clearly. As behaviors appear, rate them on two aspects—obviousness and proximity to the speech mechanism. Set performance criteria to be met before you move to the next stage, based on the two rating aspects, for example,

Highly obvious/distal behavior	100%
Moderate obvious/distal or highly obvious/proximal	80%
Mild/distal, moderate/proximal	50%

If your client is poor at these early stages, you may want to introduce contingent scheduling by using a signal or "wrong" for every miss and setting a penalty for X number of misses.

While the stutterer continues to use the mirror, have her or him concentrate on feeling the struggles and overflows while you work. Ask for descriptions of physical feelings and relate them to the visible and/or audible cues. Then move your chair beside or slightly behind the client and tell him or her to talk to you by way of the mirror (you do the same). Briefly drop back to simpler material at first. Now the stutterer is to maintain good eye contact with you. As you talk, alternate periods of time when the clients are to have 100 percent eye contact with you on every stuttering or with themselves each time. Check the client's accuracy and awareness in the two modes of contact. When the two are approximately equivalent, have the client turn away from the mirror and speak directly to you. As before, ask for good eye contact in general[1] and excellent eye contact on each stuttering. To encourage broad awareness of auditors, periodically ask the client about what you were doing (smiling, drooping an eyelid, frowning) while she or he stuttered.

By now you have a fairly complete catalog of behaviors. Also, the client is able to be aware of nearly all the obvious behaviors (and may have spontaneously inhibited some of them). Give outside assignments, starting with activities while alone, such as mirror work while reading or talking. In therapy sessions, revert to mirror work while you have the client use the telephone. Initial calls can be to colleagues or to you in another room As adequacy continues to develop, add real telephone calls for various purposes. As described before, bring in outside auditors, having the client stop and analyze with the auditors present. Move to easy outside assignments, modeling first to provide examples. Keep situations brief so the client can

---

[1]You may need to improve your own eye contact.

evaluate for you after each one. Lag behind clinic schedules, but bring telephoning and real situations into home assignments. Your overall target will be the ability of the client to be aware of and to describe struggle and overflow behaviors in any situation with an accuracy range from about 90 percent down to 40 percent, depending on the duration and obviousness. As mentioned, the stutterer will have reduced or eliminated some of the behaviors and significantly improved eye contact. Because of your various practices, there should be less sensitivity to stuttering, less avoidance of actual speech situations, and some improvement in self-concept.

ANALYSIS OF ASSOCIATED BEHAVIORS

Nature and Types

The nature and types of associated behaviors have been defined previously and discussed in Chapter 2. They include postponements, starters, retrials, substitutions, and so on. Some clinicians prefer to interpose this stage of self-analysis between basic spasm counting and the struggle and overflow analysis. They do this on the grounds that it often is easier to catch these behaviors than some of the more integrated struggle and overflow ones. Also, it is more of a holistic monitoring project since it can include many nonstuttered words as well as actual dysfluencies. Often, the clinician will use the analysis as an opportunity for early changes in speech, eliminating or at least reducing the more overt behaviors. This can be a very positive motivation factor and, so to speak, can strip away some of the underbrush masking the main stuttering. I have followed this pattern frequently. It is presented differently here because I would prefer to have the client approach these behaviors with the greater knowledge, awareness, desensitization, and self-confidence engendered by the previous section. Both approaches have their rationale.

Values

Values of analysis of these behaviors are clear. Most of them are, or were, conscious efforts to avoid the occurrence of stuttering or to escape from the spasm once it has occurred. They usually are secondary developments as a result of fear, anxiety, and guilt associated with stuttering and the environment. As such, self-analysis provides positive mental hygiene for the stutterer, especially as she or he becomes aware of the frequency with which many of the behaviors also occur (in varying forms) in the nonstuttering population. In addition, many of the behaviors are sufficiently obvious that they can be controlled or eliminated, giving the stutterer an early feeling that she or he is "really doing something" about their speech.

Basic Steps

Basic steps in self-analysis of associated behaviors involve some instruction by the clinician. The client needs to be taught about the various behaviors used by stutterers. You might want to draw on the resource list at the end of Chapter 1 or descriptions in this book. Several pages of descriptions can be given to the client, with a blank space after each category. After in-clinic teaching and discussion, the client can be told to take the sheets home and, for each type of behavior, answer the following:

Did you ever do this?
Do you do it now?
If you do, describe it and rate its efficiency.
To what degree is it under voluntary control?

Another approach is to use the stuttering behavior checklist in Chapter 2. When the stutterer has completed the list (including struggle and overflow behaviors), go over every item with her or him:

When did you begin this behavior?
Why did you start it and under what conditions did you start?
Has it changed over time, and if so, how?
In the present, how does it vary and what factors affect it?
How effective is it, and what would happen if you didn't do it?
How aware are you when you do it?
Are there reactions from auditors you have detected?

Another aspect is to take the intellectual awareness of associated behaviors and check that awareness in actual speech. From the client's speech samples in previous self-analysis activity you are already well informed, but the client may not be. After the previous exercise, take the client through the progressive series of speech activities described several times before. Move back and forth from counting and describing a single behavior or class of behaviors to counting and identifying all behaviors as they occur. Relate them to types and severities of spasms, word position, initial phoneme, and other relevant factors. Note carefully which behaviors are easiest to catch; this will be useful in fluency reinforcement or symptom therapy. Mentally classify the behaviors as being predominantly covert (to hide stuttering) or overt (to fight it), as discussed in Chapter 2. The categorization will provide insights for therapy mode, transfer, and maintenance prognosis. Be sure you learn how to perform all the behaviors, and model them as you and the client work together. As soon as possible have the stutterer telephoning and working in outside situations, with frequent solo assignments during nonclinic hours.

Behaviors such as postponements, starters, and retrials usually are easy for both of you to detect, as are timing devices. Release devices generally are easier for you to note, but harder for the stutterer because they are integrated into the spasm. Substitution and circumlocution can be either easy or impossible to detect, depending on the client. You may have to work hard on developing a sense for the gestalt of a client's overall speech pattern before you can start to "sense" a substitution or circumlocution, and sometimes you just have to rely on a client's honesty in telling you. Have the client monitor your speech for pauses, interjections, and other behaviors. In outside assignments, regularly have him or her evaluate other speakers for similar behaviors. The client may bring up the issue of when a behavior is stuttering and when it is a normal nonfluency. As discussed before, I suggest you talk it over, and in terms of early therapy goals, agree to be suspicious and temporarily classify any such behavior as possible stuttering phenomena.

Criteria for self-analysis of associated behaviors should vary with the obviousness and frequency of each type. The range can be from 99 percent down to 40 percent. You may need to use some contingency consequence procedures where certain behaviors are not caught at a level of efficiency you feel is needed. Pay attention to how the level of stress or speech complexity affects associated behaviors and awareness of them.

Reduction and Elimination

Reduction and elimination of associated behaviors is not, properly speaking, part of a chapter on analysis. However, control is so often a part of this stage of therapy that it at least should be mentioned several times. The analysis process usually is rewarding to the client, and experience in self-control and dysfluency reduction typically are very motivating. It often is easy to take an overt postponement behavior and work on its elimination while continuing analysis. Once, I just asked my "aw heck" postponer why he didn't stop doing it. He thought a moment, agreed, and never did it again. That was not typical. If you are going to use pseudostuttering (Chapter 4), you can start easily by having the client fake associated behaviors you want to eliminate. The faking heightens awareness, facilitates understanding of motor patterns, desensitizes, deautomatizes, and makes elimination of the behavior much easier.

ANALYSIS OF ATTITUDES AND SITUATIONAL BEHAVIORS

Identification of Variables

Identification of attitude variables concerns antiexpectancy behaviors discussed in Chapter 2. Attitudes, and their emotional correlates, largely determine these overall behavior patterns. It is important to develop a clear picture of a client's feelings and not blunder into modification or suppression of symptoms. Success in avoiding in order to conceal or overcome symptoms is not necessarily a valid indicator of reductions in negative feelings (Naylor, 1953), whether or not the speech is acceptable. Those who work with stutterers tend to structure their evaluations and measurements of progress around the moment of stuttering. However, the stutterer's concept of his or her problem typically extends beyond the overt speech phenomena (F. H. Silverman, 1980). Basically, we need to develop a perspective from the client's point of view, to see the client's world as the client, not the clinician, sees it (Hood, 1973). Therapy designed only to combat symptoms or to induce fluency does not meet the client's needs. The stutterer has spent years, sometimes thirty or forty, feeling and behaving on the premise that she or he is a stutterer. A simple reconstruction of the speech production is not going to alter those feelings. This is true in many other areas of behavioral alteration. Falck (1969) notes a general need to rechannel stutterers' attitudes because they tend to think like stutterers, even when they are not talking. For many clients, stuttering has become so entrenched that they will stutter when reading or speaking while completely alone (Šváb et al. 1972). The overall picture of stutterers does not support a point of view that they are seriously maladjusted, but I assume the following when considering stutterers who are beyond the early development stages:

1. "All" stutterers have attitude and general speech behavior inadequacies that speech-oriented therapy may or may not address.
2. Most stutterers have attitude and speech behavior problems that require specific attention as part of speech-oriented activity and/or as a separate concern in therapy.
3. A few stutterers have attitude and speech behavior disorders that require referral for psychological counseling.
4. A very few stutterers display serious attitude and behavior problems apparently unrelated to speech and requiring outside remediation.

Evaluation of Attitude

Evaluation of attitude is achieved through several approaches and depends on two factors—the sophistication of the clinician and the openness of the client. Clinicians will vary in the degree of their psychology backgrounds and therapy experience. Some clients resist what they feel is invasion of their inner selves and want to work only on symptoms or fluency, whereas others are relieved and thankful for an opportunity to discuss their attitudes and fears. You will adapt your approach to your abilities and to the type of stutterer. The covert types will not spend long in this section, and you will have to work hard throughout therapy to secure information and effect changes. The overt stutterer will work longer in this section and respond better to direct approaches in therapy.

A first step in analysis often can be found in the use of the autobiography (Chapter 2). If already assigned, it can be brought out and discussed, reassigned to expand or add sections, or structured for first-time use. You are not concerned with in-depth probing but with getting to know the client as a person with a personal history. For the clients, it is an easy way to begin self-disclosure and to examine written statements made about themselves. Whether or not the autobiography is used, there are additional home writing assignments that can be given. The client can be asked to write, and then discuss, answers to some or all of the following:

1. Describe your personal feelings
   a. Just before a moment when you are sure you will stutter.
   b. During the time when you actually are stuttering.
   c. The moment after you finish a stuttering and the next few seconds after that.
2. What do you think of your speech when you are not stuttering? Compare it to that of your friends in terms of rate, loudness, pitch, voice quality, and other characteristics.
3. From the time when you can clearly remember stuttering, how has your attitude toward it, and toward speaking in general, changed?
4. How do people react when you stutter? You might want to divide this answer into family, friends, strangers, and other specific persons.
5. How do you wish people would respond to your stuttering?
6. What activities or goals does stuttering seem to make difficult or impossible for you?
7. Does stuttering offer any advantages to you?

Other questions can be added, depending on the individual client.

In addition to the autobiography, other paper-and-pencil tests can be used at this early point. The Erickson S-scale or Iowa Test of Attitude Toward Stutter, discussed in Chapter 2, can be useful. They can be read-ministered as therapy progresses. You could have the client fill out either or both scales, and with a different colored pencil, repeat the scale, with the instruction to mark it ". . . the way you think a typical stutterer would feel . . . ." The results can be interesting. At times I have asked clients to fill out attitude scales for parents, spouses, close friends, employers, and strangers to see what attitudes the stutterer perceives (or projects) in his or her environment. Another approach is to have the stutterer take an attitude scale, or a situation rating scale, on an "If I didn't stutter . . ." basis. Results of such evaluations should be checked for halo effect. Research has indicated a significant drop in admitted anxiety about speech situations when the stutterer assumes absence of speech difficulty (Nuttall & Scheidel, 1965). Discuss results with the client. Some people enjoy talking to strangers; others do not enjoy it but do it for work or to be social; some don't like it and don't do it. You want to know the extent to which the stutterer's attitudes affect her or his behavior.

Situational Hierarchies

Situational hierarchies will be used again in other chapters, so their coverage here will be brief. As part of attitude evaluation, the stutterer responded to a number of "what if" situations. Now you want to concentrate on situations and rate them in terms of their effects on attitude and behavior. The easiest beginning is to use something like the Self-Rating of Reactions to Speech Situations checklist in Chapter 2, where four different evaluations (amount of stuttering, emotional reaction, avoidance pattern, frequency of occurrence) are made for a number of situations. For attitude evaluation I have found it very useful for the client to go back over the list and add situations that are met but not listed and to rate them. At the same time, situations never met (for example, academic situations for a nonstudent) can be eliminated. You now have a basic list of reactions to particular situations. Make a clean copy of the revised situation list (omitting and adding appropriately) and have the client take the list home and rank each item serially, 1 being the easiest and the highest number the hardest or most feared. Go over the list with the client and compare it to the previous reactions listed and adjust any discrepancies. Review the situations and help the stutterer look for common factors, for example,

> Number of persons involved.
> Familiarity of other persons and/or situations.
> Predictability of utterance.
> Emotional level of situation or subject.
> Ego importance of making a good (or bad) impression.
> Specific past experiences with similar situations.

You may find unique factors, such as the amount of eye contact required or the ages of the auditors. This hierarchy is extremely useful for planning clinic and home assignments, desensitization procedures, measurement of progress, and transfer and maintenance activity. Another rating-reporting format (Gottlober, 1953) provides a ten-point rating scale, with 1 being best, 5 average, and 10 worst. The form has a list of factors (number of stutterings, emotional reactions, willingness to speak, tension level, auditor's reaction, and so on) with one column for each speech situation encountered. The stutterer is to use the form for current situations met, filling in the various ratings after each one. It can be used throughout therapy by adding or deleting various dimensions to be rated.

Antiexpectancy Efforts

Behaviors utilized in antiexpectancy efforts can be measured against attitudes and reactions to situations. Empirically, I feel that the poorer the attitude and reactions in a client, the more likely there will be generalized antiexpectancy behaviors. Embarrassment or other negative feelings relate primarily to the presence of other people (Modigliani, 1971). The actual responses of auditors often have little relationship to the reactions of stutterers. McDonald and Frick (1954) interviewed fifty store clerks immediately after they were exposed to a stutterer. Only one person admitted feelings of repulsion, two each were amused or felt impatient, and forty to fifty reported reactions of curiosity, sympathy, and pity. Students in my classes, when learning pseudostuttering, frequently report reactions of overhelpfulness and sympathy from auditors. As one student said, "When they realize I have a problem they suddenly start to act like I'm mentally retarded!" It is not surprising, then, that a stutterer will attempt to control a speech situation, or speech itself, through antiexpectancy behaviors.

Antiexpectancy behaviors, discussed in Chapter 2, are divided into those directly associated with speech and those generally associated with social behavior. Examples are:

Speech: soft or loud voice, altered pitch, fast or slow rate, stereotyped inflection, rhythm, inflection patterns, timed movements of body parts, changes in positions or movements, speech respiration anomalies.

Behavior: mutism, humor, sarcasm, aggression, submission, flattery, interrogation.

As discussed earlier, these are performance patterns more or less associated with all speaking efforts and not just with specific moments of stuttering. Early in self-analysis a client might find it difficult to be aware of or admit to these patterns. As a clinician, you are evaluating the basic behavioral patterns of the individual, and sometimes you will need to keep your focus on speech and speech-related behaviors. If other aspects of adjustment concern you, you may want to consider restructuring part of your therapy to secure the client's agreement for psychological referral. I suggest you consider the previous statement carefully and not become too concerned about it. Most of us have neurotic tendencies or behaviors. So will your clients. I rarely have found behavioral problems so intrusive that therapy was disrupted and referral necessary; I may not like the client, or the behavior may be nonproductive, but that does not have to interfere with my work.

Explain, illustrate, and discuss antiexpectancy behaviors with the client. Ask her or him to analyze a list of them, as you did for avoidance devices, and discuss the results. Go through the situation hierarchy list with the client, seeing if antiexpectancy behaviors increase, decrease, or shift along the hierarchy. Other activities are these:

1. Assign homework in inspecting the behaviors closely and reporting on them.
2. Ask the client to try and find the various behaviors among nonstutterers.
3. Deliberately have the stutterer try some of the behaviors in clinic and in outside assignments. These often result in drastic reductions in stuttering symptoms. Discuss this with the client and emphasize how continued use would lead to habituation and further deterioration of speech.
4. Whatever the client's behaviors happen to be, have her or him deliberately do the opposite in the clinic and in specific situations, observing the results.

By the end of this sequence the client should have an excellent awareness of attitudes, reactions, and antiexpectancy behaviors associated with speaking and with different speech stuations.

SUMMARY

Importance of Self-Analysis

The importance of self-analysis by the stutterer has been emphasized repeatedly in this chapter. The arguments of the few who feel that control or elimination of the stuttering symptom obviates any need for the self-analysis process have been disputed. Self-analysis is a logical first step to any mode of therapy and will facilitate the acquisition and application of many techniques. When one considers that the goals of any therapy program are transfer and maintenance of performance, self-awareness and understanding become particularly important. Even the day-to-day activities of therapy are given direction and structure by the analysis. To evaluate a client's symptomatology and then move directly into remediation, skipping self-analysis, is to deny the essential uniqueness of the person who stutters.

Skills of Clinician

The clinician's skills were also emphasized, as well as the need for clinicians to be familiar with the typical characteristics of a stutterer's behavior. At the same time, clinicians need to be completely aware of their own speech behavior. The applied practice is useful, the information has value, and it anticipates the time when the clients will make the same evaluations of the clinician that they are asked to make of themselves. The values of technical skills and knowledge are of prime importance to the client, but so are interpersonal feelings of warmth, genuineness, empathy, and caring. This is particularly true in analysis procedures, where the client wants to feel secure about shared confidences.

Ongoing Nature of Analysis

The ongoing nature of self-analysis is apparent. Although it typically occurs as the first stage of therapy, many clinicians then blend self-analysis into other therapy procedures so that analysis continues as part of each session. Aside from this, analyses made at the outset of therapy will need to be repeated during therapy to measure progress, uncover unsuspected problems, and provide for differential application of therapy procedures. The client must learn to use self-analysis as an ongoing tool and let it become a significant part of growth in self-management. Clinical separation in transfer work and successful functioning in maintenance are significantly related to the habits, skills, and motivations derived from self-analysis.

Possible Problems

Problems that can occur in self-analysis are varied, as with any procedure. A few clients will resist self-analysis because they do not want to expose themselves to the clinician or see themselves objectively. Prognosis for such persons often is questionable. Rarely, self-analysis will disclose serious behavioral problems that require referral to special counselors. Most clients will present problems involving variable amounts of apathy, happy ignorance, misunderstanding, lying, and sabotage. They are just being normal. A particular problem can be the clinician who operates from a stereotype of stutterers and wants to fit every client to it. Also, the criteria or attitudes of the clinician can be projected to the client so that reality is difficult to achieve. As in most therapy, problems are surmountable, and maturity on the part of the clinician will deal with them.

ASSIGNMENTS FOR THE CLINICIAN

I will provide a number of projects, more than reasonably could be done for one class on a tight schedule. You or the instructor may wish to select certain items or add others that seem worthwhile. As before, some of the assignments will be more valuable if you perform them with a partner. Over time it will be useful if you do all the assignments, unless you already possess the knowledge or skills involved.

1. Stereotype checklist. This is to be done twice. On a piece of paper, number vertically 1 through 20, and mark an A column and a B column to rate on a

three-point scale. The scale is applied so that 1 = slightly, 2 = moderately, and 3 = very. For each of the two times you take the scale, pick the adjective that best describes the person, A or B. Then in the A or B column, mark a 1, 2, or 3 to indicate how strong the characteristic is. Do this on yourself and then repeat it on a person you know well (but who remains anonymous).

A	B	A	B
dominant	submissive	aggressive	placid
approaching	withdrawing	talkative	silent
noisy	quiet	happy	sad
confident	anxious	tense	relaxed
trusting	doubting	bold	hesitant
friendly	unfriendly	believing	skeptical
independent	dependent	courageous	cowardly
honest	devious	thoughtful	thoughtless
open	secretive	social	unsocial
hostile	friendly	secure	insecure

An interesting class exercise is to have the class evaluate a well-known public figure and to compare judgments.

2. Perform the following eye-contact activities and submit a brief report about each situation and the results:
    a. Observe at least ten different persons as they talk to other people. Rate each person on how frequent and adequate his or her eye contact is as each talks.
    b. In the same situations, observe the eye contact of the auditors. How did that vary?
    c. In three situations where you are an auditor, work at having superior, friendly eye contact; really be an excellent auditor. In each situation, after awhile, find an acceptable reason to look abruptly away. What happened while you had good eye contact? What happened when you suddenly looked away?
3. Use a mirror so that you can see yourself, as described in this chapter. Have your partner observe, out of your line of direct sight. Converse with your partner, but watch your own image, for about five minutes. After approximately each thirty seconds, stop and describe your expressions, postures, articulator movements, and so on, and compare them with your partner's observations.
4. Select some aspect of speech behavior that you engage in (for example, interjections or repetitions) and
    a. Try to monitor yourself for an entire day, keeping a running total of the occurrences of that behavior. How many did you accumulate? How many times did you forget?
    b. Tell your partner which behavior you selected. On five different occasions talk with him or her while you both monitor the occurrence of the behavior. Compare afterwards and report results.
5. Sit down with your partner and analyze behavioral mannerisms, nonspeech as well as speech. Include forehead wrinkling, eyebrow movement, lip distortion or biting, nail picking, and so on. When you have a complete list on yourself, check it with your family and/or friends for any modifications. What did you come up with, and did any of them surprise you?

6. Take the list of your partner's mannerisms, and after discussion, decide on one behavior or group of behaviors to be reduced or eliminated. By yourself, design five assignments covering monitoring, description, and evaluation. Study the sample assignments in this chapter for an idea of options. Give the assignments to your partner for review. What were her or his reactions? Reasonably modify items where it seems right.

7. Take the five assignments your partner designed for you (which you critiqued) and carry three, four, or all five out. Report on the results.

8. Fill out the Erickson S-scale on someone you know well (use instructions from the assignments at the end of Chapter 2). Then, have that person answer the S-scale. Compare your judgments to those of your subject.

9. Following are a number of speech situations. Look them over and omit any that you rarely or never meet because of no opportunity (not because of avoidance). Add situations currently met by you that are not on the list. Rank them from 1 to the highest number, 1 being the easiest. Whether a situation is 1, 2 or 3 is not important; whether it is 1 or 10 or 25 is.

NO.	SITUATION
⎯⎯	Answering the telephone
⎯⎯	Telephoning a friend
⎯⎯	Telephoning for service or information
⎯⎯	Telephoning for business
⎯⎯	Conducting a telephone survey
⎯⎯	Saying hello, in passing, to friends
⎯⎯	Talking with friends
⎯⎯	Introducing friends to each other
⎯⎯	Introducing strangers
⎯⎯	Talking with strangers
⎯⎯	Talking to a small group
⎯⎯	Leading a discussion
⎯⎯	Speaking to a class
⎯⎯	Speaking to a large group
⎯⎯	Answering in class
⎯⎯	Asking questions in class
⎯⎯	Interviewing for a job
⎯⎯	Arranging for a social date
⎯⎯	and so on

SAMPLE ASSIGNMENTS FOR CLIENTS

Since this chapter already contains a number of activities for clients, the examples in this section are reduced in number. They are presented primarily to illustrate the variety and options available.

1. In privacy, use an audio recorder while you speak. Listen to the playback and mark a checklist of stuttering behaviors each time you hear one. Do this for (select one)
    a. Two five-minute periods.

   b.   Four five-minute periods.
   c.   Six five-minute periods.

2.   Repeat the first assignment, but instead of reading, make brief telephone calls to secure information or service. Select one:
   a.   Three calls.
   b.   Five calls.
   c.   Seven calls.

3.   Make three telephone calls to friends, watching yourself in the mirror as you talk. During the telephone calls (select one),
   a.   Have excellent eye contact every time you stutter.
   b.   Have excellent eye contact on each stuttering, and be able to describe what you did.
   c.   Have excellent eye contact and, for each time you slip, add an extra telephone call.

4.   You are to count your moments of stuttering for five consecutive days in order to get a "time line" picture of your speech. Select one:
   a.   One typical situation in the morning, the afternoon, and the evening, each day.
   b.   All speaking situations that are more than a brief contact.
   c.   Every utterance throughout the day.

5.   Watch for _____ behavior as discussed in the clinic. Whenever it happens, notice the word, the situation, and your feelings. Write it down as soon as possible after the situation is over. Select one:
   a.   One situation per day for five days, each lasting several minutes.
   b.   Three situations per day for five days.
   c.   Five situations per day for five days.

6.   In therapy, you used "uh, well" to postpone speech efforts on a word where stuttering was feared. Select one of the following to do for the next three days:
   a.   Try to count how many times you do it, in all situations.
   b.   Each day, use "uh, well" deliberately twenty times before words on which you usually don't stutter.
   c.   Each time you use "uh, well" involuntarily, use it deliberately on the next word.

4

Learning to Stutter

ORIENTATION TO PSEUDOSTUTTERING

Definition

Definitions of pseudostuttering need to be considered before we look at the rationale and uses. This step is necessary because of extensive confusion and overlaps that occur. Different clinicians use the same terms, but do not mean the same things, when discussing pseudostuttering. The terms that can fall into separate categories, but tend to become confused, are these:

> *Voluntary stuttering*, by the stutterer.
> *Negative practice*, by the stutterer.
> *Pseudostuttering*, or faking, by the stutterer, as
> a tool for analysis and desensitization, or
> a means of symptom reduction and modification, or
> an adjunct to various therapy techniques.
> *Pseudostuttering*, or faking, by the clinician.

All these will be discussed in the following pages.

Voluntary stuttering is a confusing area of terminology because it combines involuntary spasms and pseudostuttering spasms in the same concept. Whitten (1938) considered voluntary stuttering to be stuttering that occurred openly and without substitutions and recommended a target of 50 to 100 such stutterings per day. Heltman (1943) viewed voluntary stuttering similarly and felt it was important for the stutterer not to avoid stuttering or to "avoid avoiding." Bryngelson et al. (1944) stated clearly that voluntary stuttering was willingness to stutter openly; they told stutterers not to try to cover up their stuttering but to bring it all out and "take a stuttering bath." They were told that this behavior would give them a better opportunity to study their stuttering and to become more objective about it (p. 111). As you can see, one attitude is to regard voluntary stuttering as encouraging the stutterer to stutter often and in various situations. Repeated exposure to feared situations is to occur. However, some clinicians feel that pseudostuttering is an integral part of voluntary stuttering. In his historical account of therapy experimentation, Van Riper (1958) noted that during the 1936 therapy year he had stutterers deliberately produce a repetition of any word on which stuttering was feared. The faked spasm was to appear real, and not the easy, repetitive bounce utilized later by Iowa therapists.

In 1971, Van Riper discussed voluntary stuttering as part of his program of symptomatic psychotherapy, regarding the activity as an open, nonavoiding stuttering. Sheehan (Speech Foundation) argued that voluntary stuttering is valuable because stuttering actually does not hurt the stutterer, and the stutterer's fluency hasn't done him or her any good in the past. Bryngelson (1935) is given credit for developing voluntary stuttering (Van Riper, 1971), combining symptomatic therapy and psychotherapy. Freund (1966) felt that this was one of the most original contributions any American has made to stuttering therapy. Originally, voluntary stuttering meant being willing to stutter openly, in any situation. Impulses to stay silent or use any of the avoidance devices were to be resisted. However, "voluntary real" stuttering became confused with "voluntary fake" stuttering. Many clinicians use "voluntary" to mean faked or pseudostuttering, and "involuntary" to mean real stuttering. However, "voluntary stuttering" can mean either, or both. Bryngelson (1935) mixed faking with voluntary (real) stuttering, and Emerick (1963) proposed a different mode of pseudostuttering on final sounds of stuttered words. In its publication on self-therapy for the stutterer, the Speech Foundation of America (No. 12, p. 170) defined voluntary stuttering as

> . . . a manner of talking in which the stutterer in a conscious way imitates a pattern of stuttering. . . . This style of talking may be used as a deliberate replacement for the usual stuttering behavior.

The self-therapy guide has a glossary but provides no definition of "faking" or "pseudostuttering," so one can assume their intention is to place all such activities under the single referent of voluntary stuttering. As we can see, voluntary stuttering, as a concept, has a structural differential.

Some clinicians mean for the stutterer to get out and stutter without avoidance. Other clinicians desire situation exposure but add fakes to the real spasms. Still other clinicians differentiate real spasms from faked ones, using "voluntary" for faking and "involuntary" for real spasms.

Another confusing factor is added when we consider "negative practice." This concept is identified with Dunlap (1942) who postulated that deliberately practicing or repeating an error can change it and reduce the probability of its future occurrence. Supposedly, Bryngelson utilized Dunlap's concepts in developing therapy to gain conscious control of the stuttering spasm, and Johnson used it to "avoid avoiding" rather than to gain symptom control (Bloodstein, 1969). Negative practice was not just being willing to stutter or faking spasms in general; it was a deliberate effort by the stutterer to reproduce either a specific occurrence preceding stuttering or the typical dysfluency pattern. It could be an involuntary spasm, a controlled fake of a real spasm, a fake that turned real, or a real spasm that was continued deliberately until it became a fake. The negative practice approach was an early therapy procedure. Fishman (1937) used negative practice with five stutterers, reporting significant failures with two and success with the other three. The failures had tonic block patterns, whereas the other three had repetition patterns. Many years later, negative practice was used by Alford and Ingham (1969) as part of a syllable-timed speech fluency program, along with a token reinforcement system. In other words, negative practice is still in use.

Faking, or pseudostuttering, according to Bloodstein and Shogan (1972), occurs when there is an imitation of a natural stuttering spasm, differing in various aspects of personal feeling and subjective experience. They differentiate this from "forced stuttering," which they define as uncontrolled spasms initiated by deliberately increased pressure of the articulators. The fake may be a duplicate of a known spasm, or it may be structured in any number of ways. The significant distinction is that the time of occurrence, duration and termination point, and nonfluency characteristics are under the control of the speaker. As we will see later on, control does not necessarily mean that the speaker does not suffer from anxiety and other emotional reactions during the pseudostuttering utterance (Woods, 1976).

Considering the foregoing discussion and confusion, I offer the following definitions, which I will adhere to in this chapter and elsewhere:

> *Voluntary stuttering*—a willingness to stutter openly without avoiding speech opportunities, particular persons, or specific situations. To varying degrees, covert behaviors are eliminated so that stuttering is as close as possible to the basic spasm struggle.
>
> *Negative practice*—a real or faked duplication, by the stutterer concerned, of a specific stuttering spasm or of the general dysfluency pattern. As, and if, changes occur in the stuttering behavior, negative practice will mirror these changes.

Pseudostuttering (faking)—the deliberate production, by any speaker, of overt dysfluencies that resemble stuttering. Any parameter can be included, varied, or omitted, and all aspects are under conscious control at all times.

Throughout the remainder of this chapter I will refer less to voluntary stuttering and negative practice and more to faking. I would not refer to the others at all except for the fact that some clinicians mix faking into them.

Opinions about the use of pseudostuttering vary. Many, but not all, of the fluency reinforcement group reject it as either unnecessary or a reinforcement of aberrant behavior. Many others have applied it, in a variety of ways. Freund (1966) felt that it was extremely valuable. A Speech Foundation of America publication (No. 9) quotes a number of clinicians advocating its use. Eisenson (1975) felt that faking was potent, both as a symptom therapy and a psychotherapy. Barbara (1965) and Starkweather (1980) also supported the use of faking in therapy. It seems to have a strong function in many different therapies. However, we also are interested in the adoption of pseudostuttering by the clinician and not just by the client.

Rationale

A rationale for the clinician's use of pseudostuttering is not difficult to develop. Mulder (1961) spoke of the hypocrisy inherent in sending a client into a speaking situation that the clinician would not enter. Freund (1966) felt it was important for the clinician to accompany the stutterer into a graded series of speech situations and demonstrate faking possibilities and potentials. This was echoed in a Speech Foundation of America publication (No. 5) on training clinicians, which routinely assumed that student clinicians would learn how to stutter imitatively. Later, Maxwell (1982) noted a frequent need for the clinician to model fake stuttering for analysis and for other therapy purposes.

Learning to stutter is a challenge that should be met by any clinician, regardless of the therapy orientation. In the first chapter, I quoted Sheehan (1970) concerning the unwillingness of clinicians to do those things they ask the client to do, and both should do. With consistent frequency, publications on stuttering therapy propose or assume the capacity of the clinician to "stutter." Van Riper (1973) recommends that the clinician imitate the stutterer's own spasms in conversation with another person while the stutterer watches. He also suggests that the clinician demonstrate a wide range of dysfluency repetitions, prolongations of varying durations, and various forms of avoidance and release mechanisms. Luper and Mulder (1964), in discussing therapy techniques for children who stutter, also recommend the production of stuttering behavior by the clinician. Again, Van Riper (1974c, p. 55) advises stuttering by clinicians:

You should do some pseudostuttering, especially in the early stages of the hierarchy, and show him you can do so fairly calmly. . . . You'll be modeling a calm and objective attitude for your client. If you find it hard to provide this model, well, you'd better learn to desensitize yourself if you want to help the stutterer.

Chapman (1959) feels that an appropriate skill level is to be able to imitate a particular stutterer so well that people who know the person can recognize him or her from the stuttering characterization.

Although there seems to be wide acceptance of the idea that clinicians should learn to imitate stuttering, it is appropriate to explore the rationale. Students occasionally suggest to me that it is a password-type torment developed by "authorities" who stutter and want to make something special out of it. I must confess I entertained similar feelings during the learning process. However, over time I came to the conclusion that inability of the clinician to produce stuttering behavior reduced the effectiveness of the clinician, the response of the client, and the effect of therapy. I felt this to be so whether the procedures used were for fluency reinforcement, for symptom control, or dealt only with communication adjustment factors. Imitative stuttering, as a clinical skill, seems appropriate for the following reasons:

1. The clinician will learn in a meaningful way the definitions of the professional terms for stuttering behavior. The words *repetition, prolongation, retrial,* and so on will be understood rather than memorized.
2. The clinician will understand better the interrelationships between the respiratory-phonatory-articulatory aspects of the dysfluent speech process and the spread of associated reactions to other parts of the body.
3. By following a hierarchy of severity, the clinician will understand better the developmental aspects of stuttering: how a simple repetition or a brief prolongation can escalate to fierce struggle with the passage of time.
4. The function of associated behaviors will be understood, and the conditioning factors that foster them will be clearer.
5. Because of faking demands on the speech mechanism control and the self-monitoring system, speech clinicians will not only improve in evaluation skills for speech dysfluency patterns of themselves but also will become better evaluators of clients in diagnosis and therapy.
6. When practice efforts are carried into real situations, the clinician will experience, to varying degrees, the frustration, anxiety, and other feelings of the true stutterer. A greater appreciation of the attitude and general speech behavior of the stutterer will develop.
7. Clinicians will be able to demonstrate to the stutterer that they not only understand what the client is doing or feeling but also can duplicate that experience for the client's observation and analysis and to help in desensitization and practice.
8. In teaching the stutterer, the clinician will be able to demonstrate techniques to the client *as a stutterer*, anticipate problems, express the client's concerns, and be better able to search for solutions.
9. The ability will increase the self-confidence of clinicians, facilitate planning of therapy, and improve accuracy of judgments.
10. The client who might be disposed to challenge therapy or the clinician will be

less likely to do so. Interpersonal relationships in therapy may be facilitated by the clinician's faking.

Learning to stutter, and doing it well, is not easy. Students in my classes regularly provide feedback indicating this observation:

"Very difficult, painful, and tiresome; have to give the stutterers credit."

"More than any of the other assignments this one really hit home with therapy and asking stutterers to do things. I can understand much better the avoidance. . . ."

"I have also learned how [stutterers] must put things off, because I avoided this assignment like the plague."

"I think that as clinicians we often forget what we are asking our clients to do. . . ."

"I was amazed at how involved stuttering can be."

"I felt 'stupid,' 'silly,' or just 'anxious' . . . made me wonder what stutterers really felt, even more, and how they deal with those feelings."

In my classroom use of faking assignments, only one student out of hundreds could not learn to do it, and none subsequently felt it was inappropriate or unimportant.

BASICS IN PSEUDOSTUTTERING FOR CLINICIANS

In learning to imitate stuttering, you must draw a distinction between being dysfluent and imitating stuttering. The goal of this technique is for you to speak in such a way that the auditor will think you are a stutterer, even if the auditor is another clinician or a stutterer. Mumbling a few repetitions and blinking your eyes is not pseudostuttering. It will be very helpful if you observe real stutterers, view films or tapes of them, or even listen to audio tapes. Try to observe a number of different stutterers and note the variations superimposed on the basic commonalities of repetitions, prolongations, and stoppages. If you are in a class learning faking, pay close attention to how others vary their dysfluency efforts, and do not hesitate to borrow from them. You will want to avoid a one-pattern form of faking since you will need to stutter in many ways for different reasons. Inevitably, you will tend to develop a particular pattern because it fits, but you should not be limited to it.

Spasm Types

A review of spasm types is the first step in learning to fake stuttering. It has been noted that there are three basic forms: repetitions, prolongations, and stoppages or blocks. Repetitions, or clonic spasms, were divided by Wingate (1976) into "elemental repetitions," which are those repetitions involving a basic dimension of length of a syllable or less. Those repetitions that involve more than a syllable length often cannot be classified as stuttering, although some stuttering does occur on syllable strings, whole words, and even on phrases. However, the core of the stuttering repetition seems to revolve around the elemental repetition as defined by Wingate. Gregory (1968) suggested using a bounce, usually on the first syllable, to fake a repetition spasm. Bryngelson (1935) also advised repeating the first sound or syllable of a word, distinctly, several times. He further suggested a variation in the number of repetitions from fake to fake in order to avoid a set pattern that will not appear to be real. Stop consonants are faked most easily in syllable form, that is, /pʌ/- /pʌ/ rather than /p/-/p/, but you can try both. Fricative and continuant consonants lend themselves easily to phoneme repetition as well as to syllable repetition. Vowels can be repeated easily. It is important to remember that many stutterers do not repeat in a studied, bouncy rhythm but are jerky in their repetition. Stuttered repetitions typically are produced with tension and effort; they do not fall effortlessly from the lips.

Prolongations refer to the extension of a sound beyond its appropriate duration (Wingate, 1976). Typically, this is an audible prolongation, but there can be inaudible ones as well. Separating a client's prolongation from a stoppage (block) can be difficult at times. Prolongations are most likely to occur on the carrier vowel of consonant-vowel pairs, on vowels alone, or on continuant or fricative phonemes. Faking a prolongation is usually easy since it simply requires a continuation of the voiced (usually) release. However, just prolonging a sound is insufficient in faking stuttering. The prolongation is failed effort by the stutterer to move on to the next sound or syllable. There needs to be strain, effort, and tension in the prolongation. Frequently, the stutterer will show an increase in volume or pitch in an effort to complete production. Continuous production uses up air, so "prolonged prolongations" are not common. A three-to-five second prolongation generally will be the longest you will care to go.

Stoppages, tonic spasms, or blocks are the third aspect of dysfluency. Whereas repetitions seem to predominate in stop consonants, blocks appear to occur more often on continuant phonemes. This may be reversed in some stutterers (Van Riper, 1982). In blocks the speaker is frozen or locked into the phonatory and articulatory postures to produce a phoneme and cannot continue. The blockage typically occurs at the point of onset of the phoneme rather than further into the production sequence. It may be completely silent or involve vocalization efforts to break through and move on. There may be efforts to try again and move forward, so there is a repetitious quality to the stoppage; but it is not a typical cyclic repetition. In such an instance the stutterer usually repeats the syllable or phoneme just prior to the stoppage point, coming to a stop each time the trouble spot reoccurs. Many inexperienced clinicians do not realize the extent to which many tonic blocks occur or initiate at the vocal folds rather than just at the tongue, lips, or jaw. In practicing pseudostuttering, you should be sure that a certain number of fake stoppages occur at the vocal fold level. When you do so, be sure to tense the strap muscles of the neck and feel the pressure and strain in the vocal area. Also, breaking the stoppage and continuing on to the rest of the word, or the next word, usually does not occur as a result of simple relaxation of the tonic state. The stutterer sounds as if the phoneme is being forced, pushed, or jerked out. You may find the opposite of this in some stutterers, where they simply stop fighting and give up. Facial muscles, expression, and eyes should show the overflow effects of attempts to push through the tonic block. Consider these aspects as you work on the assignments at the end of this chapter.

Struggle Reactions

A review of struggle reactions should follow that of spasm types. Stuttering spasms are not unchanging and isolated. Although the adult stutterer may finally settle on a particular pattern, changes can still occur. During the more active stages of stuttering development, alterations and additions may appear or disappear with some frequency. If a different behavior is incorporated into the spasm, it may progress in severity so that thrusting of the tongue in an early stage habituates and increases to become a prolonged, grotesque protrusion accompanying the speech effort. Struggle reactions tend to occur first, as just exemplified, with structures of the speech mechanism itself. Abnormalities in respiratory patterns may develop, with too-frequent and gasping inhalation, excessive exhalation prior to utterance, thorax and shoulder girdle fixation, and so on. There may be struggle phenomena in the vocal area, usually in the form of spasmodic closure of the vocal folds. The respiratory system may conflict with the vocal fold valve so that phonatory closure and expiratory pressure occur together to an undesirable degree. The oral articulators are prone to effect from the struggle overflow, so the tongue and/or jaw and lips are moved and positioned with abnormal tension or moved into postures that are inappropriate for the sound being produced. Any fixed posture in articulation is basically undesirable (see chapter on preparatory sets) since speech production is a dynamic process and not a series of static postures. Tension and struggle also are reflected in the muscles of facial expression, partly because of their labial-mandibular involvement in articulation. Lips will pucker, twist, distort, or go into tremors. The external nasal muscles can flare, narrow, or wrinkle the nose, and the forehead can show overflow as its muscle corrugates. Typically, stutterers have poor eye contact. Whether this is due particularly to muscular effort or whether it is a behavioral response is unimportant at this time. Some stutterers adopt an antiexpectancy pattern of rarely looking at their auditors (so do some non-stutterers), whereas others break contact only when they stutter. A few will actually close their eyes tightly, blink rapidly, or even roll their eyes up so the pupils disappear and they look as if they are going to faint. You will not find it difficult to have poor eye contact while faking, but it will be difficult to fake a severe spasm and maintain good eye contact in order to see, describe, and evaluate auditors' reactions.

Struggle reactions are also often associated with abnormal postures and movements of the head and neck. The stutterer may crane the head backward, drop it forward and down, or cock the head at an angle. There may be clonic-type movement, where the head jerks in synchrony to the stuttered utterance or in time with efforts to force out of a block. Abnormal physical postures may occur. They can be rather mild, such as squaring or sagging the shoulders, or go to extremes of squatting, stretching, and bending. Stutterers may present limb movements during stuttering spasms. This is discusssed further elsewhere, but may include leg flexing or extension, foot movements, finger snapping or extension, fist clenching, arm flexing, and other movements or combinations.

Associated with the various phenomena just discussed may also be variations in the phonatory and articulatory function. There can be some confusion over whether these abnormalities are just a reflection and over-flow of the ongoing struggle or whether they represent efforts to "release" the stuttering spasm, and therefore belong in a different category. Some of the actions described in the previous paragraph offer similarly dual pos-sibilities, that is, an arm movement can be struggle or it can be carefully timed to try and trigger the articulator movement and release the spasm. For our discussion, I am looking only at overflow phenomena and will consider spasm release later. Vocal changes during stuttering spasms usu-ally involve changes in pitch and/or loudness of tone. There may be a pattern to the changes, or they may just occur during the spasm. Artic-ulatory changes are less common and are more likely to result from altera-tion of one or more distinctive features of a phoneme as a result of muscle tension or deviant positioning of the articulators. Interjections of extra-neous, inappropriate sounds may occur, but these are often associated with release efforts rather than overflow struggle.

As you can see, stuttering is a complicated set of behaviors. It takes years for the stutterer to acquire all of them, and the behaviors interlock to a degree that makes unraveling them difficult. Learning to imitate stutter-ing is made more complex because of this interlocking structure; the clini-cian has so many things to do at one time just to stutter convincingly, and she or he usually is also trying to accomplish some other purpose at the same time—such as observing the stutterer, demonstrating a technique, or using some other procedure.

Associated Behaviors

Associated behaviors, or secondaries, can be found in most stutterers. The term covers many of the struggle behaviors just described and was coined by Bluemel (1957) in 1913 to differentiate between early and developed forms of stuttering, the early stages being called *primary*. He intended the term *secondary* to describe the struggle phenomena of advanced stuttering, but it has been applied frequently to speech behaviors intended to avoid stuttering. Wingate (1976, p. 48) defines secondaries as ". . . learned behaviors which are *temporally* second in appearance and reflect the stutterer's efforts to produce fluent speech." He objects to the idea that they necessarily occur secondarily or that they are learned and conditioned responses. He applied the term *accessory features* and used it to cover the previously described struggle areas. Van Riper (1982) uses both *secondary* and *accessory*; he feels the behaviors are temporally secondary and that they are learned and habituated responses in reaction to the fear of stuttering. As I have stated, I separated the struggle behavior group into two broad categories, and I regard the "associated behaviors" as being secondary to the actual stuttering struggle. The first problem is the basic core of dysfluency and the physical struggle with that core, even if that struggle developed later in the syndrome. Secondary to, or associated with, this struggle are the coping strategies developed by the stutterer, and these are our current focus of attention. The coping behaviors tend to be arranged separately in therapy planning, and I have arranged them accordingly in considering pseudostuttering. Associated behaviors may be a minor part of the syndrome, with struggle efforts predominating, or the spasm struggle may be fairly mild, with an extensive overlay of associated behaviors, or secondaries, that seem to be much more developed than the spasm would warrant.

In Chapter 2, on self-analysis, an extensive discussion of associated behaviors was provided. These were divided into two categories, avoidance behaviors and antiexpectancy behaviors. The names, literally, are interchangeable. However, I used the avoidance label to cover behaviors aimed at specific words, phonemes, or syllables. Antiexpectancy behaviors are those behaviors aimed at reducing, in general, the overall probability that stuttering will occur in a speech series. Rather than repeat the definitions and descriptions from the prior chapter, I will list the types and suggest you refer to Chapters 2 or 3 for any needed explanations:

Postponement	Release, Timing
Starter	Substitution
Retrial	Circumlocution, Revision
Omission	Trigger Postures[1]

Antiexpectancy behaviors include

Mutism

Situation avoidance

[1]Related to starters and mentioned by Van Riper (1982) as the addition of an articulatory posture or phoneme production in advance of the proper production.

Alteration of speech production parameters (pitch, rate, loudness, quality, and so on)
Alteration of other elements (rhythm, inflection, stress)
Behavioral personality patterns

Potential problems

A summary and comment on potential problems in learning to stutter is in order. The previous paragraphs have made, perhaps belabored, the point that stuttering is a complex act. The core of the stuttering spasm is the effort to emit a phoneme, syllable, or word unit, and instead, being trapped in repetition, prolongation, or stoppage. This entrapment may vary from dysfluencies that even the trained observer might miss up to severity levels that become the focus of negative attention. In learning pseudostuttering you need to be able to produce all three spasm types; to produce them at mild, moderate, and severe levels; and to produce them in combinations. Efforts to fight clear of the stuttering spasm typically create struggle reactions, which basically are musculoskeletal overflow actions. The overflow actions may involve parts of the speech mechanism directly, plus the face, eyes, head, neck, limbs, and body postures. The clinician should be able to fake thoracic fixation, premature exhalation, loss of eye contact, aberrant head movement, and other postures or movements discussed earlier. Associated, or secondary, behaviors were classified into avoidance and antiexpectancy behaviors. Avoidance behaviors are speech-specific, to avoid a specific moment of stuttering, and antiexpectancies are behavior-specific, to reduce the probability that stuttering will occur at any time. You should practice each of the avoidance devices, singly and in combination. You also should do enough practice with antiexpectancy behaviors to understand how they work and how much work it is to maintain them.

Throughout this chapter I have warned that learning to fake stuttering is not easy and can produce anxiety. I do not wish to exaggerate. Learning and using many of the skills in speech and language pathology is complex and can produce anxiety when you have to use them in therapy. Your first therapy sessions of various types, the first job, a tough examination, all can produce anxiety—but you cope with them all. If you follow the procedures in the assignment section on pseudostuttering you will rapidly acquire the skills you need. Woods (1976) reported experiences in giving faking assignments to students. He said the students typically reported considerable anxiety and reluctance to try faking and that they had a strong impulse to tell auditors, during and after an assignment, that they weren't really stutterers. He felt this was linked to the stereotyped stigma of stuttering and a desire by the students not to have the auditors think of them as belonging to that stereotype. Some students report to me that they are "starting to stutter" involuntarily. This is a combination of several things: greater awareness of normal nonfluencies, the simple practice effects of what is being attempted, and the partial deautomatization of both production and monitoring patterns. I never have had a student (nor have I ever heard of it happening) become a stutterer because of faking practice.

Every time I use faking assignments with students a few will report, with some concern, that a fake spasm became "real." This is not only possible but probable. Every speaking person has moments of uncontrolled nonfluency that briefly perpetuate themselves. In all such reports from students, inquiry disclosed that without exception, the incidents were the result of one of these two factors:

1. A student hit a real-life practice situation, panicked, and wound up in a classic approach-avoidance conflict from which she or he could not run away. The behavioral freeze and oscillation is what the stutterer experiences, but it is not stuttering.
2. A student used a fake that developed such a rhythm that it suddenly was hard to break out and finish the utterance. This usually occurs on repetition and typically involves only the articulators. It is caused by the strength of the motor feedback loop and not by stuttering. It happens to me in class several times every quarter.

If you work at the assignments sincerely, you probably will have some uncomfortable moments. Several years after I learned faking, a clerk in an office supply store reacted negatively to my faking. I panicked and spent the next three years using up a ream of yellow second sheets I had not intended to buy.

The final problem is somewhat the reverse of the fears, anxieties, and other things just discussed, but it usually stems from the same fear and embarrassment. This problem is the clinician who produces a nonbelievable stuttering fake. A "fake fake," a pseudostuttering that does not seem real, is worse than not faking at all. I do not mean that you cannot slip at times; we all do. Clients will understand and accept this. But consistent patterns of unreal fakes may damage your credibility as a clinician, unless you improve over time. I have supervised clinicians who frankly said to their clients, "I'm learning faking; will you help me?" and therapy was facilitated. I have often asked stutterers to teach me their stuttering pattern. If your *final product* is a poor imitation of the real thing, work harder. This chapter is not intended to generate a final product; it is meant to get you started and to encourage you to progress in the future.

BASICS IN PSEUDOSTUTTERING FOR CLIENTS

General Considerations

General considerations in faking for stutterers overlap in part with the earlier section on self-analysis. Faking spasms by stutterers has a variety of uses in therapy. Some of them already have been indicated in the discussions of voluntary stuttering and negative practice. Faking also can be used in the initial stages of therapy when working on spasm analysis and desensitization. It also comes into use when practicing a variety of control techniques. Learning the complexities of a particular technique on faked spasms is much easier for the client than is trying to jump right into use of the method with real spasms. Practice and rehearsal can start with easy spasm fakes and progress to more complex ones, making transfer easier. If therapy is for symptom control, pseudostuttering is the natural avenue for converting involuntary spasms into controlled dysfluencies that are acceptable as a mode of speech production. Pragmatically, stuttering can be of use as the stutterer adapts to you and the therapy situation. As adaptation occurs, real stuttering typically reduces, sometimes nearly to extinction (in the clinic). The clinician then faces the problem of having "cured" the client in the clinic only. Faking can be a valuable way of securing in-clinic spasms for evaluation and practice. Faking is less obvious in value for fluency reinforcement therapies, especially if the client is automated in a contingency response format and trained only to monitor the particular fluency control mode taught. However, I have found faking quite useful in fluency programs for analysis, study of auditors' responses, desensitization, relaxation, a punishment contingency, and so on.

An extremely important point to remember: Many stutterers do not know how to stutter. They must learn about faking and spasm components, just as the clinician did. At its worst, this could place a clinician who knows all *about* stuttering (but not how to produce it) with a client who is an expert at production but does not understand what is involved. Van Riper advocates confronting stuttering through faking, admitting and displaying it openly and objectively (Speech Foundation, No. 9). In the same source, Emerick states, "The more you stutter, the less you hold back; and the less you hold back, the less you stutter" (p. 12).

Specific Procedure

Specific procedural steps in faking will vary according to the uses, timing, overall mode of therapy, and other variables. Faking for a stutterer has engendered a wide range of interpretation by clinicians. A number of them have been noted already. In 1942, Van Riper (1958) noted that fakes, if they were close duplicates of the real spasm, often tended to become real. At first, he thought that this was unwise but then decided that it was good for tolerance, good for practice on modifications, and was "easier" to work with than completely involuntary spasms. He also felt that pseudostuttering was good psychotherapy since it turned avoidance of stuttering into approach behavior. A different view, in part, was expressed in the self-therapy publication of the Speech Foundation of America (No. 12) in that it recommended the stutterer avoid his or her own pattern at first, keep the production "low and easy" (no tension or fast rate), and concentrate on faking brief repetitions and prolongations. However, it agreed with Van

Riper that faking was an open admission of stuttering and increased self-confidence. They also noted it was a useful way of finding out how other people react to stuttering. On the opposite side again, Gottlober (1953) felt that faking should start with duplicating the real pattern and then evolve into something that was more acceptable. As noted before, Chapman (1959) had similar ideas about duplicating the real spasm. Thus we have a situation where a number of clinicians agree that pseudostuttering is useful but do not agree on how it should be used. The steps that are recommended subsequently are tentative, and various factors might call for revisions or rearrangements. The first four steps assume a particular approach to therapy, and a different therapy plan might change significantly some of the subsequent steps. The sequence proposes generally that the stutterer start by learning his or her own secondary behaviors and how to fake them, then progress to core spasms and spasm types not used or used less often, then move to specific struggle behaviors, and finally fake antiexpectancy devices only if needed.

If faking is to be used early in the therapy program, certain prerequisites need to be met. Do not start by simply asking stutterers to fake spasms. They very likely cannot because of lack of information about their own speech patterns. Certainly, the client will not like the concept. Preliminary steps you might want to follow are these:

1. Complete initial steps of introduction, acclimation, early rapport, bibliotherapy, or other beginning activities.
2. Perform any tests, evaluations, forms, and so on. Determine goals; explain general therapy plan. Find out about prior faking experience.
3. Begin the self-analysis phase (see Chapters 2 and 3) with outside monitoring assignments. As each of the stuttering levels is analyzed, the clinician fakes to demonstrate things the stutterer does or does not do. This exposes the client to the concept of faking and its possibilities. By this time you have accumulated extensive information about your client, know and understand the overall speech pattern as well as the stuttering, and so on. Typically, because of adaptation and development of confidence, the client has reduced stuttering significantly in the clinic and may even have reported out-clinic reductions. Intensive analysis usually has made him or her less sensitive about stuttering. Your repeated use of pseudostuttering has set an example, and you should be ready to lead the client into active participation in the technique.
4. When the client understands the what, how, when, and where of her or his stuttering, introduce faking duplications of secondary (associated) behaviors—postponements, starters, and so on. Start with behaviors that are temporally removed (for example, postponements) from the spasm and/or involve body areas distal to the speech mechanism. For example, work on the client's poor eye contact because of turning the head to one side, the postponement device of "well now," and the release device of gesturing with the right hand. Use these on nonstuttered words until the client is aware of them and can imitate them well (you may want to start inhibiting some of these involuntary behaviors as soon as they can be faked).

5. Progress to associated behaviors (secondaries) that temporally are closer to the core spasm and/or more proximal to the speech mechanism. There very likely will be some behaviors that are difficult at this stage, and you should be flexible. Efforts at inhibition might fail now but be successful later on.

6. By this time therapy probably has moved into desensitization or fluency activity, and faking should concentrate on in-clinic duplication of the core spasms and associated behaviors. At first, the fakes may tend to become real, but emphasize the analysis and desensitization development. Add different patterns to fake. If the client typically stutters by irregular bursts of repetitions, with the head down, you might have him or her

   a. fake the exact same pattern,
   b. fake the same pattern but use slow, rhythmic repetitions,
   c. fake the same pattern but change positions of the articulators,
   d. fake the same or any pattern, with a different head posture,
   e. replace repetitions with faked prolongations,
   f. vary the severity of the fakes, or
   g. fake the familiar pattern but end the spasm by turning it into a different dysfluency pattern.

7. Give out-clinic assignments to fake associated behaviors on nonstuttered words and to inhibit easy avoidances on real stutterings. Keep the assignments progressing in difficulty.

8. Concentrate on flexibility. Introduce a variety of easy nonfluencies and let the stutterer experiment with them.

Do not ask the stutterer to produce any fake you cannot do and are not willing to produce in any situation in which you ask him or her to speak.

Acquisition

Acquisition activities and criteria, like the procedural steps, will vary. The procedures in teaching fakes are subject to many factors. Some clients grasp faking quickly, whereas others learn slowly. Methods can include the following:

1. Have the client watch other stutterers, watch video tapes or films, or listen to audio tapes. Try to imitate examples.

2. Use mirror work extensively for the client to observe effects and to improve eye contact and monitoring.

3. Model various stuttering spasms yourself, for the client to duplicate.

4. Audio-record samples of stuttering behavior for the client to imitate.

5. Have the client evaluate your efforts to duplicate his or her spasms, correcting and modeling for you.

6. Have the client originate "new" stuttering patterns for you to learn at the same time.

7. Give out-clinic assignments in faking, starting with word lists and working up to situations.

8. Use out-clinic assignments the two of you perform together. Follow a hierarchy; *the clinician should demonstrate first.*
9. Invite other clinicians, or auditors, to sit in and observe.
10. If there is a stuttering group, assign each stutterer to learn to duplicate the patterns of other stutterers. The goal is to be so good that others can identify the person being imitated.

Different situations, ages, therapy plans, and other resources will provide a great variety in your faking procedures. Some of you may concentrate on faking as a major method in approach-avoidance therapy. Others will use faking as a subsidiary technique in the learning of other techniques. Some of you will use faking as a teaching tool but not as therapy. It is adaptable to all modes of therapy.

The criteria for stutterers' performance on faking are difficult to establish because of the many uses for the technique. In general, I suggest a median range approach, with the following as suggestions:

> *In-clinic*: production of all aspects of usual stuttering pattern, without loss of control; production of a variety of noncharacteristic patterns with control; production of usual patterns, altering them in various ways, with control.
>
> *Out-clinic*: duplication of temporally distant and/or distal behaviors of the usual pattern, with control; production of a variety of noncharacteristic patterns, in a variety of situations with a 90 percent control average; duplication of usual stuttering pattern, with a 75 percent control average.

Other criteria can be added. The percentages can be modified according to the stutterer involved. There is an assumption that a certain number of fakes will slip and become real. In many therapy techniques this is regarded as usual and not undesirable, since other techniques are taught to deal with such events.

Potential Problems

The values and uses of faking for clients have been emphasized. Learning, tolerance, self-analysis and monitoring skills, desensitization, practice values, and motivation are some of the factors discussed. Applications have been suggested for almost every stage of therapy, and problems have been referred to. Consistently, stutterers will not like faking, partly because of the stigma of the stuttering stereotype cited earlier (Woods, 1976). Clients do not wish to be more nonfluent. Czuchna (Speech Foundation) suggested that covert stutterers will resist faking more, whereas overt stutterers will be more accepting. It has been my experience that milder stutterers respond less favorably to faking, with greater tolerance occurring as severity increases. Starkweather (1980) stated that faking will be resisted unless approached gradually through identification and exploration. Shames (1953) used deliberate adaptation to minimize the "contaminating effect" of having fakes turn into involuntary spasms. Reluctance to fake can be dealt with by two possible routes:

1. Rather than introducing faking as a topic and discussing all its characteristics and uses, lead the client slowly to the concept. Session by session have her or him imitate first one and then another aspect of stuttering, keying on the dysfluency and not on the fake. In-clinic work in analysis and desensitization can be done this way. At the same time, your own use of fakes to demonstrate stays ahead of the client's level of performance so that anxiety is not increased. The in-clinic adaptation discussed earlier will make it easier to request pseudostuttering. Out-clinic use of fakes can start with the least traumatic and noncomplex aspects, and gradually escalate. Faking is treated as a vehicle, not a particular procedure.

2. When you are ready to make use of fakes, explain to the stutterer and provide some reading material (see end of Chapter 1) that discusses pseudostuttering. Discuss uses and values, and problems, with the client. Ask the client to express his or her feelings, and discuss them. Occasionally a client will draw performance deadlines, such as no out-clinic faking or faking only of mild spasms. These "will nots" are client-management problems and can be dealt with either head-on or by degrees. Usually it is best to restate your point of view about faking, temporarily accept the client's deadline if it will not prevent the therapy you plan, and inform the client that you will try to change his or her mind as therapy continues.

ASSIGNMENTS FOR CLINICIANS

Learning to fake stuttering need not be confusing. Mulder (1961) provides a series of suggestions, including use of delayed auditory feedback. He also recommends a graded hierarchy of situations to avoid being overwhelmed by anxiety or complexity. The practice assignments following start on a low level, initially concentrating on mechanical or motor patterns differentiating spasm types and then moving through progressive levels. You, or your instructors, may omit basic items or add individual variations. The sequence of assignments concentrates on levels of spasm severity and complexity, with less attention given to situation progressions. As you become competent in faking, you can advance situation factors according to your own needs and availabilities.

1. Use a mirror and tape recorder. Have a list of any fifty words and a list of at least twenty-five sentences from any source. As you read aloud, watch your face in the mirror, and record yourself on tape.

   a. Read the word list aloud. Fake a repetition on the first word, a prolongation on the second word, and a block on the third word. Repeat the cycle on the next three words. Record about ten cycles (thirty words) so that you have ten samples of each spasm type. Make the fakes all "mild" with two or three repetitions, one-to-two second prolongations, and one-to-two second blocks. You should feel tension in your speech muscles, see it in your facial muscles, and hear it on tape playback. Do not attempt severe spasms, associated behaviors, and so on. If your efforts don't look or sound adequate, repeat the ten cycles.

b. Repeat the assignment, responding to your own evaluations of the first cycle. Report on your efforts and changes.

2. Read five sentences aloud, after you have underlined three words in each sentence. Follow these dysfluency instructions. Watch in the mirror and record as before. Keep the dysfluencies mild.

   a. In each sentence, repeat on the first underlined word, prolong on the second, and block on the third. Evaluate.
   b. Read the same five sentences aloud again, but prolong on the first underlined word, block on the second one, and repeat on the third. Evaluate.
   c. Read the same five sentences aloud again, but block on the first underlined word, repeat on the second, and prolong on the third. Evaluate.

   How did sentence fakes differ from single words? What changes did you notice in different spasm types on the same words? What spasm type was easiest for you?

3. Sit down with your partner so that she or he can see and hear you. Using fifteen new words, read the word list aloud with five productions each of repetitions, prolongations, and blocks. Have your partner do the same. Evaluate each other's productions and compare them. Then move to sentences:

   a. Use five new sentences, underlining three words in each sentence. Read them aloud to your partner, cycling the productions as in 2a, b, and c. Have your partner do the same. Evaluate and compare.
   b. Each of you, in turn, talk (monologue) to the other on any topic. Talk until you have faked three examples each of the three spasm types. Evaluate and compare.

   At this point, discuss with your partner whether you look and sound like a mild stutterer with little struggle and no associated behaviors. If you do not, back up and repeat the practice steps. Inadequacies probably are due to one or more of the following:

   Not taking assignments seriously; having too much fun.

   Muscular tension level is too low.

   Feeling ridiculous and embarrassed.

   Repetitions are too easy, bouncy, and rhythmical.

   Blocks are cessations rather than "getting stuck."

   Feeling fear or anxiety over faking in front of your partner.

   Facial expressions, tone of voice, and so on are too calm and relaxed.

   In the next segment you want to include the variable of severity (in terms of duration, effort, loudness) as you fake. As in the first assignments, you will want a mirror, tape recorder, and (on some) your partner.

4. Select any five words from your reading list. Record and watch in the mirror as you read each word aloud three consecutive times:

   a. Repeat three to five times on each word with easy, normal repetitions.
   b. Then repeat five to eight times on each word, with a louder voice and visible tension.

c. Finally, repeat ten to fifteen times on each word with irregular rhythm, increased tension, and audible strain.

5. Repeat the basics of 4, using the same words, but prolong.

   a. Prolong for two to three seconds on each word with a slight increase in loudness.
   b. Prolong three to five seconds on each word, lose eye contact, and increase loudness.
   c. Prolong five to eight seconds on each word, turn or drop your head, constrict vocal folds and strain, and clench your fist as you move an arm.

6. Repeat the basics of 4, using the same words, but block:

   a. Block on each word for two to three seconds, staring at yourself in the mirror.
   b. Block for three to five seconds on each word, staring and then dropping your eyes; move your lips as if trying to complete the word each time.
   c. Block on each word for five to ten seconds, cocking your head to one side or back; move lips and jaw silently; and strain to get the word out.

Write a one-paragraph report on 4 through 6, describing your efforts, how it all went, and your feelings. This would be a good point to demonstrate progress in class.

Find a paragraph that runs 300 to 500 words and underline 30 words that start sentences or phrases and/or are significant words for the "sense of the sentence." It will help if the lines are double-spaced so you can put the code symbols below or above the underlined words. Randomly mark five words each, with each of the following code symbols, so that you have finally marked each of the 30 underlined words and have 5 examples of each of these associated behaviors:

P	=	postponement	Rs	=	release
C	=	circumlocution	St	=	starter
Re	=	retrial	Su	=	substitution

7. Read the paragraph aloud while you record on tape. On each underlined word fake a mild-to-moderate spasm of any type and add the associated behavior you have marked there. On /C/ and /Su/ you will not fake spasms. Play back the recording and evaluate.

8. Repeat 7 but make spasms and associated behaviors more obvious (not on /C/ and /Su/, but change them). Play back and evaluate.

9. Mark thirty new words on your paragraph, or use a new paragraph and mark thirty words as before, with underlining and coded associated behaviors. Read aloud to your partner, faking moderate-to-severe spasms and making secondaries obvious (see previous comments about /C/ and /Su/). Before this your partner is to set up a sheet of paper, numbered 1 through 30 (see sample), where he or she writes down the dysfluent word, identifies spasm type, identifies associated mannerism, and evaluates the combined spasm and mannerism production. Record for playback in case your partner misses any items. Note: If you are really good, your partner will have to guess at /C/ and /Su/, so your partner should not have a copy of your paragraph. Use a 1-to-5 evaluation scale.

WORD	ASSOCIATED MANNERISM	SPASM TYPE	EVALUATION
1.			
. . .			
30.			

> If your partner is objective and accurate in his or her evaluations, you have a good sampling of your progress. You should have an evaluation average of 3 or better (add up all evaluations and divide by the number of evaluations). No evaluation should be below 2, and the 3 average is minimal.

Moving to less structured situations is difficult for some persons. Others will have felt constricted and artificial with the preceding assignments. In the following assignments, the important basic is to treat them seriously. People tend to relieve stress by humor and laughter. Sometimes humor is unavoidable when we do funny things, but generally make every attempt to "be a stutterer" or to act as if the person talking to you is one.

10. Over a period of five days, talk with your partner once each day, in person or on the telephone. During each verbal contact, fake three mild-to-moderate spasms with one or more associated behaviors added. After each contact write down the results and your own evaluations, setting up a form like the one used in the previous assignment. Use the 1-to-5 rating scale. You may obtain feedback from your partner, but the evaluation should be your own.

11. During the five-day period, have conversations with a total of five people in your class (or other persons). During each verbal contact fake a moderate-to-severe spasm with two associated behaviors. As soon as possible after each contact, write down the results and your evaluations. Describe your feelings.

12. Prepare a progress report on yourself as a developing pseudostutterer. Treat it as if you were a clinician writing a client evaluation. Your goal is to sound and look like a real stutterer while being aware and able to evaluate what occurs.

If you are not satisfied with this report, go back to previous assignments where you need work and work on 12 again. On the following assignments, your partner is to be present for at least one performance of each assignment.

13. Select three telephone numbers from the newspaper or telephone directory classified advertisements. Look for services or sources you ordinarily might use. Before the three calls, write two questions you will ask in each call. Underline one word in each question to fake on. Select one of the following levels of difficulty for the three calls:

   a. Fake a mild repetition or prolongation in each call.
   b. Fake any mild spasm and an audible associated behavior in each call.
   c. Fake a moderate spasm, plus a postponement and a starter in each call.

    d. Fake a postponement, a severe block, and a retrial, and finish with a repetition in each call.

14. Stop three people on the street and ask directions to an appropriate building. Keep good enough eye contact to evaluate the reactions of the auditors. Select one of these options:

    a. Fake a moderate repetition with two associated behaviors each time.
    b. Fake a different spasm to each person and vary associated behaviors.
    c. Fake a severe repetition with two associated behaviors to each person.

    Write a report that identifies persons or situations selected, levels of difficulty selected and reasons for selections, success of efforts, responses of auditors, and your feelings. Combine your evaluations with those made by your partner.

The assignment sequence could continue, but the overall purpose was to have you learn basic skills and have the experience of using them in real situations. Further developments depend on your needs and motivation.

SAMPLE ASSIGNMENTS FOR CLIENTS

The following assignments are suggestions for practice in faking to be used with clients. The arrangement is intended to approximate a hierarchy, but clients will differ in their problems and needs, and therapy plans may necessitate rearrangement, elimination, or addition of items. Routinely (see discussion of assignments in Chapter 3) some options have been provided.

1. Make two lists of the associated behaviors we have identified in your speech. One list should be behaviors that occur in time before the stuttering spasm or involve any part of the body other than the head, neck, or face. Everything else goes on the second list. While looking in the mirror, give answers to a list of questions provided by the clinician. Read a question; then look in the mirror as you answer. Select one of the following to do on each answer:

    a. Fake one first-list behavior on each answer.
    b. Fake three first-list behaviors on each answer.
    c. Fake two first-list behaviors per answer, until you have gone through the list twice.

    Prepare a report on your results, indicating your success and the quality of your eye contact.

2. Make a list of fifty words and read it aloud. As you read, fake various associated behaviors on every production. Afterwards, write down which behaviors were easiest to fake, whether any slipped into involuntary spasms, and whether particular spasms seemed to "fit" certain words more than others. Select your level of difficulty:

    a. Read the list until each of your behaviors has been faked twice.
    b. Read the list until each behavior has been faked three times.

    c. Read the list until you have faked two associated behaviors on each pro-
duction, going through the list of words twice.

3. Take any paragraph and underline enough words so that each of your associated behaviors can be used twice. Select your option:

    a. On each underlined word, use the behavior you chose; say the word,
pause, and then repeat the word, using the same associated behavior in an
altered form (louder, softer, slower, faster, and so on).

    b. On each underlined word, use the associated behavior you chose; say the
word, and then repeat it, using a "new" associated behavior you do or do
not usually use.

4. In conversations or telephone calls that occur normally, work on your associated behaviors by selecting one of the following options:

    a. In three situations, pick any associated behavior and fake it on three
different, nonstuttered words.

    b. In six situations, follow the same pattern.

    c. In nine situations, follow the same pattern.

5. Make deliberate telephone calls to strangers, where you practice faking associated behaviors by (select one option):

    a. In three calls, use one of your audible associated behaviors and an audible
"new" behavior on each call.

    b. In six calls, repeat the same pattern.

    c. In nine calls, repeat the same pattern.

6. Make deliberate telephone calls where you practice faking associated
behaviors that you do not use. Select your level of difficulty.

    a. Three telephone calls, with one fake per call.

    b. Three telephone calls, with two fakes per call.

    c. Three telephone calls, with three fakes per call.

7. Use a tape recorder and a word list. Read aloud, selecting your difficulty level.
Evaluate your efforts. Fake a stuttering spasm on each word. If any fakes
become real, try to figure out why. Do the fakes without any associated
behaviors.

    a. Read and fake five words for each of your most common stuttering pat-
terns.

    b. Read and fake ten words for each of your most common stuttering pat-
terns, and repeat any that you fail on.

    c. Read and fake twenty words for each of your most common stuttering
patterns.

8. For a period of five days, fake your most common associated behavior on
nonstuttered words. Select your option:

    a. Ten fakes per day.

    b. Ten fakes per day, and add two more for each fake that becomes real.

    c. Twenty fakes per day.

9. For a period of two days, fake a mild stuttering spasm of any type on the first
word of a verbal contact. Select your option:

    a. In at least five speech situations.

    b. In at least five situations, and add one situation for each fake that slips and becomes real.

    c. In every situation during the day, no matter how brief.

10. Make telephone calls and try to collect real stutterings. If you cannot stutter, fake a major spasm on each call. On the next appropriate word following the real or faked spasm, fake two of your usual associated behaviors. Select your option:

    a. Two telephone calls.
    b. Four telephone calls.
    c. Six telephone calls.

11. Make telephone calls that are preplanned. In each call fake a severe stuttering spasm (any type) with two associated behaviors. If the fake spasm becomes real, make a similar telephone call and fake again on the same word. Keep doing this until the fake stays fake. Select your option:

    a. One telephone call.
    b. Two telephone calls.
    c. Three telephone calls.

12. During conversations with friends collect fakes made on the associated behaviors that follow. Do not fake any spasms. Select your option:

Number of Associated Behaviors to Fake

	STARTERS	RETRIALS	SUBSTITUTIONS	POSTPONEMENTS
a.	3	1	3	3
b.	4	3	2	4
c.	6	5	1	7

13. During conversations with friends, collect fakes on stuttering spasms and associated behaviors, selecting your option. If a fake slips, pause and try to repeat the word with an altered fake. If the second effort slips, move on but remember it for discussion in clinic.

    a. Have three mild and one moderate faked spasms, with single associated behaviors on three of the spasms.

    b. Have one mild, three moderate, and one severe faked spasms, with single associated behaviors on four spasms and a double behavior fake on one spasm.

    c. Have three moderate and three severe faked spasms, with three single associated behaviors and three double associated behaviors.

14. Stop strangers on the street and ask for directions to appropriate buildings or services. Fake spasms as indicated, selecting your option. All spasms are to be moderate to severe, and use associated behaviors.

    a. Collect five fakes.
    b. Collect fifteen fakes.
    c. Collect twenty-five fakes.

15. Go into stores or business establishments and talk with people about pur-

chases, services, and so forth. During each conversation, fake the elected number of times. Keep track of any fakes that slip, and write them down afterwards. Select your option:

a. Three situations, each with three fakes and no associated behaviors.
b. Five situations, each with three fakes and no associated behaviors.
c. Five situations, each with five fakes and at least one associated behavior on each fake.

As you can see I have not included many possible variations. Also, I have not included videotaping, clinician participation, involvement of a stuttering group, or other variables. I have tried to give an idea of a faking hierarchy. In other chapters there will be assignments involving faking, and these may help broaden concepts. Whatever form and sequence used, you will be helping your client do what must be done: ". . . your clients must touch the untouchable," their stuttering (Van Riper, 1974).

5

Relaxation and Desensitization

OVERVIEW

The dual topics of relaxation and desensitization will be discussed in the same chapter for two reasons. First, both procedures basically deal with the physiological or emotional results of a single phenomenon, anxiety. Second, therapy procedures used in both instances tend to overlap, and in some approaches, combine. Both topics have been of considerable interest for decades to psychiatry, psychotherapy, medicine, physical therapy, speech and language pathology, and other helping professions. Separate volumes have been devoted to each subject and to their combinations. Entire therapy systems have been based on either or both of the procedures. This chapter, of necessity, will be limited in its review of clinical applications and procedures. Basic approaches and uses will be indicated, but the reader intent on acquiring expertise in the two areas will need to read more extensively and secure additional instruction and supervision of practice.

Anxiety

Anxiety and its role in stuttering have been the source of considerable debate for generations of clinicians. Anxiety per se has occupied the attention of generations of psychologists. We can consider it in terms of cognition, behavior, physiology, and related emotions. Definition is complex because of the interplay of the four areas just named and involvement of other states, such as fear, anger, excitement, sexual arousal, and joy, that overlap. Anger can function as a response and also as a cause. Aspects of anxiety include phobias, obsessive-compulsive disorders, and vague or generalized anxiety. Related conditions such as somatoform and dissociative disorders also confuse the picture (Sue et al. 1981). For behavior in general, and stuttering in particular, I believe the confusion is lessened by the development of the concept of two anxiety syndromes: trait and state. *State anxiety* refers to the concern, fear, anticipation, and so on prior to and during a situation that is (or is perceived to be) dangerous, threatening, embarrassing, or otherwise negatively functional for the well-being of the human organism. *Trait anxiety* is an ongoing functional state wherein the human organism perceives more threat and stress than probably exists, is more susceptible to it when it occurs, and reacts more strongly when under threat or stress (Spielberger, 1966, 1970, 1972).

Many researchers, theorists, and clinicians have an understandable tendency to try and force human beings to fit into rigidly defined categories. This "neat niche" tendency creates declarative statements that are often, at best, generalizations. Self-serving studies are conducted to support the particular niche approach. This has happened in many areas of stuttering, and anxiety is no exception. Boland (1953) reported that stutterers are higher in general (trait) and speech situation (state) anxiety than are nonstutterers, whereas Andrews (1974a) argued the absence of a proven relationship between anxiety and stuttering. Anxiety in stuttering has been measured by palmar sweat indices (Brutten, 1963), where findings were positive; by adaptation (Gray & Brutten, 1965), where findings were negative; by EMG measurements of laryngeal muscle tension in stutterers, where findings have been negative (McLean & Cooper, 1978) and positive (Gautheron et al. 1972); and so on. Many other studies, pointing in both directions, have accumulated (Ragsdale, 1976; Sherrard, 1975; Young, 1965). As expected, results are confused. The explanation probably rests on several factors:

1. Research done with minuscule subject populations that are not always representative of their own demographic subgroup, much less of the universe population of stutterers.
2. Measurement of anxiety by criteria of physiological state changes that may or may not reflect anxiety and/or nonanxiety arousal states.
3. Measurement of anxiety by criteria of behavioral state changes that may or may not actually reflect anxiety.
4. Utilization of stimuli (audience size, electrical shock, role play, and so on) that are presumed to invoke anxiety in all and to the same degree for different persons.
5. Testing and evaluation performed in settings alien to the normal routine of the subjects, but with the results applied to daily life.

6. Statistical analysis that elevates the .05 alpha level to greater importance than "clinical significance."

To these factors we must add theoretical and experimental bias. Theoretical orientation seems to divide into three points of view (Gronhovd & Zenner, 1982). Some clinicians regard anxiety as a causative agent and preeminent factor in the origin and maintenance of stuttering. Therapy should be directed, therefore, at the anxiety first and secondly at the stuttering as a malleable result of emotion. Other clinicians regard anxiety as a significant contributory factor in stuttering, and they structure therapy to deal specifically (but not solely) with the speech anxiety and behaviors. The third group of clinicians feel that anxiety is a response to stuttering development and that reduction or elimination of the dysfluency will result in the removal of any anxiety syndrome. Sheehan (1975) particularly represents the first group, Van Riper (1973) the second, and Ryan (1974) the third point of view. For an excellent summary of these points of view, I recommend the Gronhovd and Zenner (1982) chapter. On the basis of conflicting research, logic of subgroups, and empirical reasoning, it seems appropriate to suggest that anxiety is a significant but variable factor in stuttering. Some stutterers should be trait anxiety types, some should be strong state anxiety prone, and some should be a mixture of both. The significance of levels will vary from minimal up to where the anxiety is the most important consideration in therapy. I suggest it is equally inappropriate to regard all clients as needing anxiety-reduction therapy or to assume that any type of symptom or fluency therapy obviates a need to consider anxiety. As we review various therapy procedures for anxiety effects, the reader is urged to keep an open mind.

Tension

Tension and associated neurological states tend to accompany anxiety. The autonomic and central nervous systems combine, primarily through limbic and reticular networks, to produce changes in the organism during stress. Respiration, heartbeat, vascular pressure, sweating, blood chemistry, muscle tonus, and many other factors are changed by arousal states. Sherrard (1975) suggested that anxiety also changes the attention we pay to speech feedback (auditory, tactile, kinesthetic), increasing the tendency to correct "errors," whereas Timmons and Boudreau (1972) feel that anxiety may act as a catalyst in feedback disruptions. There is no question that in a physiological arousal state, the reticular inhibition of gamma efferents of the muscle system will be reduced so that an increase in alpha motoneuron firing results, increasing muscle tension. Brain stem timing and coordinating patterns, cerebellar inhibiting and tonus effects, and spinal cord feedback loops for reflex reactions can be altered. Whether all this is positive or negative in effect is arguable. Since the status of the central nervous system is a reflection of the current status of the peripheral organism, it follows that an alteration in the status of the peripheral organism will change the function pattern of the central nervous system. Reflex inhibition postures and other physical therapies are founded on this principle. These therapies change the neural signals to the limbic system so that anxiety-fear responses are not stimulated or, if stimulated, are incompatible with the state of the peripheral organism. It also is possible to approach the CNS and ANS subcortical centers and alter or diminish the emotional arousal signals they send out. This can be done through chemical tranquilizing agents, by education to remove the fear potential of ignorance or misunderstanding, by adaptation through repeated or prolonged exposure, or by developing competitive organism responses incompatible with arousal state physiology. In this chapter we will look at one area of each of the following two approaches: anxiety control through relaxation of the peripheral mechanism, and anxiety control through desensitization to the stimuli that tend to produce anxiety.

RELAXATION

Background

Cycles in relaxation therapy have occurred in the treatment of stuttering. It was strong in psychologically oriented therapies that stressed neurotic stuttering and rejected fluency therapies (Boome & Richardson, 1931). It was regarded by these clinicians as a complex capacity or skill, but one that could improve general health, academic progress, games and sports, self-confidence, mental concentration, and physical coordination (Boome et al. 1939). As symptom therapy and symptomatic psychotherapy grew in popularity, relaxation was divided into polarized uses—by reputable psychotherapy practitioners and by quacks. Relaxation became the province both of skilled therapists in Jacobsonian relaxation (see next section), and of quacks using cheap tricks and suggestion. I am speaking of relaxation as the only therapy and not of the many reputable therapies that included relaxation as part of their programs. As stuttering therapies in the 1960s became more diverse, relaxation increased in use. Attitudes toward its efficacy were, and are, mixed. Bluemel (1960) stated that relaxation really had no theoretical basis to support it, but empirical evidence was sufficient to recommend its use. Lennon (1962) presented a detailed sequence for relaxation therapy with stutterers. A more common attitude was expressed by Bloodstein (1969) who felt that it was used primarily as a subprocedure, and not as a major therapy by any leading clinicians. This subprocedure approach was followed by Gregory (1968), who supported a brief series of procedures, starting early in therapy and continuing as part of therapy sessions, that used other techniques as the major approaches to remediation. Both in therapy and in research in related fields, there was a resurgence of interest in relaxation (Slorach, 1971). Dalton and Hardcastle (1977) expressed the opinion that relaxation, per se, was not very effective. However, they recommended its inclusion as part of an overall remediation program. Many therapies that were not "relaxation programs" routinely included some form of it. Relaxation of some sort became involved in many of the fluency induction approaches, such as airflow (Schwartz, 1976), regulated breathing (Azrin & Nunn, 1974), and fluency shaping (Webster, 1979). The ability to relax, in whole or in part, is a basic component of most therapy methods (Crystal, 1980).

Approaches to relaxation are multiple. In modern medicine there has been an explosion of chemical substances to relax the patient. A survey of the 1982 *Physicians' Desk Reference* indicated ninety-one products that could be identified directly as tranquilizing or relaxing agents, and there are many more. I will not review the drug literature on stuttering, and at the risk of overgeneralization, will say only that in too many cases drug therapy has tended to create tranquil stutterers who retain dysfluencies. Carbon dioxide therapy, which has been used as a technique, in most instances was the only, or major, treatment (Kent, 1961). Wolpe (1973) pointed out that the gas could be a powerful anxiety inhibitor, although Fransella (1972) reported it had no significant effect on stuttering itself. Falck (1969) summarized the use of hypnosis in desensitization with stuttering, and Wolpe commented favorably on the use of yoga and transcendental meditation techniques in relaxation and desensitization programs. Relaxation also has been approached in a number of therapy methods by having the client concentrate on reducing tension in the respiratory-phonatory-articulatory systems. This may be taught on a whole-system basis or concentrated on a very specific area, such as the jaw or tongue. Progressive relaxation, developed by Jacobson (1938), was a whole-body relaxation that progressively moved through the muscle groups of the body until the client could be totally relaxed. Stuttering therapies today use both the partial and the total relaxation programs in various combinations. Depending on the application, goals of relaxation may be the following:

1. Indirect relaxation by teaching breathing, phonation, or articulation procedures that relax those muscle groups.
2. Direct relaxation of tensions in the speech-production mechanism so that speech efforts can be made from a relaxed state.
3. Direct relaxation of the body wherein the speech mechanism is only a part of the total organism.

Prerequisites for the Clinician

Personal preparation of the clinician for using relaxation therapy involves several points, depending on the degree of relaxation sought and its uses. In addition to the normal preparation of a speech and language pathologist, some areas of knowledge might be helpful. A basic grounding in anatomy, to know and understand the muscle systems of the body, is useful. Division or combination of muscles into ramp-type (slow, postural) and saccadic-type (fast, precise) movers will help in relaxation approaches. Application and evaluation are facilitated if the clinician understands the concept of agonist, antagonist, and synergist functions. Of course, specific knowledge of the speech mechanism musculature and the complex interplay of relaxation and tension and agonist and antagonist in production is useful. A basic preparation in the neurology of motor function will provide a better understanding of tension and relaxation and how CNS systems affect and are affected by the peripheral organism. Instruction is useful in the psychological aspects of anxiety, fear, and other emotions related to relaxation. Finally, every clinician should *experience* relaxation. Relaxation is not always easy. You do not need to feel it so much for demonstration as to understand it, solve problems you may have with it, and be able to identify with the client's progression and problems.

Observation and evaluation.   These aspects in relaxation concern the point just cited: It can be difficult to know when a person is truly relaxed. The most efficient method involves use of instruments such as the galvanic skin response (GSR) or electromyography (EMG) measurement. Such devices can read out general or specific areas of body tension, establish a baseline for measurement of progress, and be used as part of the relaxation technique itself. Such instruments are not inexpensive, take variable amounts of time for setup and cleanup, and require provision of calibration and maintenance. Many clinicians must work without them. More often, the clinician must rely on other indicators to monitor relaxation. One source is the client's reports, if the person is reliable and has learned to recognize the feeling of relaxation. Other indicators of overall relaxation include the following:

1. Dysfluency rate—if the client is relaxed, the dysfluency rate usually drops sharply.
2. Phonatory output—pitch typically lowers, loudness decreases, vowels may be more prolonged, glottal attacks are reduced, and the voice often is breathier.
3. Rate and prosody factors—rate of utterance is slowed, stress and frequency of stress are reduced, and inflections and variations are reduced.
4. Respiration—respiratory rate will slow with relaxation. Normal, quiet inhalation and exhalation follow a two-to-three second pulse beat for each half of the cycle (Overstake, 1979). Look for faster rates and/or imbalances between inspiration and expiration times. If the client is supine (on the back), breathing predominance may shift because of the gravity effect and visceral inertia.
5. Pulse rate—a normal adult pulse rate will be 60 to 80 bpm (beats per minute) at rest, and 80 to 100 bpm during ordinary activity. However, there can be

wide variations, and you will need to know those of your client if you are using pulse rate as a measure. Pulse rate can be checked by the conventional wrist contact or by pressing lightly against the carotid artery area of the neck (usually about an inch below and slightly anterior to the angle of the mandible). Don't use your thumb or forefinger to check as you may pick up your own pulse instead, and don't press too hard as that will constrict the blood vessel and change the pulse rate.

6. Rigidity—does the person appear to be relaxed and comfortable? Are legs, arms, hands, fingers, and head in relaxed configurations? Some clients initially feel unprotected and vulnerable in a relaxation posture.

7. Tremors—watch for foot twitches, small movements of the fingers, eyelid tremors, lip movements, and so on. These usually are signals of tension, even when larger muscles are semirelaxed. Occasionally, you may encounter nonintention or resting tremors in a subclinical neurological state or with advanced age. This can be verified and allowed for in therapy, or referral may be considered if it is a significant finding.

Equipment and environments. These factors need to be considered. Special equipment, such as GSR and EMG units have been discussed. In addition, other items can be considered. The therapy room should be quiet, private, and with a light source that can be dimmed or replaced by a low-wattage lamp. If total relaxation is the aim, you will want a floor pad, mattress, cot, relaxation chair, or plinth (wood table covered in foam and upholstered for easy cleaning). In some clinic rooms for relaxation, one wall is covered with photomural wallpaper showing a forest, a beach, a sunset, or some other pleasant scene. Large wall posters, paintings, or camera slides projected on a blank wall may be used. Other clinicians simply ask the client to visualize internal images. It is possible to use sound as a background support for relaxation. Soft music, forest sounds, surf or wind recordings, and so forth can be purchased or developed. Again, some clinicians do not use such props. The clinician will want to adopt a relaxed speech pattern to instruct, encourage, and communicate with the client. It also models a relaxed speech pattern for the stutterer. As the client progresses, speech energy and tension may be increased deliberately by the clinician, but generally it is best to model what is being taught.

Procedures

General relaxation. This technique is used frequently in therapy to reduce daily tensions that a client brings to the session or the induced anxiety and tension that some clients develop about coming to therapy. The client benefits from a reduction in tension, therapy sessions become associated with feelings of security, and concomitant fluency or symptom techniques benefit from a more relaxed starting point. Some clinicians begin every session with a period of relaxation practice. Brief intervals also can be inserted during a therapy session if the client becomes tense while attempting certain procedures or while discussing certain topics. These general activities or exercises can be organized in different ways. The clinician may instruct the client as follows:

1. Sit back in the chair or lie down. Look at the picture on the wall (or close your eyes and imagine a peaceful scene). Breathe deeply several times, and then try to breathe in even, gentle cycles. Listen to the music (or voice of the clinician), and try to clear the mind of all thoughts. Let the body sag and relax.

2. Sit in the chair. Sit up very straight, exaggerating a stiff and tense posture. Grip the chair hard with your hands and press your feet firmly against the floor. Combine all these tensions and hold a deep inhalation for at least five seconds. Now, all at one time, exhale air strongly and sag forward like a stuffed toy. Feel the difference.

3. Lie down on the mat (cot, plinth, and so on). Take a deep breath and then let it out very slowly. As the air slowly moves out, try to sink into the mat surface. Repeat the cycle three times, on each exhalation trying to relax more and sink deeper into the mat as you close your eyes and clear your mind.

Many variations are possible, and adaptations for children are easy to develop (Goven & Vette, 1966; Luper & Mulder, 1964). Rustin (1978) has described relaxation procedures that can be used as part of an intensive group therapy program for adolescents.

In contrast to general relaxation techniques are procedures for reducing tension in specific muscle groups, usually speech-production muscles. Hanna et al. (1975) used an EMG unit attached to the larynx to secure relaxation of vocal muscles. The EMG was attached to a tone generator so that any increment in muscle tension drove the pitch of the generator higher. In this way, the stutterers could auditorily monitor their own tension levels. Gordon et al. (1983) also used EMG feedback from speech muscles to secure relaxation, and Treon and Tamayo (1974) compared EMG relaxation and DAF. In the latter study, they found that DAF reduced stuttering much more than did EMG relaxation, and a combination of the two was more effective than either technique used separately. Guitar (1975) used analog EMG feedback to help stutterers learn to relax lip tension and laryngeal tension. The three subjects all reduced their stuttering in this way; however, one focused on lip tension, one on laryngeal tension, and one on a relaxation of both areas. The importance of tension localization (see Chapter 3 on self-analysis of spasms) cannot be overemphasized. Van Riper (1971, 1973, 1982) strongly supported the idea of localized tensions acting as triggers for stuttering spasms. This possibly explains why Still and Griggs (1979) reported a significant decrease in stuttering during the first thirty words following a stuttering spasm; the relaxation following a completed stuttering spasm facilitates fluency. Gautheron et al. (1973) reinforced the concept of localized tension, reporting that stutterers have a longer time interval between a preceding consonant and a following vowel—resulting in higher subglottal air pressure and a need for hard glottal attacks to emit phonation. Wells (1983), in a distinctive feature analysis of stuttered phonemes, supported localizing tension; he reported that adult stuttering was most likely to occur when primary tensions and discoordinations are lingual and laryngeal and when the stutterer must shift from a (− voicing) to a (+ voicing) mode. Methods of localized relaxation will be suggested in the section on sample techniques.

Progressive relaxation. This technique, associated with Jacobson (1938), has been significant in stuttering therapy for years. By tensing and then relaxing specific muscle groups, the client progressively learns to relax the whole body. Although some clients cannot master the procedure, most learn to totally relax after only several minutes (Korchin, 1976). The client tenses and relaxes muscles or muscle groups, one at a time, beginning with the feet and traveling toward the head. The clinician cues tension and relaxation and instructs the client in feeling gradations of difference. As the client learns to monitor the sensory signals of intermediate gradations of muscle tone, he or she takes over the cuing process and develops a capacity for self-relaxation (Gregory, 1968).

Sample programs. Examples of general relaxation have been provided earlier. In this section I will give examples of localized relaxation and progressive relaxation. The progressive relaxation is a blend of Jacobson (1938), Overstake (1979), and approaches I have used in therapy. The environmental considerations mentioned earlier should be adopted, and you will need a pad or cot on which the client can lie supine.

1. Before starting the exercises, discuss relaxation with the client. Elicit discussion of things that make the client tense, what tension feels like, and how tension affects her or him. Describe the relaxation procedure. Verbally recognize feelings of oddity and reduce any embarrassment.
2. Lie down on the mat, and close your eyes. Demonstrate "settling in" on the mat and slow breathing while you relax.
3. Have the client take your place and duplicate your performance. After about thirty seconds, have the client open his or her eyes and respond to questions about comfort, physical sensation, and embarrassment.
4. When the client is comfortable and able to relax to some degree, instruct her or him to raise one leg off the mat, about ten to twelve inches, and hold it. Instruct the client to feel the weight and the tension of hip, thigh, and abdominal muscles. After about ten seconds, instruct the client to relax and let the leg drop (the client is not to *move* the leg back but to relax the muscle contraction and let the leg fall). Repeat this process with the other leg.
5. Instruct the client to flex the leg at the knee while raising the leg (hip flexion) and to ventroflex the foot (toward the knee) until the leg, knee, and foot are

maximally flexed. The client should hold briefly, relax to the mat, and repeat with other leg.

Repeat steps 4 and 5 several times. Then check relaxation by putting your hand first on one knee and then the other and slightly rocking each one in and out to see if there is resistance. You may want the client to tense briefly and resist your slight motion, and then relax on the last couple of motions. Putting your hand under one knee and slightly raising the leg also checks relaxation. You also can have the client resist and relax to this movement: You can instruct the client to flex the knee slightly (foot still on mat), resist your effort to push down on the knee, and then relax back against the mat. I do not recommend extending or flexing both legs at the same time. Such action is too strength-dependent, and could pull a muscle.

6. Instruct the client to "Try and touch your ears with your shoulders . . . pull them down as low as possible . . . bow the shoulders in an upward curve . . . relax back on the mat." This move can be done unilaterally first and then bilaterally.
7. Have the client put all three motions from 6 together and "rotate" the shoulders in a circle. Demonstration and help may be needed.
8. Have the client elevate her or his head and touch chin to chest for about five seconds; then cue relaxation. Direct the client to press his or her head strongly against the mat, hold for about five seconds, and relax on your cue. Finally, tell the client to ". . . touch your right shoulder with your chin. . . . Feel the pull and tension on your left side. . . ." After about five seconds, cue relaxation and repeat with pointing the chin to the left shoulder.

Repeat steps 6, 7, and 8 several times. Check relaxation by pressing the client's shoulders down slightly, pulling them up gently, and gently moving the head in a right-and-left direction. Feel for resistance and tension, commenting to the client.

9. Have the client supinate the forearm and hand (palms up) and flex the elbow so the forearm is perpendicular. Direct the client to clench both fists and flex the biceps at the same time, for about five seconds. The client should relax on cue. Have one forearm placed perpendicularly as before. Place your hand on the inner surface of the wrist and resist the client's effort to complete flexion; but don't overdo it.[1] Move to the opposite side of the wrist and resist extension. Cue relaxation each time. Move to the other arm and repeat.
10. Instruct the client to assume the vertical forearms position again, this time with the inner surface of the forearms facing medially and the wrists flexed so that palms are up and fingers point laterally. Place one of your hands flat on each palm of the client and press down as the client presses up. Unlike other times, tell the client to tense the whole body with effort. As before, do not turn this into a test of strength. After about five seconds, cue for relaxation.

[1]On all resistance efforts, keep the level low. Too strong an effort will overflow to other muscles and raise overall tension. Repeatedly tell the client to "let the other parts of your body stay relaxed" throughout all exercises.

Check legs, shoulders, and arms for relaxation. This exercise was performed to reduce overflow tension that built up during other activities and to prepare for final relaxation efforts.

11. The following are to be performed as a series, with each action lasting three to five seconds, terminating on your cue, "Relax." At first you will have to instruct each step, but quickly move to a key cue word and then omit the cue words as the client follows the now-familiar sequence:

   a. Tightly squeeze both eyes shut as if a bright light was shining in them. Cue word: *eyes.*
   b. Frown exaggeratedly, bringing the forehead down in wrinkles and the eyebrows down and inward. Cue word: *forehead.*
   c. Wrinkle the nose upward as if for a sneeze or a sneer, elevating and everting upper lip at the time. Cue word: *nose.*
   d. With lips together normally, produce a very exaggerated grin until the mouth corners stretch. After holding this position, reverse (on cue) to an exaggerated mouth, corners down, as if for crying or pouting. Cue words: *grin* and *down.*
   e. Pucker lips strongly as if to whistle. Cue word: *lips.*
   f. Clench mandible against maxillary molars as if biting or lifting a heavy weight. Cue word: *jaws.*
   g. With mouth closed, place the blade of the tongue (not just the tip or apex) against the hard palate and push as strongly as possible.[2] Cue word: *tongue.*

The first run-through easily can take thirty minutes or more, and you both will be more tired than relaxed. However, if there are no problems, in two or three sessions the client can run through the whole series (no repeats) in five minutes or less. Obviously, resistance exercises will be dropped. However, the client can lift imaginary weights and carry out exercise 10. Notice that the speech mechanism was left until last. When the client can run through the series without cues, and occasional checks indicate that relaxation is present, work for finer distinctions. Have the client go through the series three times. The first effort should contain just enough tension and effort to carry the movements out. On the second effort, tension should be what the client thinks is normal for her or him. The final effort should be made with maximum tension. As before, relax after each effort. As soon as the client has learned the basic procedures, give outside assignments. A useful time is just before rising in the morning and at bedtime in the evening. Clients may find the floor better than a soft bed. Those stutterers who can arrange it should practice during the day.

Progressive relaxation can be used, as has been noted, to start sessions, facilitate fluency, and enhance techniques. Many clients will be able to translate the postural movements of the exercise into less obvious forms and perform them while sitting or standing, actually practicing them dur-

---

[2]This will involve the soft palate because of *glossopalatus*, pharyngeal areas because of *pharyngopalatus*, and other muscles. Lingual attachments to hyoid will involve strap neck muscles, and probable glottal valve approximation would involve extrinsic and intrinsic laryngeal muscles.

ing tension-provoking situations. As will be seen during the second part of this chapter, relaxation also can be tied to desensitization efforts.

Problems in overall relaxation occur occasionally. Some clients do not dress appropriately, and relaxation has to be postponed or steps omitted. Most clients feel slightly "silly" at first, but that usually disappears if the clinician behaves professionally. People in our culture seem to dislike or fear being touched, which occasionally can be a serious problem since touching the client to check relaxation causes tension. If this does not disappear after several sessions, check as best you can without touching. Affectionate responses to touches are possible but rare. Such an occurrence indicates either a failure on the clinician's part to be professional or a client with problems beyond those of dysfluency. Your options are appropriate reprimands, termination of the session, bringing in an "observer," dropping relaxation efforts, confronting the client and resolving the problem, or arranging for another clinician. Never let such an event pass without a clinical response. One other problem: I once had to drop relaxation with a teenage stutterer in school; he went soundly asleep every time.

Specific relaxation procedures are those usually targeted directly at the speech mechanism. They may be aimed at the overall system and, to a limited degree, the rest of the body, or they may focus on a single structure or area. Usually they are never a total program of therapy but are taught to enhance and facilitate other procedures. Point of introduction, depth of instruction, association with other procedures, transfer goals, and other factors provide too many variables to cover adequately even most possibilities, but several samples are provided:

1. The breath-chewing techniques described elsewhere can be used to relax the linked speech-production systems by contrasting the fierce energy and tension of breath chewing with low tension states.

2. The various stages of step 11 from the progressive relaxation sequence described earlier are useful alone for various degrees of relaxation.

3. Various breathing exercises cited in this text can carry a relaxation effect that will include phonatory and articulatory systems.

4. A word list can be prepared that has various CV and VC combinations, such as *popcorn, stable, airplane, gearbox, urban, bedframe, eighteen,* and *thicken.* The client should read the list loudly and with strong tension, stressing every syllable. This may trigger stuttering; if so, make note of any consistencies on particular phonemes or syllable combinations. Repeat the word list several times, having the client reduce stress and lighten contacts each time. Discuss the changes in tactile and kinesthetic sensations as relaxation increases.

5. A word list can be prepared for the client to read (you can use words from item 4). Before uttering each word, the client should maximally tense the articulators in an anticipatory position *without* attempting to speak. She or he should then relax and utter the target word in relaxation.

DESENSITIZATION

Background

Sensitization in stuttering. This technique has been basic to many theories and therapies. As stated in the earlier discussion (Chapter 1) of stuttering development, a general picture of awareness without sensitization was common in young stutterers. As stuttering continued and met the conditioning of social interaction and self-judgment, sensitization (and stuttering) increased in a feedback loop until the two components became interdependent. Desensitization is directly involved in most symptom therapies and many psychotherapies. It is variable in fluency therapies, but they operate on an assumption that replacement of stuttering with fluency will reduce sensitivity (anxiety) in speaking situations. The term *desensitization* involves the concept that stuttering persons are hypersensitive to normal nonfluencies, stuttering dysfluencies, people, situations, specific words, and various other stimuli. Clinicians differ in what they consider to be important hypersensitivities. Gerstman (1983) makes the point that the stutterer typically is not some anxiety-bound neurotic but has problems in communication that are legitimate reason for anxiety as well as the worries that any person would feel in stressful situations. Depending on the degree of anxiety the stutterer is affected in evaluative capacity, physiological tension levels in speech production, and emotional responses to stress. Desensitization therapies, in various ways, attempt to reduce or eliminate these problems.

Anxiety in stuttering. This subject was discussed at some length earlier in the chapter. Presumably, anxiety (sensitivity) is the target of desensitization therapies. Lerman and Shames (1965) failed to find graduated anxiety levels with increases in the difficulty of structured situations, but Moore (1954) reported that "good" and "bad" topics were related to stuttering frequency and variability. Santostefano (1960), stating that research supports presumptions of anxiety in stutterers, reported on a Rorschach evaluation indicating higher anxiety and hostility in stutterers. Burgraff (1974) compared traditional symptom therapy and systematic desensitization therapy, finding no significant differences in the results obtained—which raises the question of which therapy was treating what symptoms. Adams and Moore (1972) seem to suggest that simply reducing stuttering does not eliminate anxiety. They reported a 75 percent reduction of stuttering while reading under auditory masking conditions, but with little change in anxiety as measured by palmar sweat scores. As discussed earlier, disagreement over the role of anxiety exists, as does similar disagreement over desensitization therapy.

Prerequisites for the Clinician

Psychological bases of sensitization and desensitization should be understood by the clinician. These involve knowledge and understanding of learning, conditioning, and deconditioning elements. Principles of positive and negative reinforcement, adaptation, and extinction should be studied. Generalization, or transfer, of learning is significant in both sensitization and desensitization. The effects of fear, anxiety, anger, guilt, and approach and avoidance conflicts are involved in desensitization and should be understood. Most of these concepts are covered in the usual academic preparation of speech and language pathologists, but certain areas may need review.

Experience is important in desensitization. It was suggested that you experience relaxation therapy, and you definitely should practice the various desensitization exercises. With few exceptions, most clients enjoy relaxation work; this is not true in many desensitization activities. Also, because of external factors that become involved, it is more intellectually and emotionally complex to learn. For these reasons, you should carry out at least some of the assignments suggested in this chapter. Preferably, you should secure special instruction in desensitization techniques.

Procedures

Symptom and situation desensitization. This technique is integral to many therapies. It concentrates on one or many aspects of stuttering and seeks to reduce sensitivity to the dysfluency and events surrounding it. Van Riper has been associated strongly with primary desensitization, advocating specific confrontation on subbehaviors such as establishing eye contact during every stuttering spasm (Van Riper & Gruber, 1957), and with broad directives for a sequence of therapy goals (Van Riper, 1958):

1. Be willing, temporarily, to stutter openly and without embarrassment.
2. Maintain good eye contact.
3. Stop avoiding feared speech situations and words.
4. Stop the use of postponements, retrials, and other avoidance devices.
5. Use negative practice and pseudostuttering.
6. Build barriers against anxiety and frustration.
7. Learn to tolerate others' stuttering, as well as your own.
8. Study and analyze your stuttering pattern.
9. Reduce reactions to perceived penalties from auditors.
10. Reduce anxiety and increase your threshold of anxiety.

Van Riper continued to advocate primary desensitization, adding DAF to procedures (1970). He suggested inserting DAF intermittently during periods of fluent speech, gradually increasing the frequency and duration of the insertions. Also, the clinician could use DAF continuously, at the easiest delay interval, gradually moving toward the most disruptive delay time, or start with low volume at the most disruptive delay interval and gradually increase the earphone volume. In 1978, Van Riper still proposed the need to "toughen" clients to those factors that tend to increase his or her stuttering. Faking and demonstration by the clinician were emphasized.

In psychology, Adler (1966) strongly recommended extensive use of voluntary stuttering, pursuit of speech situations, and avoidance of avoidances. He also proposed a semihierarchy of desensitization activities:

1. Read sentences. After each sentence, watch in the mirror while you paraphrase the sentence.
2. Look at yourself in the mirror while verbalizing feelings about stuttering and the value of an objective attitude. Simply stare at yourself in the mirror for several minutes.
3. Count to 100, or say the alphabet, while watching yourself in the mirror. Each time eye contact is broken, stop and start over.
4. Describe yourself to an audio recorder. Play back and count spasms. Do the same after counting to 100 or reciting the alphabet.
5. Record yourself saying, twenty-five times, "My name is _____ and I am a stutterer."
6. Record and play back your descriptions of situations that are difficult. Do the same for how you think others regard your speech.
7. Record while you read paragraphs and paraphrase them, engage in monologue, and so on. Play back and count spasms.
8. Analyze the speech of other stutterers, starting with spasm counts and working up to complete descriptions. Evaluate several stutterers and compare their patterns.
9. Study several stutterers until you can imitate their spasm patterns.

Although desensitization is regarded by many clinicians as a technique for stutterers in advanced stages, some use it with children. Luper and Mulder (1964) argue that the child must be "tough enough" to stand up to competitive disruptions, inattentive audiences, or impatient listeners. They suggest establishing a basal fluency level with the child; then raising speech pressures (response complexity, demands, interruptions, listener attitude, and so on) to, but not past, the point of disruption; and then dropping back to basal fluency. No more than four pressure cycles should be implemented in one session, and the goal is to raise steadily the child's disruption threshold. Ryan (1971) has reported the use of programmed desensitization activity in hierarchical steps (mainly length and complexity of response) in parallel with fluency reinforcement therapy. Another desensitization technique is that of emotional flooding, or implosive therapy (Stampfl & Lewis, 1967). This desensitization approach begins with maximally disturbing stimuli to develop the highest anxiety levels possible (in the clinic). The client is asked to duplicate the recall exercises at home.

The theory is that as the client recalls and examines the cues that called forth the anxiety flood, extinction laws will begin to apply. Adams (1982a) has published a case report of flooding in stuttering therapy. Real or remembered situations are used to elicit strong emotional reactions, in any stage of therapy. Adams has stressed that extinction is not necessary or realistic. A significant reduction in crippling emotions may be enough to allow implementation of either symptom or fluency techniques.

Desensitization of primary behaviors, rather than for social interaction (see later), can involve many formats. However, I believe all formats can be divided into two basic approaches:

1. Desensitization to stuttering by repeated exposure to stuttering in a variety of modes and situations.
2. Desensitization to fears of stuttering by exposure to a hierarchy of situations, ranked for their anxiety-causing, stuttering potentials.

The two frequently are mixed but also are applied separately. The pure form of the first is the "stuttering bath," where a combination of evaluation, adaptation, and objectivity development reduces spasm frequency, severity, and complexity while increasing tolerance and objectivity. The pure hierarchy format tries for relative symptom control, fluency practice, or transfer of in-clinic learning, with steps of progressive difficulty. Webster (1970), comparing hierarchical and repeated exposure desensitization, felt the second approach was preferable because of reduced dependency of the client on the clinician to control his or her activities.

Through evaluation (Chapter 2) and self-analysis (Chapter 3), the clinician and the stutterer should have a thorough knowledge of the client's speech pattern, stuttering characteristics, word or situation factors, behavioral avoidances, and attitudes. Frequent references, in both chapters, were made to the desensitizing effects of the activities necessary to collect the desired information. Since the timing, combination, and predominance of desensitization can vary greatly, I will not provide a set program. However, assignment samples will be offered at the end of the chapter, and the following general suggestions are made:

1. Have adequate information about the client and the speech before using desensitization.
2. Always explain, provide rationales, and demonstrate to the same level at which you expect the client to function.
3. Be alert for problems (see end of desensitization section) that can occur.
4. Provide opportunities for ventilation by and feedback from the client.
5. As much as possible, assign solo out-clinic activities that already have been performed under your guidance.

Systematic desensitization. This technique has been described already. Technically, it is desensitization wherein the experiences are arranged systematically (usually in a hierarchy). However, from clinical history, "systematic desensitization" has been associated with the psychotherapist Wolpe (1958), who structured it to combine progressive relaxation and reciprocal inhibition.[3] The technique has been used most widely with phobic fears (Korchin, 1976) but has been applied to stuttering as well. The pairing of a physiologically incompatible response (relaxation) with a feared stimulus (stuttering or stutter-prone situations) inhibits stuttering or its anticipation. This actually inhibits the emotions and physical tension that trigger stuttering, not the stuttering itself (Bloodstein, 1979). The sequence described by Brutten and Shoemaker (1967) is typically Wolpe-style therapy:

1. Teach relaxation procedures to the stutterers.
2. Make a hierarchical list of feared speech situations.
3. Starting with the easiest situation, have the client recall and visualize it in detail, while maintaining a relaxed state.
4. Help the client maintain relaxation.
5. When stable relaxation can be maintained during recall, move to the next situation on the hierarchy list.

A similar system was used by Poppen et al. (1977) as part of a therapy program including rhythm techniques and regulated breathing. Thirty-three sessions were spent on a Wolpe-type program, followed by an equal number of sessions devoted to free conversation. They reported that stuttering frequency went as low as 3 percent and never above 6 percent, but there was little transfer on an out-clinic basis. Using a different organization, Lanyon (1969) spent about three sessions on relaxation and then went to a hierarchy list, reporting good results. Gray and England (1972) used the method on thirty stutterers, divided by state and trait anxiety patterns. They reported a reduction in frequency and severity of stuttering spasms and lowering of anxiety levels in both anxiety groups. Conture (1982) supported efforts to influence the tolerance level for disruptors rather than tolerance for dysfluency. He stressed the variety of factors that can be disruptors (auditor eye contact, group size, facial expressions, certain words, topics, and so on). In contrast, Starkweather (1980) expressed a preference for desensitization to the primary behaviors rather than to the affecting factors.

Some clinicians have reservations about systematic desensitization in highly structured programs. The inherent irrationality of speech situations makes a systematic hierarchy unrealistic, and relaxation rather than desensitization may be the more effective therapy (Muckenhoff, 1976). Azrin et al. (1979) compared the effects of two three-hour sessions of relaxation and desensitization (r/d) with that of regulated-breathing therapy of equal

---

[3]Reciprocal inhibition involves pairing incompatible responses to a stimulus so that there is an inhibition of one (undesired) response by the second (desired) response.

duration, finding that the latter reduced stuttering (on follow-up) by 97 percent, whereas the former program showed a 10 percent dysfluency reduction. The authors considered the equivalence of the methods to be artificial and the r/d therapy actually to be a placebo condition. However, their article does not reflect this. At least we can be sure that "Hurry up and relax!" therapy isn't particularly effective. Boudreau and Jeffrey (1973) found r/d therapy effective after ten sessions and verified it with a twenty-month follow-up. They noted that stutterers with higher initial dysfluency counts showed the best results. A comparison between r/d therapy and Ellis Rational-Emotive Therapy[4] resulted in a claim that the latter was more effective in reducing stuttering, anxiety, and negative attitudes (Moleski & Tosi, 1976). In a different approach to desensitization, Berecz (1973) linked punishment (not relaxation) to recall of stuttering behaviors. After visualizing stuttering behavior, the client self-administered a painful electrical shock and then immediately re-reviewed the recalled behavior, changing it until it was a successful, positive memory. Several variations in Wolpe-type therapy include using a GSR-signal device to monitor relaxation while recalling aversive memories and having the client ride an exercise bicycle (incompatible with generalized tension) while viewing video tapes of actual situations in which the client participated (Yonovitz et al. 1977).

A specific application of r/d procedures is presented by Wohl (1966), who criticizes in-clinic r/d methods because they teach the client to relax, modify anxiety, and adopt altered speech patterns " . . . and then he is sent out into the normal social situation virtually unrehearsed in combining his new behavior patterns with the acute fear of speech in the social situations" (p. 67). Wohl follows this plan:

1. There are twenty sessions of general relaxation and recall of pleasant experiences.

2. Personality evaluations are made to rate situations by anxiety level, separation of sensitivity from anxiety levels, and construction of a hierarchy.

3. Starting with the easiest situation, the clinician verbally reconstructs the scenes (sounds, smells, colors, people, movements, and so on).

4. The patient is asked to speak when distress is felt, and the person usually stutters. She or he then fills out an analysis form on the situation. This avoids " . . . long, hypochondriacal litanies . . . without opportunity to indulge his desire to feed on sympathy . . ." (p. 69).

Wohl moves into other therapy after r/d is established, favoring a metronome-based procedure. Gendelman (1977) could have used Wohl's indictment of in-clinic-only r/d therapy since she skips over direct speech

---

[4]RET was founded by Albert Ellis. In this therapy, the clinician is very directive and tells the client what to do and how to think in order to improve. Irrational thinking causes emotional problems and work on thinking logically will change the internal belief system, which in turn will eliminate or reduce the problems associated with the emotional state (Rubin & McNeil, 1981).

techniques and stresses real-life situations controlled by the clinician. In the first stage, Pre-Confrontation analysis, particular situations are analyzed for the form, type, and severity of stuttering, along with affecting factors such as topic, situation, and auditor. The structure of who says what, why things are said, and where (in speech) stuttering occurs is analyzed. Finally, the stutterer is led through an in-depth analysis of feelings and thoughts before, during, and after stuttering instances. This analysis is repeated and practiced until the client is adept at it. Gendelman states that usually two response patterns are disclosed:

1. Anticipation of response—approval or rejection.
2. Anticipation of inability to control hostility toward others and fear of its results.

After sufficient practice on significant situations, the client can move to the Confrontation stage, in which persons and situations from his or her environment are ranked in a fear hierarchy. The clinician, starting with the first (lowest) fear on the list, arranges a meeting between the stutterer and the feared person. The client then discusses with the person all the attitudes, relationships, fears, and so on involved until issues are resolved and attitudes change. Some persons may need to be seen more than once. Clients may resist at first, requiring negotiations and progressive alternatives. The clinician then moves to the next person on the list. This procedure was used with forty stutterers. Four were not helped. Thirteen improved, and twenty-three were dismissed. On follow-up (two months to three years, average about six months), nine had improved, thirteen were stable, and five showed a "slight relapse" in speech.

As you can see, desensitization comes in many forms. It can be paired with different inhibiting reactions or used alone. Some therapies use it as the only treatment mode, some to facilitate learning acquisition, some in transfer facilitation of skills, and others in maintenance stabilization. There is a range from "sink or swim" to carefully gradiated desensitization. With this extensive variety in mind, let us consider some of the problems involved with desensitization.

Problems in desensitization. These tend to relate to the problems of sensitivity. If sensitivity is attacked directly, there is often resistance because the person is "sensitive" to the attack. If it is attacked indirectly, there is a problem of transfer from simulation to reality. Desensitization through systematic in-clinic procedures is not difficult to achieve, but transfer is a doubtful variable. Desensitization by repeated exposure, flooding, and so on transfers well but can be very difficult for the client to tolerate. Quarrington and Douglass (1960) suggested that nonvocalized stutterers are particularly liable to resist eye contact, faking, and other overt activities. A particular problem with in-clinic procedures is the degree to which the stutterer's self-perceived desensitization fails to match the actual level when he or she meets real situations. Clinicians sometimes tend to use desensitization procedures as an aid to other techniques, and they fail to plan or monitor transfer as carefully as they should. As a result, the adequately learned skills in symptom control or fluency production break down in real situations (either by erosion or under a crisis) so that the major skill is lost because a supporting skill was faulty.

ASSIGNMENTS FOR CLINICIANS

The following assignments are designed to sample various techniques of relaxation and desensitization. Some of them must be done alone and others involve the use of a partner. As in other chapters, you or your instructor may want to add to, subtract from or alter the list of assignments.

1. Remember or review the definitions of trait and state anxiety. All of us have both characteristics to varying degrees and with variations over time.

   a. In general, what is your overall level of trait anxiety? Consider your posture, movements, sleep patterns, mannerisms, health, and so on as you answer.
   b. How does your level compare with that of other family members or persons you know well enough to evaluate?
   c. As best you can, evaluate your partner, your roomate(s), and several friends.

2. Rate yourself for state anxiety by comparing yourself to your peers. Copy the following situations and fill in your self-ratings on a scale of 1 to 5, where 1 = unresponsive, 2 = very relaxed, 3 = average anxiety, 4 = tense and anxious, and 5 = overreaction and high anxiety. Then ask someone who knows you well to rate you, without knowing of your ratings.

SITUATIONS	EVALUATIONS	
	BY SELF	BY OTHER
Asking/answering questions in class		
Speaking before a group		
Telephoning parents to report loss of wallet		
Talking with a blind date		
Taking an oral examination		

3. Prepare a hierarchy of situations as described in Chapter 3. To each situation assign an anxiety level (1 to 5) that you think you would feel. Have your partner go over the list and enter her or his self-evaluations next to yours. How do you compare?

4. If possible arrange to use a GSR or EMG unit, with your partner. After attaching contacts, calibrating, and so forth compare your readings to those of your partner while you

   a. Close your eyes, relax, and visualize a very peaceful scene, and then switch your thoughts to any recent personal experience.

    b. Talk with your partner for several minutes about some current interests or occurrences.
    c. Read aloud.
    d. Read or talk under DAF.
    e. Simulate anger, sadness, and joy in talking to your partner.

    How did the readings vary and compare?

5. Take any paragraph of 300-to-500 words and read it aloud as you record on tape. Turn the recorder off. Follow any one of the three sample relaxation procedures on page 126, or devise your own. As soon as you have completed the exercise, try to maintain the relaxation level and record the same passage a second time. Compare the total talking times, wpm rates, nonfluencies, loudness, pitch, inflection, and other variables.

6. With your partner, go through the complete progressive relaxation procedures described on page 127. If necessary, go through them again. When you are the "clinician," use all cues, directions, questions, and comments that would be appropriate in a real situation. After you have performed adequately, progress through the routine again while your partner observes. What were your reactions? Were there any problems? How relaxed did you become? Note: Practice sessions are often stiff, embarrassing or amusing; try to overcome this reaction, and treat the session as a real situation.

7. For a week, practice the full progessive relaxation sequence once each day, alone—at bedtime, just after getting up, or any other time of day. What were the results, effects and problems?

8. With your partner, carry out the localized relaxation exercise 4 on page 130. Report on your own reactions and changes in speech production and those of your partner.

9. Take any mannerism or behavior you have (clearing throat, arranging hair, wetting lip, biting nail) and for an entire day, double its use. That is, every time you do it automatically, do it again deliberately. Inform your partner, roommate(s), and friends of the behavior and ask them to monitor for any you miss. This is not desensitization, per se, but it will help you appreciate the difficulties in self-monitoring activities.

10. Go back to the anxiety and fear hierarchy you developed earlier and review it with your partner. Consider time, availability, and other factors, and choose some situations in the mid-range of the hierarchy. Then go into the situation five separate times, as consecutively as possible. Have your partner observe or wait nearby for an immediate report. Write a summary of your experiences and feelings, adding your partner's evaluations.

11. Repeat 10, using a different type of situation. However, first go through a progressive relaxation exercise. Then visualize the anticipated situation, have your partner describe it, and re-create it while monitoring your relaxation. Work with your partner until you can remain relaxed while recalling every aspect of the situation. This may take several sessions. When prepared, go into the real situation while you attempt to re-create and maintain relaxation. Report on the results.

12. If available, use a DAF unit while you talk or read aloud. Follow the sequence below:

    a. Go through a relaxation procedure, general or progressive.
    b. Prepare a DAF unit, with your partner running it. If necessary, rerelax.
    c. Read aloud, or talk, in your relaxed state. Your partner should set the

DAF at maximum disruption delay time and volume at zero. As you speak, she or he slowly increases the volume to the point where disruption just starts to occur.

d. Hold the volume level, keep talking, and reestablish relaxation until you are fluent again.

e. Turn the volume up slightly until disruption occurs.

SAMPLE ASSIGNMENTS FOR CLIENTS

These assignments are in no particular hierarchy. They are meant to test different procedures and varying levels of relaxation and/or desensitization. Instruct your client:

1. For a period of five days, perform the general relaxation exercises we practiced, using them morning and afternoon. Each day write a short summary describing your speech right after each exercise and as time passes.

2. Practice progressive relaxation exercises every evening for ten days. On the first five days do them while lying down. For the next three days, practice while seated. On the last two days, practice while standing. Report on your progress.

3. Make telephone calls to strangers, requesting services or asking questions. Before each telephone call, quickly go through a progressive relaxation sequence and try to carry the relaxed feeling during the call. Select your option:

   a. Three telephone calls.
   b. Five telephone calls.
   c. Seven telephone calls.

4. Voluntarily enter or participate in several extended speech situations. During moments when you are not talking, practice the relaxation exercises you learned in the clinic. Evaluate the effects on your speech.

5. Take the attached list of twenty-five words and read it aloud in your normal fashion. Read the list a second time, using maximum effort and tension on each word. Read the list a third time, trying to relax your chest, throat, and mouth as we have practiced. What were the results in terms of stuttering and ease of production?

6. Make brief telephone calls to ask questions or request service. Prewrite your utterances (you can reuse material). Before each call, practice uttering the messages in a relaxed fashion. Report results.

7. Take the attached list of twenty-five words. On each word, underline the phoneme or syllable on which you probably would have trouble if you stuttered. Now read the list aloud in the following ways:

   a. Read a word aloud in your usual fashion.
   b. Without attempting speech, form the underlined phoneme or syllable with strong pressure and tension.
   c. Relax the tension.
   d. Immediately utter the word while you are relaxed. If you stutter or are not relaxed, repeat that particular cycle again.

8. For the next two days, relax approximately every thirty minutes by using the localized exercises we practiced. Timing is approximate and subject to condi-

tions. How completely you perform the exercises is also subject to conditions, but at least perform its covert parts, evaluate your tension level, and try to feel relaxed. How did these affect your speech and your overall activity?

9. Teach progressive relaxation to a family member, spouse, or friend. Demonstrate, monitor, evaluate, and do all the things I did in the clinic. Report on the results of your teaching.

10. In the clinic you estimated that you stuttered _____ times per day, on the average. For the next three days, enter more situations and speak more often until you collect one of these spasm totals:

    a. 50 percent over your usual average.
    b. 100 percent over your usual average.
    c. 150 percent over your usual average.

11. Between now and the next therapy session, monitor your stuttering closely. Each time you stutter and do one of the listed behaviors, immediately fake a spasm on the same word. The behaviors are postponement, starter, release, retrial, breaking of eye contact.

12. Over the next five days, make 100 telephone calls to random strangers, asking each person, "Is this the _____ restaurant?" Keep track of your stutterings and reactions.

13. Contact five strangers on the street and ask directions. If you stutter, stop and say, "Let me try that again." Try to have good eye contact at all times, but especially during the second attempt. Report on your speech, eye contact, feelings, and auditors' reactions.

14. Make a short speech describing your stuttering history and your therapy activity, responding to questions afterward. Select the group you will talk to:

    a. The new stutterers group.
    b. The monthly clinic staff meeting.
    c. The Introduction to Communication Disorders class.
    d. The Mothers' Health Conservation Club.

15. Take the fear hierarchy list you drew up in the clinic and deliberately enter the first (easiest) situation. Remain in that situation or reenter similar ones until you achieve your option:

    a. No stuttering.
    b. No avoidance of any kind.
    c. Excellent eye contact and evaluation during every stuttering spasm.

    If you do not stutter in the first attempt, repeat the assignment. If you still do not stutter, move to 2 on your hierarchy list, and so on.

In order to avoid repetition, I suggest that reciprocal inhibition (systematic desensitization) assignments be structured by the use of activities such as those described in assignments 3, 6, 12, 13, 14, and 15. Before each situation the client should practice the relaxation and recall exercises until relaxation can be maintained. If the client cannot achieve relaxation and recall, or if the real situation results in loss of tension control, the client should not make further attempts but should report to the clinician so that problem solving and practice can take place in more therapy situations before transfer is attempted again.

6

Delayed Auditory Feedback

OVERVIEW OF DAF

During this century, engineers in radio stations had the problem of delay or reverberation introduced into an audio circuit, to the dismay of on-air personnel. However, it was not until this generation that Lee (1950a, 1950b) published reports concerning the effects on speech of delaying the transmission of orally produced speech to the ears of the speaker. Delayed auditory feedback (DAF) was born, and it has fascinated us ever since.

In its initial use, DAF was produced simply. A magnetic tape recorder was altered so that the separate record and playback heads contacted the audio tape simultaneously, the record head being first in line. An audio signal thus would be played back a split second after it had been recorded, the delay before playback depending on the speed of the tape and the distance between the two electromagnetic heads. The person speaking wore earphones plugged into the output jack of the tape recorder, and the unit's volume control would be set on high to overcome the airborne speech signal that the headphone cushions might not attenuate. All over the country, old tape recorders were adapted to produce DAF effects. I encountered my first set in 1953. Its playback head was mounted on a crank-operated wormscrew about 24 inches long, so that very extended delay times could be achieved.

Actually, *delayed auditory feedback* is a misnomer. When we speak we normally receive auditory feedback through two pathways—through the body and through the air. Delayed auditory *feedback*, as we use the term, actually is delayed auditory *sidetone*, since the delay machine does nothing to the temporal sequence of our body-conducted feedback. In addition, both body-conducted and airborne feedback are normally delayed anyway. The sensory feedback from neurons has a conduction velocity that is different from either of the auditory vibration signals (body and air), and the two auditory vibration signals do not travel at the same rates. In other words, delay-*s* (not delay) of the feedback signal is the norm for speakers, but we are not aware of it. Nevertheless, DAF has a significant effect on speech, and we undoubtedly will continue to call it DAF and not DAS.

Modern DAF units generally produce a delay by electronic means, rather than by mechanical realignment of the electromagnetic heads. In a way this advance is regrettable. The cost of the electronic units runs into hundreds of dollars, as opposed to "cannibalizing" an old tape recorder. Also, the tape recorder type recorded the speech output as the tape ran by the heads, and if desired, this tape could be played back for the speaker to listen to. With modern units a separate audio recorder usually must be used. If restructured appropriately, the converted tape recorder could provide delay times far longer than those available on many electronic units, as well as delay times in between the typical ones on many units. On the other hand, modern electronic units generally weigh under ten pounds, provide a cleaner signal than many of the tape units, and can be combined more easily with other electronic components. Nevertheless, if you have some older tape recorders in a storeroom, it might be worthwhile to find out what an electronic service shop would charge to revise the old recorder into a delay unit.[1]

Effects

The effects of DAF, when a person speaks, are impressive. The auditory monitoring process is disrupted, with significant effects on speech output. Lee (1951) noted that delays of 100 to 150 milliseconds (msec) resulted in disruption changes in rate, rhythm, and other speech aspects so that a speaker displayed blockages, prolongations, repetitions, and other nonfluent speech behaviors. He coined the term *artificial stutter* (1950b) to describe this behavior. Later, authors called this the *negative Lee effect* (Lotzmann, 1961). Fairbanks and Guttman (1958) identified the articulatory and fluency disruptions as *direct effects*, and the disturbances in vocal pitch and intensity, pauses, and emotional stress reactions, *indirect effects* of DAF. In using DAF with a class studying fluency disorders, I noted that their repetitions (200 to 250 msec delay) in conversational speech

---

[1]In current research (spring 1985) I have returned to DAF tape use because of greater flexibility and accuracy.

increased several hundred percent, and their prolongations were even more noticeable. Stoppages and other errors also increased greatly. Words per minute rates (reading) dropped by 9 percent to 51 percent, with a median reduction of 29 percent (one student increased the wpm rate). In general, there were syllable and sound repetitions, rate reduction, vowel prolongation, increased loudness level, and reduction in the variability of pitch and loudness. Black (1955) reported that reading under normal auditory feedback (NAF) showed a slowing of speech below the speaker's normal rate. This effect, which has been experienced frequently since that time, has applications for therapy.

Individuals seem to vary widely in their reactions to DAF (Beaumont & Foss, 1957). In a seminar, I asked each student to talk while undergoing DAF. Out of fifteen people, two were almost unable to talk; four had serious difficulty; eight had variable problems but performed adequately; and one person only blinked twice, ignored the delay, and continued to talk in an almost normal fashion. Spilka (1954) suggested that responses to DAF may relate to the degree of a person's dependence on internal or external cues. Cherry and Sayers (1956) hypothesized that attention to the production of physical sounds is more important in monitoring than is the meaning of what is said. They also noted that there was little adaptation of speech disruption under DAF (see the later discussion comparing DAF stuttering and real stuttering), a point raised by other studies. However, a more recent study (Venkatagiri, 1980) analyzed dysfluencies under repeated DAF readings. The count of total dysfluencies, disrhythmic phonations, and revisions was reduced significantly over time. Part-word repetitions were reduced, but not significantly. Venkatagiri concluded that DAF interferes with speech elements at or below the syllable level (see discussion on critical delay times). Bachrach (1964) noted that females seemed to display different response patterns. (Children's delay times will be discussed during consideration of critical delay times.) Timmons and Boudreau (1972) suggested that individual reactions rested on internal and external feedback interruptions because of variable physiological characteristics of different individuals. They felt that anxiety about DAF effects created physiological correlates (tension, tremor, and so on) that could act as a catalyst for feedback disruptions.

Delay Intervals and Loudness

Critical delay intervals and levels of loudness were early concerns of researchers. Black (1951) evaluated eleven time intervals, from no delay (NAF) to 300 msec delay, finding that disruption effects seemed to peak at 180 msec. He speculated that the peaking was related to phoneme duration, although sound variability in association with syllable units (plus individual differences) make such speculation fragile. Fairbanks and Guttman (1958) found 200 msec to be more disruptive than 100, 300, or 400 msec.

Similar critical points in the 180-to-200 msec range were reported by other investigators (Ham & Steer, 1967; Zalosh & Salzman, 1965). However, most of these studies centered on young adults.

Research with children has produced interesting variations. Very young children, six to nineteen months old, were studied by Belmore et al. (1973), who reported that 46 percent showed changes in vocal duration and loudness, effects the researchers felt were attributable to DAF. Chase et al. (1961) found that a 200-msec delay time had less negative effect on children in the age range of four to six years, compared to those seven to nine years of age. MacKay (1968) counted speech dysfluencies of children during various delay times and reported that children four to six years of age showed peak effect at 750-msec delay, whereas the maximum disruption for seven-to-nine-year-old children was half that, at 375 msec. Timmons and Boudreau (1972) also reported that younger children were more affected by longer delay times than were older children. A study by Siegel et al. (1980) compared college students, older children (mean age: 8 years) and younger children (mean age: 4.8 years) on NAF and various DAF time intervals. In general, the younger children showed more effects from DAF than did the other two groups, and the authors concluded that auditory feedback reliance decreases with age. They suggested that age brings a high level of automaticity in monitoring so that immediate auditory feedback is of low significance. The effects of DAF, then, have more impact on children who still are less sure of production and who monitor more closely. Whether this fact can explain response variations in adults' degree of reliance on auditory feedback in DAF is not clear. On the other hand, Smith and Tierney (1971) stated that older adults (forty-two to sixty-eight years) experienced more disruption from 200-msec DAF than did young adults twenty-two to thirty-eight years) or adolescents. Perhaps we have a bimodal curve in age and sensitivity. Leith and Chmiel (1980, p. 269) felt that the youths' discrepancy and sensitivity to prolonged delay intervals was significant for clinical applications:

> Since age is a factor in speech reaction to DAF, stuttering treatment programs should take it into consideration in determining either the most disruptive delay time or the fluency-enhancing time for the particular program being used.

In addition to interest in critical times of DAF conditions, researchers and clinicians have been concerned with the loudness level of DAF. Routinely, DAF is delivered through earphone headsets, although Leith and Chmiel (1980) reported effective clinical use of low loudness, free-field DAF with children. In general, however, the loudness level of auditory sidetone generally has been set to outweigh the effects of bone-conducted feedback and the attenuated oral feedback is permitted entry to the middle ear by the headset's ear cushions. Ham and Steer (1967) used earphone levels of 30, 45, 60, and 75-dB SPL (Sound Pressure Level) above SRT (Speech Reception Threshold), finding that wpm rates changed from an average of 170 at normal to 180 in the first condition, and then sloped back toward 170 by the final level, in normal speakers. Stutterers, on the other hand, moved from an NAF measure of 120 wpm irregularly upward until reaching 160 wpm at 75-dB SPL. Interestingly, the NAF wpm rates for subjects with articulatory and phonatory problems were 145 and 135 respectively, well below that of the normal-speaking subjects. Results, overall, suggested that loudness increases in self-feedback do not produce the same results as equal levels of noise, tone, or other voices. Also, the reactions of normal speakers were not consistent with many of the reactions of persons with speech disorders. Tiffany and Hanley (1954) investigated decade increments (to 50 dB) above individual SRTs during DAF, and reported progressive "effectiveness" of the delays as loudness increased. Because of the Lombard Voice Reflex to increasing loudness, clinical use of amplification has tended to be pragmatic rather than technical. Some clients respond satisfactorily at + 10 dB, and a few require a very loud signal before they succumb adequately to the altered sidetone.

Theories

Theories of DAF effects have preoccupied a surprisingly small number of persons, concerning the stutteringlike nature of the effects. Leith and Chmiel (1980) provide some review and consideration of the theory behind DAF reactions. They hypothesize that speakers operate from ASF (auditory sensory feedback) and OSF (oral sensory feedback) systems. If the two systems are not in synchrony, breakdowns will occur, and people differ in their sensitivities to asynchrony. Leith and Chmiel suggest that stutterers tend to rely on OSF cues, whereas normal speakers incline to ASF monitoring, thus explaining why the latter are disrupted by DAF whereas the former become more fluent. It also would seem possible that DAF simply introduces a delay in the rate of production that allows the stutterer to time utterances more effectively, with less interference from stress and other prosodic elements. Wingate (1976) reviews a series of studies, suggesting that auditory functions (sound localization, auditory dominance, and so on) are different or at least inconsistent, compared to nonstutterers. However, he feels that there is insufficient evidence to support an "auditory theory" of stuttering. At present, we simply have no acceptable explanation, in a theoretical model, for DAF effects in general; for variable responses to DAF; for effects of frequency, loudness, and variables in delay intervals; for age differences; and for differences between stutterers and nonstutterers. There is an effect, or combination of effects, and it varies according to the influences of a number of factors.

DAF AND STUTTERING

Comparison

DAF dysfluencies compared to stuttering were common in early publications. At first, DAF speech was called *artificial stutter* (Lee, 1951) and many theorists hoped for a mechanically manipulable model of stuttering to do research with. However, studies finding differences rapidly accumulated. Neelley (1961) compared stutterers and nonstutterers during NAF and 140-msec delay, reporting that judges could differentiate stutterers' NAF speech from nonstutterers' DAF speech. Yates (1963) attacked Neelley for comparing lifetime stutterers and first-time DAF talkers, ignoring the basic issue of whether or not DAF speech and stuttered speech were comparable. Langova and Moravek (1964) compared stutterers and clutterers under DAF, finding a sharp improvement (increased fluency) in the stutterers and near-equal deterioration in the speech of the clutterers. Subsequently, Wingate (1970) specified that DAF tended to cause increases in vocal intensity, syllable duration, and phonation time in stutterers and nonstutterers; but the latter tended to become more nonfluent, whereas the former typically increased in fluency. Also, the nonstutterers typically were dysfluent only after several words had been uttered, whereas the locus of NAF stuttering tended to fall among the first three words of an initial utterance. Code (1979), on the basis of one stutterer and a control, concluded that EMG results verify a difference between stuttering and artificial DAF stuttering. However, it was noted that two other stutterers were eliminated from the study—one because of rapid adaptation to DAF, and the other because DAF caused no speech-production problems. Venkatagiri (1982a) compared stuttering to DAF dysfluencies produced at 200-msec delay. Both dysfluency types occurred more on longer than on shorter words and more on content than on function words, and both showed a large number of syllable and sound repetitions. Stutterings occurred more on vowels, whereas DAF dysfluencies were more equally spread across vowels and consonants. As already noted, stuttering occurred more often in the early parts of sentences, and DAF dysfluencies were more prominent in the later parts of sentences. In summary, there appears to be no question that DAF speech and stuttering, although both occurring as interruptions in the forward flow of speech, are dissimilar in their overt effects, not to mention the covert patterns of feeling and behavior.

Effects on Stuttering

DAF's effects on stuttering were somewhat ignored at first, but Naylor (1953) reported a highly significant negative correlation between judged stuttering severity and oral reading time under DAF; that is, as stutterer severity increased, there was greater improvement under DAF. Ham and Steer (1967) noted a similar relationship in a study of ten stutterers in 1955. Leith and Chmiel (1980) reviewed several studies from 1958 to 1961, indicating greater interest in the concept that DAF could be used as a facilitating rather than as an aversive influence on reducing nonfluencies. Lotzmann (1961) reemphasized that stuttering severity was a factor, the most severe subjects showing reduced or eradicated stuttering, smoothed breathing, and reduced or eliminated mannerisms. However, some stutterers (especially mild ones) had a "negative Lee effect," or increased dysfluency. As delay intervals went past 200 msec, the severe stutterers began to slip into negative Lee patterns. Webster et al. (1970) reported that 100 msec (not 200) was most beneficial in reducing stuttering but otherwise followed the pattern cited previously. Gibney (1973) compared combinations of delay time and loudness level, failing to find an interaction effect between delay time and speech measures (dysfluencies and rate), but finding a significant relationship between volume and the measures. Stark and Pierce (1970) also reported that high intensity levels on DAF induced more errors in stuttering subjects. Hutchinson and Burke (1973) found that stutterers (compared to clutterers and normal speakers) had fewer errors at 100- and 200-msec delay.

Prolonged delay times (150, 300, 600 msec) were investigated by McCormick (1975), who found that at the longest delay, loudness became significant in vocal changes; diagnostic values to be researched were suggested. Burke (1975) reported that the 50-to-150-msec range tends to facilitate fluency for the stutterer, with severity and facilitation highly correlated. The age factor, variability across stutterers, and the fact that some stutterers do not show improvement were cited among the variables needing further research.

Hutchinson and Norris (1977) compared DAF fluency effects to those of metronome rhythm and simple noise masking. DAF lowered dysfluencies overall, but with greater variability than did the metronome. Adamczyk (1975, 1979) compared DAF and reverberation as dual effectors, finding that although both types of alteration reduced stuttering and lowered rate, DAF was more effective on both measures. An upsurge (slight) of stuttering beyond 200-msec delay was reported. Hayden et al. (1977) stated that at 200-msec delay there was a significant decrease in stoppages, a significant increase in prolongations, and relative stability of repetitions and interjections. However, E. M Silverman (1978) failed to find significance between NAF and DAF difference scores at 113-, 226-, 306-, 413-, and 520-msec delays. Martin and Haroldson (1979) compared baseline dysfluency to five different fluency-inducing conditions. DAF was effective, reducing stuttering by an average of 50+ percent and average spasm duration by almost 40 percent. However, metronome and TO (time out) conditions were much more effective in terms of the measures cited. More recently, Andrews et al. (1982) compared DAF to an expanded version of

Bloodstein's list (1950) of conditions under which stuttering is reduced or absent. In a comparison among the fifteen conditions, they found that a majority of them were accompanied either by an increase in phonation duration or a lowering of the speech rate. DAF was the only condition accompanied by both changes. The fifteen conditions were simultaneous talking and writing, singing, dialect speech, choral reading, shadowing, talking to an animal, talking alone, talking alone with topic cards, speaking while relaxed, response contingent speech, masking noise, slow rate, talking while arm swinging, syllable timed speech, and DAF plus vowel prolonging.

Various studies have focused on the effects of DAF with stutterers. The results indicate that stutterers often improve their fluency under delay, although some do not. Also, reactions to particular delay times seem to be individualized, raising a question about the so-called critical delay phenomenon. The mechanisms that seem to operate here are those of rate reduction and phonation duration increase. Wingate (1976, p. 239) summarized this consideration that most external conditions (not just DAF) that dramatically improve stuttering are shown to operate primarily through

> . . . an induced emphasis on phonation, implemented most effectively by increase in duration . . . through slowing down and commonly involving modulation of stress controls; in brief, changes in prosodic expression.

In the following pages we will observe ways in which DAF has been applied to stuttering therapy. We have already seen that DAF can be used to produce stress and dysfluency (aversive) as well as more fluent speech (facilitative) through the mechanisms cited previously. The next section will discuss various uses of DAF in stuttering therapy, including aversive applications, and then DAF as the therapy program itself, or as the major component of it.

DAF AND THERAPY

General uses of DAF with stutterers have been varied, and early credit is hard to assign. I used it myself in 1954, but I had learned the procedures from a clinician who had used it one or two years previously. In early times, DAF was used in a variety of ways, and there was general agreement that it could be of value as part of an overall program (Gregory, 1968). Adamczyk (1959) used it as primary therapy with fifteen stutterers for two to three months, at 250 msec. He reported great improvement in thirteen of the cases. Initial use often was aversive, in which DAF was used as stress or punishment, a mode objected to by Sheehan (1968). However, many individuals reported that DAF reduced stuttering dysfluencies and slowed speech rate to a point where stutterers could appreciate and practice self-control of fluency. There may also be a persistence effect on the rate and the dysfluencies of stutterers after DAF is turned off (Soderberg, 1969b), although personal research did not verify such persistence in normal speakers after DAF exposure of five or thirty minutes, with measures immediately after, one hour later, and twenty-four hours later (Ham et al. 1984).

Webster (1970) confirmed decreases in the duration of stuttering spasms at 100, 200, 300 and 400 msec, noting that the shorter times seemed most effective. Watts (1971) used DAF in group sessions for clients to learn to slow their speech rate (about sixty wpm) and then to increase it. Any regression toward dysfluency was treated by extra DAF time. Ingham and Andrews (1973a) used DAF as part of an overall program to instill and shape prolonged speech. Treon and Tamayo (1974) suggested that facilitating DAF effects were enhanced when combined with GSR biofeedback, and MacKay (1969) reported that having the stutterers speak with a strong nasal twang (!) during DAF would significantly reduce stuttering. Ingham and Andrews (1971) felt that DAF was superior to syllable-timed speech in that the latter allowed retention of more secondary symptoms, limited optimal rates, and resulted in more errors when optimal rates were exceeded. Dalton and Hardcastle (1977) stated that DAF produces prolonged, not timed, speech and therefore makes it easier for the client to speed up and come back to normal-sounding speech. Shames (1975) recommended DAF because it has quick effects, makes the user aware of production, fosters monitoring, provides for forward and backward movement, facilitates motivation and positive attitudes, and fits well into a total program. He did note, however, that it can delay self-perception and self-responsibility, cause overdependence on the instrument, and is expensive.

Van Riper's (1970) discussion of DAF use in stuttering therapy still has relevance. Believing that many stutterers, especially the more severe ones, speak with much less dysfluency under delay, he listed a variety of possible uses for DAF:

1. Can be used early in therapy by the clinician or others to demonstrate to the client that "anybody" can stutter, and he or she is not alone. The stutterer also can observe tension, struggles, and anxiety in others as they talk under DAF.
2. Demonstrates that it is possible for stutterers to be dysfluent in a variety of ways and, therefore, they can aspire to changes in their own stuttering pattern.
3. Fluency can be reinforced by finding a delay interval that facilitates it. At an appropriate stage in therapy, the delay interval can be moved gradually toward more disruptive times in order to help the stutterer deal with direct speech stress under controlled conditions.
4. Pressure on speech can also be applied by having the stutterer read and talk under NAF, with an intermittent, disruptive DAF time interval for brief durations.

5. Another application of stress can be made by setting the unit at a disruptive delay interval, with no amplification. As the stutterer reads or talks, volume slowly is increased to a point where disruption occurs, and then the volume is attenuated. This application can be repeated to try to build resistance in the client.

6. With direction and instruction or demonstration, the stutterer can be encouraged to concentrate on tactile and kinesthetic feedback from his or her own speech mechanism and reduce dependence on the semiautomatic monitoring by audition.

Van Riper (1973) also suggested that DAF, at maximal delay time, can be used to allow the stutterer to hear and evaluate efforts to alter modes of production, preparatory sets, pullouts, and cancellations (assuming that the DAF is not limited to a ceiling of 250 msec). He felt that DAF can be used diagnostically to assess the sensitivity to speech stress and (through observation) the ability to use proprioceptive cues. Before this application of delay, the clinician might want to use masking noise, or an electrolarynx, to determine how effective the client is in terms of awareness. Van Riper noted Sheehan's (1968) aversion to punishment (supposedly synonymous with incompetence by or neurosis of the clinician) but said, for his own part, that he feels DAF either is not punishing or, at most, only mildly so. Wingate (1976) also questioned the attitude that DAF is aversive. Van Riper warned about the development of a "DAF voice" (laborious, slow, lacking inflection, lowered pitch, reduced variability in loudness, loss of stress) and the tendency of a stutterer, in some cases, to become dependent on the DAF unit for fluent speech. Wingate (p. 235) expressed a similar concern:

> . . . the significance of DAF therapy for stuttering does not focus on the auditory function per se . . . therapy should not rely upon, let alone emphasize, modification of audition as the therapy technique in itself, and adequate or appropriate means of treating stuttering . . the projected aspiration to develop a portable DAF apparatus is groundless and misguided.

The main thrust so far is in the direction of different ways to use DAF as one component of a much larger program. In the next section we will consider DAF used as a major component of therapy to achieve a reduction in rate and to provide a vehicle for other control methods.

Rate Control

Rate control through DAF has developed rapidly. As pointed out earlier, many clinicians reflect Black's (1951) report of an increase in phrase duration and feel that speech rate reduction, through an increase in syllable duration and phonation time, is the most critical effect of DAF. Watts (1973) felt that rate reduction was the most important factor in delay. Bloodstein (1975a) confirmed that efforts to overcome DAF tend to result in a slowed rate of speech as well as in overarticulating increases in loudness, and concentration on proprioceptive and tactile monitoring. He felt that DAF's effects did not, however, prove perceptual theories but fitted in with anticipatory struggle hypotheses in that the slower rate of speech simplified motor planning for the stutterer (1972). The orientation of many clinicians was toward an enforced facilitative use of DAF by the stutterer. This facilitative move to have the stutterer adopt a rate and pattern that would avoid DAF disruption (and stuttering) received strong impetus from behavior modification clinicians who approached therapy from an operant view and stressed the establishment of fluency rather than the control of dysfluency. A recognized forerunner in using DAF behaviorally to modify stuttering was Goldiamond (1960, 1965), who defined DAF as an aversive contingency that operated as a negative reinforcer of stuttering. In an attempt to avoid the "punishment" of negative reinforcement, and to increase the positive reinforcement of fluency and the clinician's approval, the stutterer would alter her or his speech pattern in such a way that speech patterns of fluency predominated. This rather ingenious explanation of DAF's effects has never dealt with the question of how it affects only the dysfluent (and minor) portion of otherwise fluent speech, and never defined the basis for calling it aversive. Indeed, Sheehan (1968) spoke to this point, in objecting to aversive therapy in general, when he said, " . . . if punishment were in any way effective, stuttering would have been cured in childhood" (p. 132). Nevertheless, Goldiamond had stutterers read under 250-msec delay, with instructions to prolong and slow their speech until coincidence with the delay interval was reached (about twenty-five wpm) and fluency achieved. When a stable reading fluency was established, the delay interval was reduced and the fluency stabilization process repeated at the faster rate. This cycle of delay decrements was repeated until the client could read fluently under the NAF condition. To help the stutterer transfer DAF fluency to daily speech, Goldiamond (1967) experimented with a portable DAF unit and ear insert for the client. Webster and Lubker (1968) removed Goldiamond's response and contingent use of DAF and let it run continuously during reading.

Curlee and Perkins (1969, 1973) published a DAF-based method of therapy called Conversational Rate Control Therapy. It considered Goldiamond's earlier work and also included aspects of TO (time-out) techniques, along with reciprocal inhibition, covert conditioning, and implosion methods. The therapy program was organized in three phases. This therapy actually is a combination of rate reduction, prolongation, easy onset, continuous phonation, and other factors. The DAF is used to force the client into the altered patterns, and as control is learned, DAF can be phased out.

Phase I.   The client and clinician converse on any topic (or read at first) in order to establish baselines, provide reinforcement, and describe procedures. DAF is then explained and introduced at 250 msec, with loudness at the highest level the client can accept. Delay is continuous, and the client is instructed to slow the rate by prolonging syllables and by using phrase lengths that are short enough to accommodate to the delay, until utterance rate and DAF return coincide (about thirty to thirty-five wpm). The client and clinician converse until both agree that the client has been stutter-free for two cumulative fifteen-minute periods. At any step, more than two stutterings in a five-minute period results in the client being stopped, returning to the previous step, and achieving stabilization there before proceeding.

The client is to maintain a thirty-to-thirty-five wpm rate while the delay interval is reduced to 200 msec. Stabilization is regarded as a mutually agreed-on achievement of two cumulative fifteen-minute periods of fluency. Still maintaining the thirty-to-thirty-five wpm rate, the client is subjected to 150 msec delay until the two fifteen-minute stabilization periods are met. This step is repeated, holding the same wpm rate, in 50-msec decrements, until 0 msec delay (NAF) is reached. Delay now is set at 200 msec, but the client is instructed to readapt her or his prolongation and phrase rate until coincidence with the new delay interval is reached. Using this slightly faster rate, the client goes through the 50-msec decrement cycle just described, with the same stabilization criterion. The entire cycle is repeated, starting at 150 msec delay, with appropriate prolongation and phrase rate adjustments. Cycle replications starting at 100 msec and at 50 msec complete the sequence, with the same stabilization criterion. At the final 0-msec delay, the headphones are removed and the client is counseled about using slow rate, prolongation, and phrase length to maintain fluency.

Curlee and Perkins regard this phase as establishing in-clinic fluency with conversational speech. They feel it is superior to reading-based programs because it is less boring, avoids the issue of reading skills, and reduces transfer problems. The subsequent stages of this program shift completely to rate-control orientation—without use of DAF.

Phase II. The client and clinician sit in a room with a single light source, reasonably shielded from outside light. They talk about any topics while the clinician monitors for stutterings, a too fast rate, phrases that are too long, or any other unacceptable speech behaviors (based on earlier analysis and discussion of the client's speech pattern). On each and every occurrence of the unacceptable items, the clinician turns out the room light, and for thirty seconds, the two persons sit in the dark without speaking. When the TO period is over, the clinician turns on the light and conversation resumes. When both persons agree that the client has been fluent for two cumulative fifteen-minute periods, the TO interval is decreased by five seconds, and the cycle is repeated. The TO interval is reduced in five-second steps until it is eliminated. As in the DAF stage, more than two unacceptable speech behaviors in a five-minute period result in repetition of the preceding cycle.

This stage weans the stutterer from any dependency on DAF and allows practice of conversation in the safe confines of the therapy room. In the next phase, attention is focused on transfer.

Phase III.   The clinician is concerned with transfer of fluency to a wide range of situations, dealing with anxieties, and laying some foundations for posttherapy maintenance. Sites of communication and degree of social complexity are altered by the clinician. The client is counseled about maintaining control over rate, phrase length, and so on. An abbreviated sequence follows:

1. Change to another therapy room.
2. Introduce a third person to the session, and over several sessions, increase that person's verbal participation.
3. Introduce other persons into the sessions in order to have a fluctuating number and variety of personalities.
4. Bring in friends and family members of the client. If possible, introduce some stutterers who are at about the same level of progress.
5. Together, the client and clinician go into selected social situations that are normal (and easy) for the client.

Curlee and Perkins reported a 75 percent to 95 percent decrease in the frequency of stuttering, with less severe residual stuttering. Subsequently, Perkins (1973a) reported that more than half the stutterers treated by the approach showed significant deterioration in their speech after dismissal. In the next publication (1973b), Perkins reported on a clinical procedure which can be expected to produce "normal" fluency in over 70 percent of adult stutterers during treatment. However, only about half will be likely to maintain normal speech permanently. The portion of this program most concerned with DAF will be described, with other aspects briefly indicated. The first goal, in three phases, is to achieve normal speech in slow motion, optimistically in about six therapy sessions.

Phase I.   The client is instructed about slow rate, prolongation, and short phrases. DAF at 250 msec is used to establish an approximate thirty-wpm rate. Reading is preferred here, but conversation can be used. All utterances in therapy are to be under DAF, and the client is advised not to use the new speech pattern outside the clinic. Perkins points out, as do others (Helps & Dalton, 1979; Shames, 1975; Watts, 1971), that it is possible to teach "DAF speech" without using a DAF unit.

Phase II.   The target is breath control, and it can be started in the first session. It should not be delayed past the second session (see breath-control procedures in other chapters). The client is to limit phrase length to three to eight syllables at the approximate thirty-wpm rate. A continuous airflow is to be maintained on utterances so that several consecutive short words sound like one word. Hard glottal attacks are illustrated and discussed. The client is directed to use easy vocal onset, even to the use of an aspirated /h/ preceding initial consonant sounds.

Phase III. Normal prosody is stressed as breath control is developed. The rhythm and stress pattern are worked on. The client is to vary inflection, duration, and loudness to produce the equivalent of normal stress. All the normal prosodic elements are present, but they are slowed and elongated, as if a recording was played at a slower speed.

Phase IV. In this phase the clinician works with the client to have him or her take responsibility for the rate of therapy progress and for self-evaluation. Three criteria are provided, with the injunction to drop back to a client-selected prior therapy level if any one of the following are not met:

1. Must be able to regain slow-rate speech pattern within three to five phrases after the error(s).
2. Must be able, within one therapy session, to regain any loss of self-confidence in ability to control speech at the appropriate level (even if fluency has been maintained).
3. Must be able, within two therapy sessions, to return to and be comfortable with the appropriate slow-rate pattern after having felt pressured to speed up inappropriately.

These criteria apply at all levels of therapy and are intended to be client-applied, with early discussion and guidance from the clinician. Shames (1975) has criticized these criteria as possibly presenting problems of judgment and ambiguity.

Phase V. If early phases were initiated through reading, this phase also can use reading initially and then shift to slow-normal conversation. A DAF time interval of 250 msec is used, and the client works on elimination of avoidance tactics during the use of slow-normal conversational speech.

Phase VI. This phase is applied at all appropriate times and is aimed at psychotherapeutic needs of the client. It is based on the recommendations in Shames et al. (1969) concerning thematic content modification procedures. The clinician is advised to continue psychotherapeusis throughout therapy, to the limit that training and competence permit.

Phase VII. The client, consulting with the clinician, is to pace decrements in DAF time intervals to return progressively to normal rate. The first decrement is to 200 msec, to increase rate to 45 to 60 wpm. When self-evaluation criteria are met, the DAF interval is decreased to 150 msec, along with increased phrase length, so that the number of syllables per phrase increases. If the client attains a stable rate of 90 to 120 wpm at this stage, and meets the criteria, successive DAF steps can be omitted. Otherwise, DAF is reduced in 50-msec steps to either 150 or 100 msec—whichever provides the best rate (100 to 150 wpm) for the client and satisfies the three criteria.

Holding at the 100 (or 150) msec-delay level, the clinician gradually reduces DAF volume. Intermittently the volume is to be increased. If the client has increased the rate too much, this either will slow rate automatically or disrupt fluency so that the client must slow down. The clinician and the client now agree on a "home base" rate for the client, one that is slow enough to promote fluency, fast enough to sound acceptable to the client, and meets the evaluation criteria.

Phase VIII. The clinician turns off the DAF unit but leaves the earphones in place while the client converses. Conversational speech is continued while first one, and then the other, earphone is removed. Evaluation criteria are applied at each step.

Phase IX. In this phase, the clinician analyzes the stutterer's general vocal attributes. Any weaknesses are to be remedied by standard voice therapy procedures.

Perkins completes the therapy sequence by a three-phase pattern to generalize the stutterer's speech into daily life. Stress is placed on self-evaluation and methods to deal with regression or accidents. Although not covered in this chapter on DAF methodology, its content is worth your attention. Ingham (1975a) praised the addition on breathing, prosody, and so on but felt the program was not described sufficiently for replication. He noted that prolonged speech has shifted from the status of a byproduct of other methods to being a specific method and major approach.

Ryan (1971, 1974, 1978, 1979) with Van Kirk (1971, 1974) have been active in operant approaches to therapy and advocacy of "speak fluently" methods. In 1971, Ryan reported on DAF therapy programs for an eight-year-old male (Curlee and Perkins had suggested a lower limit of fifteen years for their program). The stutterer was taken through three speech modes (reading, monologue, conversation) during fifty-one forty-minute therapy sessions spread over a period of fifteen months. The sessions were divided as follows:

1–3	Base-level sessions; client's stuttering average of 10 SW/M.
4	Introduction of DAF, creating an average of 0.7 SW/M in all three speech modes.
5–16	Goal of 0.5 or less SW/M achieved and held through session 16.
17–51	Efforts to secure maintenance of fluency.

The first goals were for the child to "catch" or identify stuttered words and to achieve a slow rate through prolongations under DAF. The criterion in each speech mode was 75 percent accuracy over a period of five minutes. When this criterion was met, the stutterer could go on to DAF speech. As fluency was achieved on DAF, the delay interval was decreased by 50 msec. Fluency was defined again as 0.5 or less SW/M, plus slow rate, for ten minutes and had to be met at each speech mode at each delay interval.

In 1974 Ryan and Van Kirk reported on a twenty-seven-step program to reach established fluency, followed by twenty to sixty steps in a transfer program and a four-step maintenance program lasting twenty-two months. Delayed auditory feedback was the primary component in the fluency program, and the first twenty-seven steps were as follows:

1–6	To reach criteria of one minute and 90 percent accuracy in identifying stutterings, in reading and monologue.
7–13	Reading under DAF, starting at 250 msec, using the prolonged, slow speech pattern. Verbal reinforcement was "good" and success was five minutes of fluency (0.5 or less SW/M). When fluency was obtained, the delay interval was decreased by 50 msec, and the process repeated.
14–20	Same procedures as in steps 7 to 13, but with monologue.
21–27	Same procedures as in steps 7 to 13, but with conversation.

Clients were requested to hold their speaking rate down and continue with prolongations (that is, not increasing rate as the DAF interval decreased) until the transfer phase was reached. Also, varying amounts of home practice were used. The twenty to sixty steps of the transfer program were very similar to those described by Curlee and Perkins (1969), and maintenance consisted of sampling stutterers' speech on a decreasing scale over time and providing special assistance if needed. The complete programs can be found in the publications cited at the end of this text.

Shames (1978) describes a typical DAF response-contingent program where the stutterer is penalized a ten-second TO each time stuttering occurs. Once the new fluency pattern (slow rate, vowel prolongation) is stable, DAF is faded out. It can be reintroduced if necessary. Shames deliberately developed rate increases by use of a tachistoscope (although a reading rate machine probably would be better) on words and sentences. When the speech rate reaches conversational levels, therapy is expanded to cover self-control, environmental change, and other facilitations of speech and social behavior.

The Shames and Florance study, *Stutter-Free Speech* (1980), presents an extremely detailed program of DAF therapy for stuttering rehabilitation with adults and children (in school or other settings). There is the usual 250-msec delay acclimation, with specific instructions for having the clients slow their speech rates and speak with continuous phonation. Efforts must be made to avoid monotonous, stereotyped speech patterns, but the primary target is the accumulation of thirty minutes of stutter-free speech (individually or as part of a group). From 250 msec, the delay interval is dropped to 200 msec and then progressively down as the fluency criterion is met at each step. At all delay intervals, the delay unit is turned off briefly so that the client uses the target speech without machine support. As the delay interval decreases, this is done more frequently. After each thirty-minute criterion point is reached, the client speaks for several minutes without DAF, and the clinician checks for self-control and confidence. Once the delay interval decrement cycle is completed, various delay time intervals are randomly switched in and out as the client talks. The authors provide suggestions for working with prosody (starting at 150 msec), extinguishing struggle and avoidance behaviors, using penalty contingencies, keeping records, and adapting the program for various uses. Extensive attention is paid to transfer, and it is explained in easily understood behavioral modification terms.

Leith and Chmiel (1980) describe a therapy approach they call "shaping through DAF," rather than "fading DAF." Initial use appears to be a standard rate reduction approach, with explanations and modeling by the clinician. In order to stress oral sensory feedback cues, the client is instructed to concentrate on "enunciation." Pre- and para-DAF recordings are analyzed to determine the variables creating fluency—typically slower rate, careful enunciation, easy onset, and continuous flow of air. These are embodied in the REEF acronym (rate, enunciation, easy onset, flow of speech) as a behavioral goal. A cognitive awareness of the target goals is stressed so that the stutterer is not induced to fluency but instructed in its attainment; thus DAF is an implement, not an effect.

Other Uses

Other uses of DAF have been limited only by the ingenuity of clinicians. It has been applied to individual or dialect rate problems and to slurred or lalling speech. Many clinicians have used maximal delay times to provide articulation to clients with delayed repeats of production efforts, for ear training and evaluation work. Lozano and Dreyer (1978) used DAF, to no great satisfaction, with five dyspraxic patients; but Hanson and Metter (1980) applied it successfully in portable form to midbrain-damage dysarthria and noted its use by others in aphasia and apraxic disorders. Downie et al. (1981) tried portable DAF units on eleven Parkinsonism patients. The akinetic and very mild problems seemed to benefit minimally, but two patients with festinating (rapid, tumbling) speech did very well—as long as they used the units. They tended to revert when the units were turned off or removed. I have used DAF to help family members of stutterers experience uncontrollable dysfluency. It has been of value in demonstrating involuntary dysfluency to groups and stuttering classes, although some clinicians today have been so oriented to fluency facilitation they have forgotten that DAF, if contested, can be a significant fluency disruptor rather than a facilitator.

CLINICAL USE OF DAF

Technical Procedures

Technical procedures in DAF are simple. Most DAF units are not complicated and require less skill to operate than the usual stereo set. The limitations of commercial DAF units have been noted earlier. We have compared one such unit to a unit of laboratory quality. Although the clinical unit's frequency response, delay time accuracy, earphone quality, and loudness equivalence all were inferior to those of the laboratory unit, judged speech output (that is, DAF effects) was not significantly different with the two units (Ham et al. 1983). On the other hand, you may have access to a tape DAF unit or can have one produced for you from a standard tape recorder. In such instances, you will need to be able to calculate delay intervals and mark the more common ones on the machine (typically, the record head is fixed and the playback head is moved linearly). Calculations of delay time can be made by letting A equal the distance between record and playback heads, B equal the tape speed (in ips), and C equal the delay interval. If you know A and B, you can obtain C (delay time) if you divide A by B. If your tape speed is 7½ ips, and the separation distance A is, say, 1.5 inches, 1.5 divided by 7.5 is 0.20, or 200 msec delay. If you set the tape recorder speed control to 3.75 ips instead of 7.5, you would then automatically double the delay time since 1.5 divided by 3.75 is equal to 0.40, or 400 msec.

The equation can be solved for any third contingent, as long as you know the other two. For instance, if you want to have a delay of 250 msec but don't know the needed head separation difference for that delay time, calculate $B \times C = A$, or 7.5 ips $\times$ 250 msec = 1.9 inches (rounded off) of head separation. Similarly, head separation distance, A, divided by the delay time interval, C, would provide the tape speed needed for that delay time.

With so many different instruments available, I cannot tell you how to run a particular DAF unit. However, certain basic procedures can be followed. If you are using a reel-to-reel unit, degauss (erase) the tape with a bulk degausser after every few hours of use, to eliminate built-up background noise. On any unit, check the volume control on yourself and several others to determine proper settings for maximum tolerance levels. Use the best earphone speakers and cushions you can get. Ear cups, so-called doughnut cushions, or modern stereo cushions are best. They will attenuate airborne sidetone and reduce the earphone loudness level needed. In fitting the headset, be sure you adjust for a snug fit, and don't become entangled with long hair or earrings. I once worked with poorly fitting earphones, and the amplified (delayed) voice of the client was picked up again by the microphone, redelayed, and delivered a second time to a very confused client. Also clients will tend to pull back from the microphone as delay and loudness hit them. The easiest control for this is a boom microphone attached to the headset, or lavaliere and clip-on microphones can be used. Also, you can tape or band the microphone on a ruler at the six-inch or nine-inch measure and have the clients rest the end of the ruler against their chins as they talk.

Reactions

As we have seen, sex and age can affect reactions. Also, individuals may show sharp variations in response to DAF in general or to particular delay intervals. You need to find out about your own reactions by reading at the various delay intervals, using several loudness settings each time. What are your emotional responses to DAF? Record your speaking DAF and then analyze it thoroughly for dysfluencies and prosodic characteristics. If you happen to be a person who is thrown into verbal confusion by DAF, do not let this stop you from using it. It is not a clinical handicap to be vulnerable to DAF. At the worst, your client might feel a little superior, and that can be useful.

Practice

It is wise to practice with DAF and also use your associates to gain experience in explaining it to others, preferably using those who have never been exposed to it before. You will need to be certain of routine procedures for headset fit, microphone distance, and instrument settings. For the first time it usually is best, after the explanation, to instruct the subject to say nothing while you are completing the instrument setup and activating it; if they start talking and are caught by the delay, things can become confused. Set the delay time at maximum interval and tell the client to read or repeat single words. Use short words and space them so the client can receive each feedback completely before starting to say the next word. Instruct the client to speak only when responding to your direct stimuli. Now, use longer words or short phrases for the subject to repeat, and finish by having the client read several consecutive sentences. At this point you may want to turn the unit off, or switch to NAF, and have the subject express any first reactions to DAF. Then reactivate the delay and work with the loudness setting to determine the maximum acceptable loudness for the client. When it is achieved, temporarily remove the headset and check the loudness with your own ears. If the level seems unusually low, discuss this with the client and see if you can negotiate a higher volume, within safe limits.

When an agreeable loudness level is set and the subject is aware of what DAF is like, you are ready to move on. If you have not, inform the client about different types of speech disruption effects and instruct the client to "just try and talk normally." Starting with maximum delay time, have the client read aloud from printed sentences. From the delay time set, move down in time decrements after each series of sentences. Look and listen for the point of maximum disruption, rechecking to make sure. Perform an analysis of the speech characteristics displayed. Terminate the DAF, remove the headset, and again query reactions and feelings; be alert for those who seem to be unduly surprised, upset, or depressed by the experience.

Previous sections involved observation of more-or-less spontaneous reactions to DAF. However, much of DAF therapy involves teaching the stutterer to alter her or his speech pattern in order to conform to the delay interval and, hence, avoid disruption and/or stuttering. This usually is done by slowing the spm (syllables per minute) rate, which is achieved mainly by prolonging vowels, increasing pause duration, using shorter phrases, and slowing down. Prolongations also can be used on semivowels and continuants, and even consonants in the strong-movement pattern described elsewhere. Set the DAF unit on a long delay (250 msec or more) and then have the client read aloud, to establish the disruption pattern. Then work at shortening phrases, slowing down, and so on, until reading rate and delay time coincide. Record efforts and play them back for evaluation. Once you have established a talking rate and pattern that eliminate disruption, change the delay setting and have the client read several paragraphs, recording them, while the acquired speech pattern is maintained. Play the recording back and compare it to the controlled speech in the initial establishment. Back on DAF, have the client deliver a monologue or talk to a friend, practicing the rate control. Record and evaluate some samples. As before, terminate the DAF and try to have an extended conversation while the altered speech pattern is used, resisting rapid bursts of syllables or other vagaries of speech. Be sure that you and the client can converse thusly at several different spm rates of speed. As noted earlier, struggle with and accommodation to DAF tend to produce speech that is deficient in prosodic elements, as well as having slurring or other undesirable aspects (Lechner, 1979; Perkins, 1973b; Shames & Florance, 1980; Van Riper, 1970; Wingate, 1976). Listen to the recordings of your own rate control speech and that of your practice client, and if possible, the recordings of others who are practicing the procedure. Take some of the stimulus materials and repeat them with the same rate of speed control, but try to improve the liveliness and quality. The analogy to a slowed-down record (Perkins 1973b) is a useful one, and it may help initially to exaggerate some of the stress and inflection patterns. Again, the preceding instructions should be carried out by yourself to experience the DAF methods, and then you should "teach" it to one or more normally speaking persons for practice.

Reference has been made to "beating DAF" rather than slowing or accommodating your speech to the delay interval (Van Riper, 1970, 1973).

This is somewhat optimistic as a description since any change in your speech pattern is some form of accommodation to DAF, and the usual fighting technique involves a slowing down or speeding up, volume changes, and so on. Basically, resistance to DAF involves an attempt to ignore the auditory signal and force one's way through the delay interruption. Novice speakers may sharply increase loudness in an unconscious effort to try and overcome earphone cushion attenuation of the airborne signal (this also can be a response to the loudness effect). Separately or simultaneously they may draw back from the microphone to reduce the headset signal volume. Neither of the techniques are acceptable and may be regarded as avoidance devices of the "artificial stutterer." Attempts to fight DAF can be used before or after rate control speech patterns have been developed or not used at all. Why people vary in their response is not known. There may be a conscious effort not to respond to the auditory input, an emphasis on response to proprioceptive feedback, or something else. Each of us knows people who can listen to auditory stimuli and do other things at the same time, whereas others must focus their attention on auditory input in order to "hear" it. Variability of response to DAF is a fact, not a conjecture. You may or may not be proficient at overcoming DAF, and it is not particularly important. After hearing hundreds of persons speak under DAF, it seems clear that everybody reacts in some way to the interference with their temporal feedback pattern.

Use with Stutterers

This will be a brief section since so much detail was provided in earlier sections concerning specific DAF procedures. Similarly, the section on assignments for clients will be brief. Delayed auditory feedback has been significant in stuttering therapy for only approximately twenty years. As a therapy approach it has been used as a response-contingent stimulus to reinforce stuttering negatively and to facilitate fluency, as a stress producer to build up resistance to disruption, as a diagnostic device in evaluating coping behaviors or separating stutter types, and as a delayed response mode to improve self-evaluation and performance. For some it occupies a small portion of the therapy agenda, others apply it intermittently during therapy, and for some it is the basic program of therapy. It even can be made portable.

In the section on practice procedures I indicated a need to practice explaining and demonstrating delay to other people. This ability is important for working with some stutterers. They may be anxious about the clinic, about you, and about therapy in general and particularly uncertain about being attached to a strange machine. They have lived for years with a precarious hold on the fluency they have, and a fluency-disrupting device may not be their all-time favorite example of technology. You should be thorough in your explanations, but avoid lecturing. Identify clearly the purposes for which you are going to use the unit, and predict initial responses that are liable to occur. It will help if you demonstrate the unit on yourself. If you are aiming toward a goal (for example, slow rate or resistance to stress) demonstrate before-and-after states for the client. Solicit questions, ask for a recapitulation of your statements, and offer opportunities for the clients to express their feelings. As you go through a procedure, be sure to check for questions and reactions on a regular basis. This will be stressed again later.

Before using DAF it usually is wise to know thoroughly the speech patterns of the stutterer. This includes nonstuttered as well as stuttered speech. DAF usually will change the dysfluencies significantly, but it will change other aspects of the speech pattern as well, and you should be familiar with the pretreatment speech patterns in order to assess the impact of delay. You will want to determine baseline dysfluencies per minute in order to measure DAF effects and to have meaningful posttreatment measurements. Throughout the use of DAF you should evaluate and chart your clients dysfluent behaviors at each session. Apply similar record-keeping procedures to any work you do on respiration, phonation, inflection, and so on. Such records are easy to draw up, but Perkins (1973b) and Shames and Florance (1980) have useful examples.

I would urge you not to feel strictly bound to any sequence of the various programs that have been suggested or that you find; but introduce modifications and additions based on your experience and the needs of each particular client. Many prepackaged programs predict outstanding results, but it may be hard to replicate their suggested outcomes. Not surprisingly, many of the programs have a relapse rate that runs as high as 70 percent (Owen, 1980), and many stutterers can become cynical and doubtful about therapy. I do not intend to criticize DAF therapy but to caution against its unthinking, unplanned, mass use as if all stutterers can benefit from one approach. DAF therapy, by itself, is going to meet the needs of few stutterers, and it should be regarded as one of the possible parts of an overall therapy program where stability, self-direction, normal speech, and behavioral adequacy are the goals.

Problems

Problems with DAF use do exist. First, it is not cheap. Modern microelectronics have brought costs down significantly, but an initial investment of about $500 (including accessories) would not be high. After that expense will come the question of continuing maintenance and repair costs. This also raises the problem of downtime, when the unit needs repair and must be shipped back to the factory while you wait. Having a spare unit is wise but adds to the expense. I already have discussed the possibility that a client will be seriously upset by DAF. Nearly all will learn to cope with it in a fairly short period of time, but I have seen a few people who were unable to tolerate it. Also, the work by Hutchinson and Burke (1973) on differential responses of clutterers and stutterers should be kept in mind. Aside from initial reactions, working under DAF is not pleasant for the stutterer. Some programs require extensive time under delay, and the stutterer (especially if working alone) can become bored, feel depressed, feel coerced by the machine, and resent its inanimate and nonhuman consistency. One adult stutterer (McCabe & McCollum, 1972) reported his feelings under a rigidly programmed DAF sequence. He frequently felt anger and depression at the persistent demands of the machine for fluency and the possibility of punishment for nonfluency. Even as he improved, and knew he was, he was aware of feelings of resistance toward DAF work. He urged that clinicians help stutterers by providing opportunities to express their feelings and release some frustration, noting that it might keep in therapy some clients who otherwise would leave.

Another problem with DAF therapy is too-early attempts by the stutterer to transfer improved fluency patterns outside the clinic—usually with negative results. The clinician needs to support and counsel the client in this area. Intensive programs can have an advantage here since fluency is reached quickly while the stutterer is under close control and available for counseling and stabilization work as part of transfer activities. Some stutterers can develop an overdependence on DAF and "DAF speech," being anxious about moving into non-DAF situations or progressing away from the safety of artificial speech patterns. Another problem can be the DAF speech itself. What the clinician needs to remember is that, for some stutterers, the noticeable differences of DAF speech are security signals for them, and efforts to move speech back toward normalcy will generate anxiety and even resistance. After all, when the stutterer came to the clinic he or she talked normally except when stuttering occurred (not quite true, but the client will think so). In the clinic, a nonnormal overall pattern was learned in order to be fluent, and as the clinician tries to shape speech toward a normal character, this can create fears of returning to the triggers of stuttering as well. Further counseling may be required in this area. Finally, transfer and maintenance may be particular problems in DAF therapy because

1. Fluency comes so quickly that the client is not prepared for it psychologically.
2. The client has no feeling that he or she did anything to achieve fluency. It was "done to me" by a machine, and feelings of adequacy may be threatened.
3. Something that works in the safety of the clinic may not work as well outside, where there are fears and other pressures.
4. The stutterers' family, friends, and peers may not be ready for his or her fluency, especially if it does not sound particularly normal.
5. The stutterer has lost the best alibi in the world for failure or for not trying.

Transfer and maintenance are the rocks on which therapy will build or on which it will founder, in the long term. Every bit of attention we can give to it is needed, especially where rapid induction of fluency techniques are used.

ASSIGNMENTS FOR CLINICIANS

As in other chapters, you may not want to cover all the assignments in this section, and your instructor may want to add to or alter them. Following instructions from the procedures section of this chapter, familiarize yourself with the unit you will use. Make sure you understand dial settings, adjust the headset fit, set microphone distance, and establish the desired loudness level.

For the first project you will want to arrange a report form to record the total talking time, wpm rate, and the following types of errors: repetition, prolongation, stoppage, other. You will want to make these measurements and counts at the following time intervals: NAF, 250 msec, 200 msec, 150 msec, 100 msec, 50 msec, and NAF (a second time). You will use this outline four times (phrases, paragraph, monologue, conversation) in the different speech modes. See Chart 6-1.

1. With the headset on and delay at 0 msec (NAF), read and reread the following phrases while turning up the volume, until you reach a tolerable loudness level. With the volume set at the acceptable level, record yourself on tape as you read the phrases aloud at each of the time intervals prescribed, starting and ending with NAF, pausing as you stop and reset the DAF dial for each interval change. Perform the measurements and counts, following the procedures from Chapter 2. Enter the results on the form suggested. Use the incomplete phrases listed, and time them as one unit of speech. There are forty-one words, but count any words you omit or add—except that whole-word repetitions are not counted as extra words.

    Where ever you go
    There is no possibility of surviving this terrible
    Six men cannot survive without help from the

CHART 6-1

CONTENT/TIME INTERVAL	TOTAL TALKING TIME	WPM RATE	DYSFLUENCIES			
			Repetition	Prolongation	Stoppage	Other
Speech Mode: ____ Phrases ____ Paragraph ____ Monologue ____ Conversation						
NAF						
250 msec						
200 msec						
150 msec						
100 msec						
50 msec						
NAF						

About every sack is gone although I have tried to contact the
Give your utmost effort to the important task of catching the

2. Using the same format and procedures as in 1, record as you read aloud the following paragraph at each of the seven time intervals. There are seventy-six words in the passage.

> Whenever I see people acting in a silly way, I am reminded of my best friend. She always tried to be very dignified, but her sense of humor betrayed her. When my Aunt Helen proudly announced that she was descended from the time of the French-Indian Wars, my friend giggled and asked her from which side she was descended. Aunt Helen was furious and her cry of rage sounded very much like a war whoop!

3. Conduct a monologue for one minute at each of the seven time intervals and record them. While you talk, have your partner categorize your dysfluencies by type, writing them down for you to compare with your own analysis later. You must talk for at least one minute, without stopping too long to try to think of what to say (DAF-caused stoppages are acceptable). Choose your own topics. Analyze and report as you did in 1.

4. Conduct a conversation with your partner while under DAF at each of the seven time intervals. Have your partner time you so that you talk slightly over one minute at each interval. If pauses not DAF-caused are too long, start that particular time interval over again. As before, have your partner count and identify your production errors for later checking against the tape recording. Analyze and report as you did in 1, 2, and 3.

5. In assignments 3 and 4 you and your partner have worked together and listened to one another. Write a brief report comparing your different and similar speech reactions (from the report forms) and also your personal reactions.

6. Check your previous reports and select the delay interval that caused the most disruption in your speech. Set that time up and then read aloud any material while you work on vowel prolongation, phrase length control, and slowing rate until your rate coincides with the DAF return and you can talk without disruption. Practice until you can read for three consecutive minutes without a DAF-caused error. When you are able to do so, record three minutes of reading. Play back and analyze the reading for wpm rate and evaluate your pitch, loudness, quality, inflection, pausing and phrasing, and general reactions.

7. Without the DAF unit, record and play back three minutes of paragraph reading while you attempt to duplicate the rate control pattern *exactly* as you did in assignment 6. Perform the same analysis you did in 6. If your wpm rate varies from that in 6 by more than ± 10 words, repeat the exercise.

8. Talk with your partner for at least thirty minutes, in which both of you say everything at the slow rate you practiced in assignment 7. Place a signal device (light, bell, clicker) between you. Whenever one of you judges that the other has lost rate control, used too-long phrases, does not prolong adequately, and so on, signal the other to stop. Turn out the light and sit without speaking for thirty seconds. Turn the light on and resume the conversation. The TO periods, laughter, side comments, and so on do not count as part of the thirty minutes. If either of you or both of you accumulate more than three TO periods, add five minutes to the total time required and maintain this criterion throughout. Afterwards, write a report describing the session, summarizing your reactions and feelings, and your personal evaluation of this technique.

SAMPLE ASSIGNMENTS FOR CLIENTS

As stated previously, this section will be brief since the clients' activities with DAF are described at some length in other parts of this chapter. Also, the varied uses of DAF make it difficult to cover all possible uses of delay and anticipate in what sequence they might be used. Instruct your client as follows.

1. Set the DAF unit at the delay interval that has caused the most disruption in your speech, but set the volume level at zero. As you perform each of the following tasks, gradually turn up the volume during each one until the delay begins to interfere with your speech. Leave the setting there and try to overcome the disruption by concentrating on the tactile and kinesthetic sensations from the speech mechanism. Do this each time, while you

    a. Read sentences from a list.
    b. Read a paragraph aloud.
    c. Talk in monologue about preselected topics.

2. If assignment 1 was successful, repeat it with the volume setting slightly higher than before. Continue this cycle until you have reached the top of your comfort level or a level at which you cannot overcome the DAF effect.

3. Prepare a list of monologue topics and talk about each one. As you talk, switch from one delay interval to another so that you must adapt your rate and phrase lengths to the different delays. Be sure the loudness level is high enough to be disruptive. Your criterion of success is to have no more than one fluency error per minute. Accumulate at least five minutes' fluency time at each delay interval. If you fail at a particular interval, set the volume down slightly, practice for awhile, and (setting the volume back) try again.

The previous assignments were examples of what the stutterer can do alone or with the clinician "available." Be sure the client has had enough experience with DAF to be able to perform adequately. The assignments should help in learning to resist stress, become more flexible in fluency, and increase attention to nonauditory feedback channels. Again, instruct the client.

4. Preplan brief telephone calls, prewriting your dialogue as much as possible. With the DAF unit, rehearse each telephone call, using the slow-rate speech. Then make the calls. If you fail to control your speech on a call, make a similar call while using the DAF unit (slide one earphone so you can use the telephone receiver). Report the results of the calls and the auditors' reactions. Select your options:

    a. Three telephone calls.
    b. Five telephone calls.
    c. Seven telephone calls.

5. Use a list of twenty sentences and tape-record this assignment. At each delay interval (250, 200, 150, 100, 50), read a sentence so that your delivery coincides with the delay factor. Turn the DAF unit volume to zero and read the next sentence in the same fashion, but without the assistance of DAF. Do this for four sentences (two under DAF, two under NAF). Move to the next delay interval and repeat the performance. Play back the twenty-four sentences and evaluate how well you could match the DAF control voluntarily.

7

Cancellation

OVERVIEW

The concept of cancellation, as a technique of therapy, has had its share of controversy, interpretation, and variant applications. The controversies and deviations have been varied according to how individuals looked at and perceived cancellation. Part of the problem in perception stems from the fact that cancellation is intended, generally, to be a part of a three-technique sequence in which it develops certain behaviors and skills that are prerequisite to the two subsequent methods. At the same time, cancellation depends very much on several procedures that should precede it. How these preceding methods are developed will affect what can be done in cancellation. How *well* these preliminary methods are taught and mastered will determine the efficacy of cancellation and, therefore, the results of the techniques that follow cancellation. When cancellation per se is analyzed and argued over, the result is analysis and argument about an incomplete topic. We will look at cancellation in isolation but will continually stress its integration into overall therapy.

Cancellation has been utilized as the primary method in several therapies, so some clinicians look at it as if it were the equivalent of an entire program rather than a technique within a program or a free-standing technique. In this chapter I will discuss definition and descriptions of cancellation and some of the various applications. More extensive coverage of the evolution of cancellation and the current methodology by Van Riper will be considered. A brief coverage of cancellation's relationship to other techniques will precede criterion measurements and will be followed by ways for clinicians to learn cancellations for themselves. Following that, a recommended synthesis for teaching cancellation to stutterers will be discussed. The chapter will end with practice assignments for the student clinician and suggested model assignments for clients.

A definition of cancellation appears simple at first (Stein, 1967):

Cancel (kan s l) 1. to make void; revoke; annul. . . . 3. to neutralize, counter-balance, compensate for.

This definition omits facets of cancellation in its general language usage (for example, perforation of postage stamps and closing a bank account). However, the basic concepts are expressed: Either something is terminated so that it no longer exists or functions, or the effect of some thing is neutralized so that it no longer can be significant. Both aspects apply to cancellation in stuttering therapy, but other factors also intervene. Exactly what is being canceled, why cancellation is being used, and how it is applied differ according to the attitudes and practices of those using it.

Cancellation, according to Bluemel (1957) is a time for the stutterer to smooth out speech blocks by thinking of the trouble word, ". . . quietly and clearly in his mind and thus 'cancels' the block. . . ." The stutterer is to do all this internally, and the word is not repeated aloud or even subvocally. Bloodstein (1975a) viewed stuttering cancellation as both a tactical (production) and a therapeutic vehicle, calling it a basic for self-confrontation, and giving the stutterer ". . .opportunities to battle for control of his fears, malattitudes, and abnormal initiation and release of sounds. . . ." The various definitions generally agree that an individual, first, stutters so that the spasm is allowed to finish and the word is completed. As a second step, there is a pause and, third, a reutterance of the previous word. Gregory (1968) indicated that cancellation is a difficult technique for the stutterer to use. Wingate (1976) stated that cognitive function by the stutterer is integral to cancellation, along with deliberate speaking as a means of emphasizing appropriate speech movements. This requires the stutterer to eliminate fear, or at least resist it, during cognitive function. The pause following the stuttering spasm has been compared by Yonovitz and Shepherd (1977) to the TO function in some stuttering therapies that are operantly based. In their research they measured reactions of stutterers and nonstutterers to TO periods and noted that stutterers, as expected, were most tense during speech but most relaxed during the greater part of the TO period, more so than were the nonstutterers.

Van Riper (1973) argued that stuttering was self-reinforcing and that cancellation attacked this aspect. The stutterer supposedly would anticipate stuttering, building fear, increasing tension, and developing struggle. The struggle of the stuttering spasm would rise to a peak, the word would be completed, and the stutterer would find that once more it had been possible to say the word *because of the struggle*. Van Riper, and others, felt that the relief, tension reduction, fluency on the subsequent words, and other reinforcements could be perceived by the stutterer as being the result of the stuttering struggle itself.

Regardless of the mechanism, it is clear that the occurrence of stuttering makes it less likely that subsequent stuttering will occur in the word strings nearest in time to the previous stuttering spasm. Hence, stuttering becomes a contingency in the reinforcement of stuttering. In cancellation, where the postspasm pause denies surrender and delays continuation to the following words, reinforcement presumably is reduced. In learning theory, it is accepted that reinforcement loses contingent effectiveness if it is delayed too long. Therefore, some view cancellation as an intervention in the total behavioral pattern of stuttering. Sheehan et al. (1962) evaluated forty-eight stutterers' feelings before, during, and after stuttering spasms. Guilt feelings were identified at all stages, especially after the spasm. However, tension was lowest during the postspasm period. The stutterers showed a wide variation in the types and strengths of response, suggesting the possibility of reinforcement differences in the postspasm time for different stutterers.

General applications of cancellation have been varied. Luper and Mulder (1964) describe cancellations as ". . . one of the most fundamental tools in stuttering therapy. . . ." They are strong advocates of its use with children who are "confirmed stutterers." In their application sequence, they provide extensive coverage of the steps and procedures.

1. The child is to stutter to completion, without giving up.
2. As soon as the spasm word is completed, the stutterer is to stop further speech effort for a variable period of time. During this pause, he or she is to relax tensions and analyze where the tensions were and the points of fixation in the speech mechanism.
3. After the pause, the child is to say the word again. It is preferable for the second production to be fluent, but stuttering (at the start) a second time is acceptable. It at least would be better to stutter in a different pattern.

These steps are worked on until they can be performed adequately and consistently. The sequence then is changed so that reutterance of the word, after a pause, is to be in the form of a controlled dysfluency. Luper and Mulder suggest dysfluency modes such as bounce and light consonant contact and a deliberate slowing down of the tremor rates of the articulators. Particular values perceived in cancellation are the following:

1. Modification of personal (negative) reactions to stuttering.
2. The development of negative practice, or faking, as a tool in therapy.
3. Providing the child with a feeling that he or she is "doing something" about stuttering.
4. The development of a variety of dysfluency patterns, breaking down the child's own stereotyped patterns.

Luper and Mulder warn that cancellation is not a complete stuttering therapy in or by itself (as some have suggested), and they recommend its use only to the point where other skills can be picked up—although some clinicians use cancellation in other programs and/or as an adjunct to maintenance procedures. Starkweather (1980) describes cancellation as being appropriate when the client has good control and can stutter with or without tension. The sequence is to repeat each stuttered word by stuttering again in a way that is less struggled and tense. At first, any variation is a target. Then the client should shape the variations in the direction of less tension and struggle.

A different approach to cancellation is found in Ryan's operant programmed sequence (1971, 1978). The client first practices intensively to develop skill in catching or counting spasms as they occur. At the various levels of language complexity, this step is worked on until 90 percent accuracy is achieved. Then the client can progress to cancellation itself. The clinician models catching a spasm and then repeating the word in a prolonged manner, either on the vowel or on the consonant of the first syllable. The client practices by imitating the clinician ten times in succession. When she or he can produce the prolonged utterance satisfactorily, catching or counting is expanded to add cancellation in the form just described. The clinician provides 100 percent reinforcement, verbal or tangible, for each success. Pause time is not emphasized and is not utilized for analysis or for planning. The word is repeated only in the prolongation pattern described. This difference from the Luper and Mulder programs (and others described later) is appropriate in view of Ryan's belief that "Cancellation in itself is not critical; it is only a step on the way to fluent speech." He also warns that there will be a false indication of fluency in charting measurements from a reduced SW/M measure, because the cancellation practice can reduce sharply the WS/M, which functions as a base reference for several of his fluency measures.

Shames and Egolf (1976) applied operant structuring with cancellation somewhat differently. To begin, a baseline is set during which the utterance of 1,000 words, or more than 5 percent SW, is elicited. The client is then directed not to repeat words or phrases, while the clinician rewards and punishes appropriately until a criterion of 1 percent or less is reached. In subsequent steps the client, after each stuttering occurrence,

> Repeats the word.
> Repeats the first syllable three times and then says the word.
> Same as above, but continues repeating the syllables and words until they are spoken fluently.
> Same as above (see the following).

Positive reinforcement is offered on every effort for the first two steps, in the third step when the word is finally repeated fluently, and in the last step when the word is repeated fluently on the first effort. In all the steps, the criterion for progress to the next step is 90 percent success. From this, Shames and Egolf bypass pullouts (see later) and move directly to preparatory sets. Each of these steps involves at least forty minutes talking time, and if SW drops below 5 percent at any step, the authors recommend trying to jump directly to an attempt at "no stuttering" fluent speech.

Shames (1978) prescribed that the client be asked to pause after every stuttered word and then repeat the word. There is to be reinforcement, even if the second effort is stuttered also. Then the client is to pause after a stuttered word and repeat the word, " . . . while prolonging the first sound." Each effort is to be reinforced. Like Ryan's program, no further development is made with cancellation, and therapy moves on to the next phase (in this case, pullouts). Another description of cancellation is presented by Perkins (1980, p. 447), in which he states,

> Van Riper's third procedure . . . is what the stutterer does as soon as the instance of stuttering stops. He pauses, then stutters again, but this time he uses a modified version of his stuttering that is simpler. These include his new pullouts and preparatory sets.

As we will see, Van Riper does not now arrange cancellations in the preceding sequence, and modifying the self-pattern of stuttering is only one of several approaches he uses in cancellation production.

A different approach to cancellation is provided by Falck (1969), although close similarities to other methods will be seen further on. In his technique, Falck has the stutterer repeat " . . . the initial stages of a block as accurately as possible and then stopping without completing the word or phrase." After this pseudospasm partial production, the stutterer is to produce the word or phrase again, using "easy way" production. This is relaxed production, with emphasis on continuous, free-flowing phonation. When the stutterer can repeat the word or phrase in an easy way, the next step is progression to "pattern modification." In this approach, the previous stuttering spasm is repeated exactly as in the original, except that one significant factor (for example, eye contact) is selected for cancellation or correction. As this is learned correctly and consistently, a second significant characteristic from the spasm is canceled, then another, until all such factors have been dealt with.

The following procedure, published by the Speech Foundation of America (No. 12) will complete this section. It essentially is Van Riperian in approach and leads to the next section on Van Riper and cancellation. The following instructions are given to the stutterer:

1. First, finish the particular stuttering spasm.
2. Come to a full stop in your speech efforts and rest, resisting any time pressure to continue talking.
3. Relax the muscular tension of your speech mechanism, especially in the throat. You may find it necessary to do specific things in order to make yourself relax.
4. Use your prior skills in self-analysis, from earlier therapy stages, and review the just-completed stuttering spasm to determine exactly what you did.
5. Review what you can do to reverse or change errors slowly.
6. Mentally rehearse, or silently mimic, each mechanism movement needed to modify your usual stuttering spasm and move through the word.
7. Repeat the word.
8. Articulate the sound on which you previously stuttered, in a smooth, flowing, prolonged manner. Keep your voice flowing to facilitate transition to the next sound.

The stutterer is advised to master this process completely before trying the next stage of therapy. Amplification of many of the steps will be found in the next section.

CANCELLATION AND VAN RIPER

One of the difficulties faced by significant contributors to areas of human behavior is the attribution of beliefs or practices to them, tagged with their names, that they have changed or dropped over time (not to mention views they never supported in the first place). Particular points of view are published or uttered at a certain time, and often are germane for only a limited time, but keep popping up years afterward as the current belief of that person. Although he did not originate the concept of the basic practice, Van Riper is associated with cancellation in the cancellation-pullout-preparatory set sequence as no other clinician is, and he has shaped it significantly over the past years.

In general comments on cancellation, one of the points made by Van Riper (1973, p. 319) is that many clinicians have not understood that ". . . cancellation is designed primarily as a vehicle for learning new responses to the stimuli that trigger abnormal stuttering responses. . . ." It has other values, which will be noted, but the basic rationale for using it is to break the reflexlike spasm patterns and associated behaviors and to learn new response patterns to replace them. The repetition of the word after stuttering is important as a contingency replacer and a practice opportunity for a different type of dysfluency (not normal speech). "We see very little value in merely saying a stuttered word again fluently" (p. 319). The pause between stuttering spasm and word repetition is important to Van Riper. You must insist on a real pause but be realistic and set criteria variably, depending on the situation. At the outset, pauses usually are too brief to be useful, but an overly long pause seems to promote fluency less effectively. Yonovitz and Shepherd (1977) found that the TO (pause) interval relaxation of stutterers started to disappear as the time for the next utterance approached; a prolonged pause would give greater opportunity for anticipation to build up. Relaxation during the pause is promoted and should be discussed with the client. However, Van Riper feels that specific procedures or exercises to secure intrapause relaxation work no better than "relax" or "be calm" types of advice. He opined that most stutterers develop some kind of covertly verbalized self-suggestion to achieve relaxation. Finally, in reference to the perceived external pressure created by a pause, Van Riper felt that a calm pause and attitude by the stutterer actually will promote listeners' acceptance and objectivity, whereas rush and embarrassment on the part of the stutterer will elicit less accepting attitudes from listeners.

In his discussion of twenty years of stuttering therapy experimentation (1937 to 1957), Van Riper (1958) touches cancellation several times. In the 1942-1943 report he referred to a technique called *varying* or *dropping*, in which the stutterer is to vary the characteristic stuttering pattern by subtraction, alteration, or addition—possibly an early variant of cancellation. The next year, cancellation is referred to in a client's self-report, talking of "canceling" a failure of several weeks past. This was done by entering three similar situations and performing successfully. Another stutterer's daily report simply refers to having performed ten to twelve cancellations (undefined). In the 1945-1946 summary, Van Riper reported that cancellations (and pullouts and preparatory sets) were used, although they had not been used consistently or emphasized in previous years. After that cancellation appears consistently as part of each year's therapy program and was published (1947, 1949). The pause and preparation that soon became a requirement of cancellation was, at that time, described as part of the process for the preparatory set. If the preparatory set failed, "When he finds himself stuttering in his old way, he attempts to bring his symptoms under control before effecting a release." (1947, p. 370). This describes a pullout attempt. Then, on the same page, the stutterer is advised to cancel the failure by pausing and doing a better job of preparation before repeating the word. By 1949, the familiar sequence was well established. In general, it appears that Van Riper used cancellation intermittently and in variable forms from the 1930s on, but without the developments and refinements that occurred later. When I was a graduate clinician in his 1953-1954 program, cancellation was a very significant technique with carefully delineated steps and qualitative criteria. In many ways it was similar to the procedures we know now.

Cancellations were to occur first in the learning of the triad sequence. They were regarded as foundation for the next two techniques. Bloodstein (1969) regarded cancellation as something to use when preparatory sets or pullouts were not successful, and he suggested that the teaching sequence was preparatory sets, then pullouts, and cancellation last. He noted that ". . . Van Riper frequently begins with cancellation, and proceeds systematically to pull-out and then preparatory set" (p. 252). I question Bloodstein's reversal of the teaching sequence, although situational use should follow exactly that sequence in a fall-back series of control options.

In his 1973 reference on stuttering therapy, Van Riper discussed cancellation extensively. The stutterer must have developed high ability in knowing his or her own stuttering pattern in all its forms and variations. One must know not only the gross aspects of spasm types, location, avoidance devices, eye contact, and so on but also the subtler components of articulatory postures, laryngeal tension, tremor characteristics, and transitional cues. The client should be able to derive this information in a wide range of situations. Tolerance is important in that the stutterer must be willing to stutter, or at least be able to bear it, and then increase the period of dysfluency with the cancellation. During preceding therapy the stutterer should have experimented with altering various aspects of the spasm, real or faked, and in trying alternate forms of dysfluency. If the stutterer does not "know" her or his stuttering, either because of ignorance or because of panic under stress, then an adequate precancellation analysis cannot be conducted. If desensitization has not developed some degree of tolerance for anxiety and frustration, the client cannot pause adequately and/or analyze and plan effectively. Finally, if the stutterer has not experimented with other dysfluency forms, there are no resources to plan with in preparing the cancellation. Van Riper (1971) earlier described the ready-for-cancellation stutterers as having more mental and physical ease when stuttering. They have developed interest in and curiosity about fluency and dysfluency. Along with increased tolerance for frustration, their general insight has improved, they are in better contact with themselves and with the listener, their personal feelings make sense now, and they have experimented with interpersonal relationships. Functionally, the stutterer has a recent history of at least partial success in self-acceptance and control and is realizing there is less need for support of the clinician and/or of a peer therapy group.

Spasm Period

The spasm period of cancellation is an important first step. The client is strongly advised to stutter completely and finish the spasm. Many will want to shorten the spasm, give up, and get to the cancellation. This cannot be allowed. The entire routine of stuttering behavior for that particular utterance must be endured, or the subsequent cancellation is incomplete. The TO punishment value of the following pause will be reduced. Tolerance not only will fail to be reinforced but also will probably be weakened. Analysis of a partial spasm is, ipso facto, incomplete analysis, and therefore, not valid. Planning for a cancellation, similarly, is incomplete and does not meet its purpose. Clinicians must watch stutterers closely for premature termination of a spasm and encourage clients to complete the intended word.

Postspasm Period

During the postspasm pause the stutterer is to accomplish several things. The interword pauses will be long at first and will seem, to the stutterer, to last forever:

1. First, the clinician duplicates in pantomime a shortened version of the real spasm; it is not a faithful msec-by-msec copy, but it should be accurate in its time compression. Stutterers may stick here for awhile until they realize what was done during the real spasm and have enough tolerance to approximate it in pantomime. This makes the client confront the maladaptive behavior head on. Also, the auditor will realize what the stutterer is doing and usually respect it. "We need no electric shocks or blasts of 100 decibel tones . . . to produce a decrement of stuttering" (Van Riper, 1973, p. 324). This process makes communication continuance contingent on a revision of the maladaptive behavior, so the revision (cancellation) is reinforced and not the maladaptive behavior (stuttering). If necessary, the clinician can apply negative practice principles and have the client pantomime the spasm duplication many times before moving on.
2. The stutterer then pantomimes a revision of the prior utterance, one that is not emitted with normal speed or tactile-kinesthetic levels. The client is to use ". . . a highly conscious, deliberate, slow-motion pantomimed rehearsal of the motoric sequence which comprises the word" (p. 325). Note that this exaggerated production encompasses the whole word and not just the phoneme or syllable stuttered on, although that is the focus. The stutterer is to start with the correct articulatory posture but concentrate on shifting from one movement to the next, with strong (but not tight) movement. An effort should be made to feel the sequence of movements and contacts as they occur in succession. The stutterer is not, at this point, to say the word aloud, but the auditor should be able to recognize easily that the stutterer is rehearsing a different way to attempt the word a second time.
3. In therapy training, stutterers should progress to a point where they are doing the reduplication and rehearsal in ". . . a soft, almost inaudible whisper so that airflow can accompany both" (Van Riper, 1973, p. 326). This is felt to be a necessary transitional step prior to canceling audibly.

Production of Cancellation

Production of the cancellation follows certain steps. When the stutterer shows an ability to pantomime a reduced version of the real spasm, a pantomime repetition of the word is added. As the second step is mastered, the stutterer is permitted to add just enough whispered vocalization to establish the timing of the airflow release with phoneme utterance. The stutterer is ready to cancel.

1. The clinician should gradually fade out the pantomime process duplicating the spasm and the pantomime rehearsal. However, the pause time for analysis and planning should be retained.
2. The stutterer should repeat the word aloud, after the pause, using the strong, deliberate, slow-motion utterance described under step 2 previously. At first, it is acceptable if some of the original stuttered behavior reoccurs, as long as the cancellation is "better" than the original spasm. Whatever the format, the cancellation should always be nonfluent and not just a reproduction of the word.
3. It may be necessary to work the cancellation in steps, shaping the cancellation product progressively. A stuttering spasm may be too complex to cancel completely at first, or a particular stutterer may be too bound up in certain spasm components to cancel all of them initially.

   a. First, the stutterer should smooth out the repetitions so there are a few, slow, prolonged ones or just a strong, slow movement through the word.
   b. Second, the stutterer should relax the facial muscles and present a normal expression.
   c. Third, as tremors slow, the stutterer should eliminate accompanying head jerks.
   d. Fourth, as the head posture returns to normal and facial muscles relax, the stutterer should ensure eye contact so that he or she can see and evaluate auditors.
   e. "The case is not to try to say the word without stuttering . . . even if he can say it without having any symptoms, he deliberately does some pseudostuttering . . ." (Van Riper, 1971, p. 1,003).

OTHER ASPECTS OF CANCELLATION

Postcancellation Activity

Postcancellation activity depends on the therapy program being used. Van Riper (1973) felt, as has been indicated, that cancellation was only one step in a process. However, it was so comprehensive in its production requirements that it was not unusual for stutterers to make maximum progress during its phase. "We have seen many stutterers who needed very little additional therapy" (p. 327). Nevertheless, he did not propose cancellation as a terminal point in therapy, much less as a program of therapy by itself. It is a technique, albeit a useful one, and should be in an appropriate context. This is particularly true when a stutterer does not respond well to cancellation and/or is in the moderate-to-mild severity range.

With Children

Cancellation with children is not frequent, although it was discussed earlier. Despite a strong advocacy (Luper & Mulder, 1964) of cancellation with children, Van Riper (1973) was not persuaded that it was consistently applicable. He did not, however, feel that it was an inappropriate technique. He suggests analogy-type teaching procedures, such as using an oversize pencil eraser to "erase" verbal mistakes symbolically. By using analogy and some game structure, tolerance for and understanding of cancellation often can be gained. However, he commented that "In their pell mell hurry to communicate, most . . . children find it very hard to cancel" (p. 442). He also quoted Goven and Vette (1965) in providing cancellation explanations for an older child and noted that operant procedures such as Ryan's (1971) system sometimes are very suitable for children.

Other Relationships

Reference already has been made to cancellation as part of a trio of techniques. Cancellations provide the basic skills and procedures needed for pullouts and, subsequently, preparatory sets. However, the linkage goes beyond this point. Cancellation teaches the stutterer that the appropriate responses to stress and fear are not tension, not anxiety, not struggle, and not avoidance. It penalizes these behaviors and weakens reinforcement values associated with them. Subsequent work in any other technique is supposed to benefit from cancellation. Theoretically, it could be followed by a classical fluency reinforcement program, and that program could be enchanced by the knowledge, tolerance, self-control, and skills developed during cancellation. However, most of the cancellation procedures outlined in existing programmed sequences are sorry excuses for the real thing, and they should either be revised drastically or receive a different label since their goals are different and their procedures only a partial shadow of what has been described in this chapter. In other areas, cancellation would support self-monitoring skills in a maintenance program. It also is linked to the earlier stages of some programs in that it takes desensitization, tolerance, and analysis and carries them to a higher level of speed and adequacy. Cancellation is a single technique, but it has ramifications for other techniques. It also has implications for theoretical constructs in considerations such as approach-avoidance resolution, antifragmentation, and rehearsal and scanning time in organic breakdown theories. However, at this time, speculations are too hypothetical and must await future growth.

Criteria

Criteria in cancellation should be considered beyond the limited coverage earlier. When has a stutterer made sufficient progress to move to the next stage or technique of therapy? When is a client ready to move from one phase of cancellation to the next? Ryan (1978), in his pseudocancellation, provides a very clear criterion in that the stutterer must be at a 90 percent success level before moving on. His use of cancellation seems to be limited to in-clinic sessions, and as noted, he regards it as a noncritical technique intended for temporary use in fluency reinforcement therapy. Gregory (1968), on the other hand, feels that cancellation is a difficult technique to learn: "Thus, when the stutterer cancels 50 percent to 70 percent of his blocks in the clinic, this is judged to be proficient" (p. 120). A more general criterion is supplied by Van Riper (1974a): "Once your stutterer is willing and able to cancel his old abnormal responses and do so with some consistency, it's wise to move on . . ." (p. 71). What he means by "willing and able" and by "some consistency" is open to debate. In other words, we do not seem to have a generally accepted criterion, in the clinic or out of the clinic. Add to this complicating variables of mild, moderate, and severe spasm differentials; effects of easy, average, and high stress; aspects of different types of stuttering spasms to be canceled; the important factors of clients' motivation and attitudes; variation in the abilities of clinicians—and the criterion becomes more difficult. Later on I will make some suggestions, but they reflect my situation and biases, and you may well need to develop your own standards.

CANCELLATION FOR CLINICIANS

Personal Attitudes

Personal attitudes toward cancellation will vary. If cancellations are difficult for stutterers to learn, they are not easy for a fluent person to acquire. First, you must be able to fake stuttering spasms in a variety of ways, and do it well. Next, you must be able to retain full awareness of what you did when you faked, how you did it, and other variables. You have to be able to pause after a faked spasm, use the pause meaningfully, and resist pressure to move on. Finally, you should be able to model a dysfluency for the stutterer to imitate, evaluate, or otherwise respond to. Beyond this basic series, you will want to duplicate accurately your client's cancellations so that she or he can be aided in self-analysis. Students learning cancellations in my classes have responded as follows:

> This was harder than learning faking. . . . I chose telephone calls because I just couldn't face a store clerk. . . . I had such a feeling of achievement! . . . I

talked to a store clerk; she suddenly turned sympathetic, understanding, and overly pleasant. . . . I can see where motivation is one of the most important aspects of this stage of therapy.

All the students reported high levels of anxiety, avoidance of difficult situations, concern about auditors' reactions, and other normal feelings. My most recent class generated about fifty contacts in cancellation, and none of them experienced overt rejection, challenge, cruel humor, anger, or other strong negative reactions from auditors. I will make further comments about anxiety later on.

Prerequisites

Prerequisites in learning cancellation need review. I feel a number of skills are important, and you should examine your abilities before starting to work.

1. Do you have the basic self-monitoring capacity to know what you say and how you say it? How did you do on self-listening in the earlier assignments? If you cannot rate yourself as adequate or average in this area, you should practice before continuing.
2. Can you stop after any particular word that you utter, but especially after the initial word of a sentence or phrase, after stressed words, or after words that are significant for meaning? If not, or if you don't improve quickly, further practice may be needed.
3. If you are able to stop after words, can you remain calm and continue to pause for five seconds or more? The urge to continue will be strong, but you must be able to resist it. As a corollary, how accurate is your sense of time on the length of pauses? You don't need a stopwatch, but you should be able to pause for variable periods of two to four, six to eight, and ten to twelve seconds and be fairly close to those times. You can develop this ability as you work on cancellations.
4. Can you fake stuttering spasms within and across these various combinations?
    a. Repetitions, prolongations, and tonic stoppages.
    b. Struggle reactions of mild, moderate, and severe degrees.
    c. Various secondaries including grimace, eye contact loss, head jerk, and limb movements.
    d. Various avoidance devices such as postponement, starter, and release.
5. Can you generate these fakes in outside situations where strangers who hear you will assume you really are a stutterer?

The final item concerns a point made several times before—the importance of the clinician doing anything that the stutterer is asked to do. I have expounded on the value gained if the clinician models techniques and acts as a reference for the client, the motivation factor involved if the clinician shows the stutterer that a technique really is possible, and the reliability of actually observing the client in real situations. I will mention all such points again in other sections and chapters. One can teach cancellations without having mastered any of the skills personally, but I seriously doubt that the client will be receiving the best therapy possible.

Anxiety

Anxiety, or even fear, can enter into the use of cancellations. I am speaking of your anxiety and fear, and not those of the client. As you get into the assignments, you will find that some of them involve faking and canceling in real situations. These tend to set up a basic approach-avoidance conflict, where you have the desire to learn cancellation skills but would like to avoid the situations in which you have to practice them. This is similar to the approach-avoidance feelings of the stutterer who wants to communicate with people but wishes to avoid the penalizing effects of anticipated stuttering. You will have an avoidant feeling or attitude based on anxiety about possible failures, listeners' actions and reactions, being thought of as a stutterer, and looking ridiculous. The stutterer has very similar feelings, only they are increased exponentially by many past failures and by the fact that the stuttering is not voluntary; stuttering occurs despite every effort not to do so. The approach-avoidance feelings are very normal. You probably never will be free of them completely. After thousands of cancellations over the years I still become nervous in real cancellation situations.

If you cannot resolve your approach-avoidance conflict, it is possible to rely on packaged programs that excuse you from active modeling, and you can hope your stutterer will conform to the therapy. You also can be a passive clinician in describing, but not modeling, required activities and skills. However, you can deal with your approach-avoidance problem just as you might ask a stutterer to deal with it. You can sit down and sift out the elements that contribute most to your anxiety. As you consider them, be sure that your concern is not over whether or not you have the necessary basic skills. Your concern should focus on your ability to perform the skills in particular situations. Take basic skills, such as self-monitoring and pausing, and concentrate only on them in real situations to be sure that you can do them. If they are satisfactory, check on your ability to fake (not fake and cancel) until you are satisfied with it. Set yourself a really large number of small fakes to be collected, and when that is done, repeat the process with slightly more obvious fakes. Working on the pseudostuttering will be your biggest source of desensitization, but you must do a lot of them. Doing just a few usually will only reinforce any anxiety you have. Set yourself a goal of, say, fifty fakes a day for a week or three fakes in every conversation for a week, or pick certain common words and fake every time you say them. When you can do that task, start increasing the severity level again. As I have said, you may always hold a certain level of anxiety, but you should become secure in knowing that

1. Mechanically, you can do it.
2. When you did it, you performed and survived.
3. Auditors typically showed few or only brief negative responses.

Move from pseudostuttering only to faking spasms and then pausing, followed by a normal repetition of the word. Now build this up with bigger fakes and longer pauses, especially longer pauses. Some of your assignments stress this aspect. As you gain control of pauses, start repeating the word with controlled dysfluencies and you will be on the last lap of cancellation.

Earlier chapters have discussed some of the attitudes concerning stuttering and the apparent stigma of stuttering perceived by many clinicians. They do not want to be thought of as stutterers by other people in the environment and, stuttering labels or not, do not want to look "silly" in front of other people. I believe that some clinicians have developed theoretical objections to faking, cancellation, and similar techniques largely as a defense for their own unwillingness to experience the anticipatory, apprehensive, hypertonic, avoidance reactions of (voluntary) dysfluency in public. I require my classes never to inform strangers that they were "just practicing" unless it is necessary. It is quite possible not to use cancellations for good clinical reasons, and not because of fear and anxiety, but you should not teach these skills if you cannot perform them.

CANCELLATION FOR STUTTERERS

Earlier pages have described several procedures for developing cancellation skills. The following plan utilizes some of these steps, omits some, and adds a few. The final product is not necessarily the best, or only, way to teach cancellation. You will have your own opinions on the subject and may want to introduce some variations for each client. As part of the initial stage, the stutterer should receive an explanation of what is going to happen, and why. The theory of cancellation should be explained, the pressures identified, and the steps described. Simply having the stutterer learn to cancel on demand is inadequate. If possible, use video or audio recordings of stutterers who have learned to cancel well. The clinician should be able to model fakes and cancellations in a variety of forms with a high level of realism. If there are junior therapists or observers, this would be a good time for them to learn cancellations, along with the stutterer.

Preliminary Information

Preliminary information and criteria need to be assessed in teaching cancellation. The section on clinician skills described preliminary abilities and information needed for cancellation development. The discussion will not be repeated extensively here, and emphasis will be on the specific areas needed or the procedures involved. If past therapy has already involved analysis, desensitization, and pseudostuttering, the requisite preliminary areas should be adequate, or nearly so. Nevertheless, it is wise to recheck, especially if the skills were learned in therapy at other times.

1. Can the stutterer stop, however briefly, after a stuttering spasm? If not, you can start in-clinic exercises to develop this ability. Then provide some out-clinic assignments to assure that stopping can be done in real situations (observe at least some of these). Approximate performance criteria for the ability to stop after stuttering spasms are as follows:

	SPASM SEVERITY (%)		
SITUATION	MILD	MODERATE	SEVERE
In-clinic, general	60	90	100
Out-clinic, average	50	70	90
Out-clinic, stress	30	50	80

2. Is the stutterer's knowledge about the stuttering pattern generally good over-all? This includes secondaries, antiexpectancies, attitudes, and less common spasm patterns, as well as typical behaviors. Request the client to submit a written summary describing the overall stuttering pattern. Ask him or her to describe verbally the overall stuttering behavior to another clinician, client, or observer. Have the client record a description of the overall pattern, play it back, and evaluate the description with your help. The performance criterion in this area should be "excellent," with no incorrect statements about her or his stuttering. Omissions should involve only minor or occasional items.
3. Is the stutterer able to use the knowledge identified in 2 in a timely fashion to describe the components of any particular stuttering spasm right after it occurs? This assumes awareness while stuttering and the capacity to organize the awareness into a description. Check in-clinic ability while reading to or talking with you, describing each spasm. Also, in the clinic, have the client make telephone calls and then subsequently describe each spasm (tape-record the calls for comparison). In brief, out-clinic tasks such as asking directions or buying small items, have the client describe and evaluate after each situation. Model as needed. Finally, set up several difficult situations where spasms can be collected and described later. Possible criteria are these:

	DESCRIPTION QUALITY (%)		
SITUATION	FAIR	ADEQUATE	COMPLETE
In-clinic, reading	0	10	90
In-clinic, telephone	0	30	70
Out-clinic, easy	10	40	50
Out-clinic, hard	20	50	30

Your evaluation should concentrate on the most significant parts of the spasms and whether they are described well. The client should improve as work progresses.

4. Can the stutterer pause after a spasm? You do not like long pauses in your speech, but they are particularly productive of pressure for the stutterer. Stutterers want very much to get away from the moment of stuttering, and they must learn to fight the impulse to flee. Pause capacity indicates tolerance for (of) stuttering, as well as providing time for planning cancellations. The client should be able to pause following either voluntary (faked) or involuntary spasms. Suggested pause lengths and criteria are provided, but they will need to be adjusted for each client:

	PAUSE TIME (%) OF AT LEAST		
SITUATION	3–5 SECONDS	7–10 SECONDS	12–15 SECONDS
In-clinic, practice	90	90	90
In-clinic, telephone	90	70	50
Out-clinic, easy	80	50	30
Out-clinic, hard	70	40	20

The long pauses may be needed at first in order for the stutterer to relax, analyze, and plan; but experience typically will allow the stutterer to perform in briefer times. However, the client should be able to use and tolerate longer times.

5. Can the stutterer fake a variety of controlled dysfluencies such as light consonant contact, bounce, easy onset, prolongation, and strong articulatory movement? You may wish to teach them as part of cancellation, or you may want to concentrate only on one form. I prefer to have a number of dysfluencies to use and let the client gravitate to the type(s) he or she prefers. Teaching such controls too soon in therapy can lead to misuse by the client and the risk that the controls will become habituated as avoidance devices.

These preliminary criteria assure you that the stutterer has most of the basic skills needed to add cancellation to control efforts or to use them as backup if fluency production efforts fail.

First Stage

The first stage of cancellation is intended to take basic skills described previously and put them into a sequence that leads to complete cancellation. In addition, the client will be increasing the tolerance for time and dysfluency pressure.

1. Have the stutterer read word lists, sentences, and paragraphs and converse with you. During these times, she or he is to try to catch 100 percent of the spasms, and after each spasm, pause; visibly, overtly relax, using a mirror if necessary; describe out loud to you everything done in the spasm.[1] At first you may insert questions and add information, so "pauses" may last for sev-

---

[1]To avoid confusion, any stutterings during discussions need not be canceled.

eral minutes; have the client state aloud what is going to be canceled and how it will be done. You will want to give suggestions, limit efforts at first, ask questions, model possibilities, and generally provide support; then the client is to produce the cancellation, pause briefly, and repeat it, as much like the first cancellation effort as possible; evaluate and discuss the whole effort before going on to the next attempt. It is possible that six to eight cancellations could take thirty minutes in this early stage, and the client may find the pace frustrating. Encourage expression of feelings, reinforce efforts, and motivate him or her to continue. Your criteria are that the client is "adequate" in each of the substeps and catches most of the spasms. This first step can be completed in one session, or you might continue it for any number of sessions until you are satisfied.

2. Have the stutterer read word lists, sentences and paragraphs, and converse with you. While doing it, he or she is to try to catch 100 percent of the spasms, and after each spasm, pause; visibly and overtly relax, using a mirror if necessary; fake, without voicing, the stuttering spasm in duplicate (at first you may correct the client, model what was missed, insert questions, and so on); pantomime (no voicing or air release) a cancellation (refer back to 1 for comments about variability of performance); produce the cancellation with airflow and easy voice, using the desired dysfluency; and discuss and analyze each time.

3. Have the stutterer read word lists, sentences and paragraphs, and converse with you. She or he is to try and catch 100 percent of the spasms, and after each spasm, pause; silently analyze what occurred during the spasm (on about 20 percent of the spasms—after the cancellation is completed—request a report on the results, to remind the client not to become careless); silently plan the cancellation (also check on this periodically); produce the cancellation, using one of the dysfluency forms; and discuss and evaluate the length of the pause, degree of relaxation, the analysis, how well the cancellation canceled the spasm, and how successful the effort was overall. By this time the stutterer should have made significant progress in the basics of cancellation. You now should have a very good idea of his or her cancellation behaviors, strong and weak points, and attitudes. Any extra practice or attitude encouragement can be planned as needed. Now the stutterer needs further practice on basic skills.

4. Have the stutterer read word lists, sentences and paragraphs, and converse with you. In each of the modes have the client fake spasms. In reading you can premark spasms if you wish, but regularly ask the client to fake X number of spasms in a task (since stutterers often tend to elect in their own probability pattern). Be sure a variety of spasms are faked, even if some are not typical of the usual pattern. After each spasm, the stutterer is to pause (you may preset pause lengths), silently analyze the fake, plan a cancellation, and produce the cancellation. Rather than evaluate every cancellation, watch for errors, bad habits, lack of variety, and so on, and you can discuss several cancellations at a time.

Stress the need to practice and acquire smooth skills. If it can be arranged, have the client take a cassette recorder home and practice cancellations in the forms presented in 4. When you are satisfied with 90 percent of the fake/cancellation combinations, the stutterer is ready to move to the next phase.

Second Stage

The second stage of cancellation is to transfer the stutterer from the in-clinic to the out-clinic situation. It also, deliberately, is to transfer responsibility for the technique to the stutterer, although you may have started that aspect near the end of the first phase. This is very important because the stutterer must believe not only that cancellation can work but also that he or she can make it work. Your involvement, modeling, and participation are vital in transfer.

1. Have the stutterer make a series of telephone calls; you model several first. Have the stutterer stutter and cancel. Start by requesting one spasm cancellation per call or a fake and a cancellation of one spasm per call; watch relaxation, pause length, and cancellation closely (see criteria section later in this chapter). If any cancellation fails, discuss it thoroughly, and then have the client use the same word again on the next call (faking if necessary) and cancel it. Keep this up until the client achieves 70 percent to 90 percent adequacy; move to telephone calls, where all involuntary spasms are to be canceled; observe, analyze, and discuss as before. If the client has adapted to a very few spasms, use more faking; have the stutterer call friends (or arrange an auditor) in order to have typical conversations; have the client talk until X number of spasms (real or faked) have been emitted and canceled, and evaluate as before. Give the stutterer some assignments to make solo telephone calls, including some to you and others you can check.

2. Go with the stutterer on outside assignments. In several different, easy situations, model fakes and cancellations while the client observes. Then have her or him complete several brief situations while you observe. Evaluate and discuss after each situation. Vary the requirements, as in earlier stages. If there are few real spasms, have the client fake. Your criterion here should be one of adequacy in the 50 percent to 70 percent range, depending on the stutterer.

3. Move to longer and more difficult situations. Concurrently, the client is receiving solo assignments to practice in easy situations and report to you. As before, model some difficult situations for the client and secure his or her evaluations. Then have the client perform, followed by evaluation and discussion. Your criterion here should be at about the 50 percent level, with reexposure for any outright failures.

4. The stutterer is now ready for further solo assignments. Periodically, you should verify progress by taking the client on some out-clinic activities or by arranging other checks.

The form of cancellation is left vague in this section. Earlier summaries of other clinicians' plans provide specifics on cancellation movements, as do other chapters on the various dysfluencies. The different stages presented here were to help take the stutterer through skill and pressure levels of learning. Also, I have backed off significantly from using cancellation as a major desensitization device, as some clinicians do. I feel that cancellations, used as cancellations, require considerable desensitization and that assigning thirty-second pauses, using out-clinic pantomime rehearsals, using very severe fake spasms in canceling, and so on are not sufficiently productive.

Evaluation

Evaluation of cancellation efforts is carried out continuously. Throughout the various stages and tasks, criterion levels have been suggested. As noted, they are subject to variation according to situations and individual stutterers. In general, criteria for unacceptable cancellations will be based on one or more of the following categories:

1. Failure to complete the spasm, so true cancellation is impossible. The effort usually is hurried and tense so that the resulting cancellation is stutterlike rather than a controlled effort. There is a high probability that the cancellation will be abortive, and the stutterer may jerk into another involuntary spasm.
2. Inadequate preparation, practice, and pacing by the clinician, so the stutterer is not ready for the skill or the pressure demands.
3. Inadequate analysis by the stutterer. This may be caused by the next item (pause time), by relying on probabilities rather than on sure knowledge, and/ or from inability to tolerate stress.
4. Inadequate pause time, creating insufficient relaxation, analysis, and planning. Pause time always is a problem, even when the client becomes proficient at cancellation (see final comment on temporal movement).
5. Failure to plan an appropriate cancellation. This may be due to poor analysis, poor information, inadequate practice, susceptibility to stress, or "automatic" cancellations.
6. Hurried, tense cancellation efforts that tend to slip out of control; token, murmured dysfluencies without real cancellation of the failed behavior.
7. Vulnerability to pressures of the situation can occur easily if the clinician has restricted supervised practice to the quiet, relaxed safety of in-clinic sessions.

Many stutterers, as they become proficient in cancellation, will start to shorten their pauses and still produce good cancellations. This often leads to a spontaneous development of pullouts (see next chapter) and should not be permitted.

Cancellation is a difficult technique to master, but I hope I have not exaggerated its complexities. The clinician needs to be a good salesperson, explaining linkage factors clearly to the stutterer and modeling successful cancellations for learning and motivation. If the client is at all inclined to slack off in therapy, to lie, sabotage, or otherwise undercut clinical activities, it is most likely to occur on cancellation. Mild stutterers may feel that the treatment is worse than the problem and refuse to do it or resist carrying it out. A very insecure stutterer, at any severity level, may express similar feelings and require extensive support. You must judge each client as he or she reacts, and decide accordingly. As a general comment, I would suggest that the more symptom therapy you do, the more you are going to use cancellation—and this may also be true with certain fluency reinforcement modes of therapy.

ASSIGNMENTS FOR CLINICIANS

The following assignments are designed to take you step by step through the early stages of cancellation skills. However, you may start at any point you feel is appropriate and delete, add, or alter assignments. Your instructor may wish to vary what is used. A number of the items necessitate a partner, and you should make appropriate arrangements.

1. Record on a cassette recorder fifty to sixty sound signals at irregular time intervals, with no interval less than five seconds. For the sound, use a bell, clicker, audiometer pure tone—anything to provide a brief, clear signal. As you perform the tasks that follow, play the cassette tape at a comfortable loudness setting. Each time the signal occurs, finish the word you are saying, pause for a slow mental count of 1 . . . 2 . . . 3 . . . 4 . . . 5, and then continue. If a signal occurs between words, during an inhalation, or while you are counting, ignore it and respond to the next signal. Failure to respond to a proper signal is defined as not finishing the word you were saying at the time you heard the signal or saying any part of the next word that would have followed the signal.

   a. Read a list of thirty words aloud. If you fail more than twice, start over. Read at a normal rate and recycle until you have at least ten efforts.
   b. Read the same list again at a faster rate, pausing as instructed each time the signal occurs during a word. If you fail more than three times, start over. Read until you have at least ten efforts.
   c. Read a 300-to-500 word paragraph aloud at your normal rate. When you hear a signal during a word, finish the word and pause. If you fail on more than 10 percent of your efforts, start over.
   d. Look at yourself in a mirror and talk about how to explain cancellation. On each signal during a word, pause. If you fail on more than 20 percent of your efforts, start over.

2. Repeat the first exercise, only use your partner instead of taped signals. Your partner should provide the signals in an irregular pattern until you accumulate at least ten efforts in each of the four tasks (reading, fast reading, paragraph reading, monologue). In the last task you should talk to your partner, not a mirror. Your partner should try to mask signal movements so you will not have a warning of a coming signal. Criteria are the same as for each task in 1.

3. Use the cassette tape while you and your partner converse. Pick your topic ahead of time and have a normal conversation. Keep talking and pausing until each of you have a base of twenty pauses (rewind the signal tape if necessary). For each signal you fail on, add one more effort to your base requirement of twenty. However, if your requirement total goes over thirty (that is, if you failed more than 50 percent of your efforts), stop and repeat the first two exercises, and then try 3 again.

4. Underline ten words from any paragraph. Read the paragraph aloud, and after each underlined word, pause for a mental count of one through ten;

then repeat the underlined word slowly, evenly, and strongly. Repeat the exercise and record it. On playback, time your pauses to see how long they actually lasted and how consistent they were. If you were not pausing for at least five seconds and if any pause differed by more than two or three seconds from your average, do the exercise again.

5. With your partner, make up a list of ten questions in which the subject is clear; for example, "What is your favorite kind of *pie*?" In your answer (complete sentences, please), use the subject word. When you finish saying the subject word, pause for at least five seconds and then repeat the entire word with a slow, deliberate utterance on the complete word. Failure is not pausing, pausing too briefly, or sounding too normal on the repeat (partner judges). Penalty is for your partner to repeat, and you to answer, the same question two more times.

6. Read the following words aloud to your partner, faking the indicated stuttering spasm and pausing for at least five seconds. Then repeat the word in the prolonged, slow, strong movement used before. Your partner should evaluate the quality of the fake, the accuracy of the duration of your pause, and the quality of the repeat. Use a scale of excellent-good-average-poor-terrible when judging. If more than three words are rated below average, repeat the entire assignment.

WORD	SPASM TYPE
party	short, easy repetitions
entire	tonic stoppage on initial vowel
new	prolongation, grimace, struggle
I	severe tonic block, loss of eye contact
service	10 to 15 hard repetitions, struggle
you	moderate repetitions, head jerks
Julie	tonic blocks changing to prolongation
group	mild repetition, head bobbing
Donald	severe tonic block, gesture release
hello	prolongation, eyes shut, retrial

7. Select five words that occur regularly in your everyday speech. Over a period of three to five days, use each word at least three times each day. When you use it deliberately, pause immediately afterward for three to five seconds and then repeat the word, slightly prolonging and increasing the strength of the articulator movements. Do not identify your efforts unless an auditor asks what you are doing. Write a brief report on the words you picked, the situations you selected (and didn't select), the adequacy of your pauses, the quality of your repeats, auditors' reactions, and your feelings.

8. Prewrite three questions to ask in a single telephone call. Underline one word in each question on which you will fake a spasm. Pause for three to five seconds after each spasm, and then cancel by repeating and "improving" your fake. Write a brief report with the same type of information requested in the previous assignment. Select your option: one phone call, all spasms mild; one phone call, all spasms moderate with some secondaries; two phone calls (write new questions if needed), all mild spasms; two phone calls, all moderate spasms with secondaries; one phone call, all spasms severe with struggle, retrials, and so on.

9. Have your partner present while you talk in general terms with another person from class or with a friend. Explain to the auditor what you are trying to learn and why. As you talk, fake a variety of spasms with differing pauses

and different types of cancellation dysfluencies (bounce, light contact, easy onset, strong movement, and so on). Your partner is to use the five-point scale suggested earlier. Any rating below average is a failure. Select your option: six efforts, repeat assignment if more than one failure; ten efforts, repeat assignment if more than three failures; fifteen efforts, repeat assignment if more than five failures. There may be some difficulty in having your partner judge you since there can be peer pressure toward not "criticizing" each other. You should be completely objective, as if you were in the clinic. Also, I suggest that a sample of these assignments should be repeated in class, to stimulate work and objectivity.

10. Ask strangers for directions to particular buildings or places. In each situation, fake a moderate spasm with loss of eye contact, use of a postponement, and head drop. Then pause for three to five seconds, reestablish eye contact, and cancel with your preferred dysfluency mode. Have your partner along, and immediately after the situation, exchange evaluative comments. Write a brief report on the areas suggested earlier. Enter either three, five or eight situations (your choice).

11. Enter a commercial location where you can ask directions, seek aid, or purchase an item. Fake two moderate tonic spasms in which you shut your eyes and jerk your head downward, and have a retrial on one. Pause for three to five seconds, visibly relax, establish eye contact, and cancel with three or more easy, slow, rhythmical bounces. Have your partner along and evaluate as before. Do this in either two, four, or six situations.

Write a brief overall report on the last two situations, summarizing your fakes, pauses, cancellations, auditors' reactions, personal feelings, and the adequacy of your partner's evaluations. What is your feeling toward cancellation as a technique? What problems do you have with it? What more do you need to do? The assignments stop here, but most of you will need further practice in cancellation if you are going to use it. Added skill can be gained by repeating and varying some of the previous assignments, and also by drawing from the sample assignments for clients in the next section or by using some of the steps described earlier in this chapter by other clinicians.

SAMPLE ASSIGNMENTS FOR CLIENTS

Tell the client the following:

1. At home, underline thirty, fifty, or seventy-five words in a newspaper or magazine paragraph; look for words you might be more liable to stutter on. Read the paragraph aloud and fake an easy spasm on each underlined word. Pause after each fake. During the pause, deliberately tighten and then relax your speech mechanism, feeling the relaxation. Then repeat the word with an easy prolongation of the first sound or syllable. Note what sounds or syllables are easier or harder to prolong than others.

2. Underline twenty-five words in any paragraph. Using a recorder, read the paragraph aloud, faking a moderate spasm on each underlined word. Try to fake different types of spasms. After each fake, pause and silently practice the movements of the cancellation you will use. Then cancel out loud. Use all the

following dysfluency modes, five times each: easy prolongation, strong artic-ulatory movement, bounce, light consonant contact, airflow, and continuous phonation. Play back your efforts and evaluate. What types worked best? Were any better for some sound combinations than others? Evaluate your fakes, pauses, and cancellations.

3. Take the word list you were given and say each word aloud while watching yourself in the mirror. After each utterance, pause and pantomime a slow, strong, continuous production of the word. Exaggerate slightly so that you can see and feel the movement. Do this on twenty-five, fifty, or seventy-five words.

4. Take the word list you were given, plus a tape recorder and a mirror. On each word fake a severe stuttering spasm with struggle and secondaries. After each spasm, pause and relax for five to ten seconds, looking at and feeling the relaxation. Then cancel each fake with the strong movement described ear-lier. Play the tape back. During each pause, look in the mirror and silently mimic the spasm and then, aloud, try to repeat the cancellation along with the one on tape. Do this on ten, twenty, or thirty words.

5. Using classified notices in the newspaper and/or telephone directory, make brief telephone calls. In each call cancel all the spasms you can catch—pausing and analyzing your spasm and then repeating the word, either with a slow, easy bounce or with the strong movement pattern. If the cancellation slips, let it go, but analyze the errors afterward. Do this on five, ten, or fifteen tele-phone calls.

6. Repeat task 5, only cancel either by slow, easy prolongation or by light con-sonant contact. This time, if the cancellation slips and becomes a real spasm, penalize yourself by adding another telephone call to your list.

   The last two assignments should be evaluated in terms of how many spasms were missed, how tense you felt, whether any spasms slipped and why, auditors' reactions, your feelings, and comparisons of the different dys-fluency modes.

7. Discuss with your clinician topics you can talk about during telephone calls that are to last ten to twenty minutes. During the call, cancel involuntary spasms by having a good pause and using your preferred dysfluency mode(s) on the repeat. In addition to canceling involuntary spasms, fake five moder-ate spasms and cancel them to preference. Select the number of calls as follows: to the clinician and to one friend; to the clinician and to two friends; to the clinician, to two friends, and to someone the clinician selects.

8. By yourself, or with the help of the clinician, prepare a five-question form and use it to call and interview people selected at random from the telephone directory. During the interview cancel all spasms with your preferred dys-fluency mode(s). Tape-record one or two calls to bring to your next clinic session. You will make three, five, or eight calls. An easy format is to identify yourself as calling for the XYZ Speech Clinic and to ask five questions about speech problems in general, or stuttering in particular.

9. Stop strangers in the street and ask directions. Cancel all spasms with strong, slow movement. If you have no spasms, fake a moderate one in each situation. Observe your auditors closely for reactions, and report on your success and your feelings. You will talk to ten, fifteen, or twenty-five persons.

10. Repeat the content of 9, but do it with persons in business establishments, changing your requests appropriately.

11. Over the next _____ days you are to collect a certain number of fakes and real cancellations each day. The situations are up to you, but they must involve other persons. Make your fakes in the moderate-to-severe range. At all times, evaluate your degree of relaxation, the fake or real spasm, the pause, the cancellation, and reactions. If you cannot meet your target of real spasms, substitute fakes on a two-to-one ratio. You will collect five real and five fake spasms, five real and ten fake spasms, and two real and twenty fake spasms.

12. With your clinician, plan a conversation with a friend or with some person the clinician selects. Prolong this conversation until you collect the number of cancellations elected. You may fake if needed, but all fakes must be of the severe variety. You will talk until you collect ten, fifteen, or twenty cancellations. Evaluate as before.

8

Pullouts

A background to pullouts was introduced in Chapter 7, where I discussed the techniques that typically are linked together—cancellations, pullouts, and preparatory sets. Cancellations occur temporally after a stuttering spasm is finished, allowing the stutterer to regain control of failed speech behavior and then to compensate (cancel) by repeating the word in such a way that the previous behaviors are nullified. Pullouts are a logical temporal extension, wherein the cancellation skills and controls are moved into the stuttering spasm itself. This chapter will discuss pullouts as part of the linked sequence and as a technique in its own right. There is, perhaps, less need to justify pullouts (compared to cancellations) because they are less controversial and, emotionally and mechanically, less difficult. Mechanically, they are not actually easy, but if the previous learning has been adequate, mechanical problems should not be serious. Pullouts precede preparatory sets, the third step, and have the same temporal and functional relationship to them as did cancellations to pullouts. This chapter will review the definition and origin of pullouts and some of the considerations and applications involved. Prerequisite skills for pullouts, criteria for evaluation, learning by the clinician, and acquisition by the client will be discussed. As usual, the chapter will end with a practice assignment series for clinicians and suggested model assignments for stutterers.

Definition

A definition of pullouts is not difficult. Basically, they are a technique in which the stutterer, during an involuntary spasm, regains control of his or her speech pattern and completes the word with a controlled dysfluency pattern. Perkins (1978, 1980) defines pullouts as what a stutter does to extricate him- or herself from stuttering spasms: "Instead of gasping, jerking pull-outs, he learns to ease himself out of difficulty with smooth controlled prolongations" (1980, p. 477). You will see other variations in this definition, as I report on various clinicians' use of the technique, but the predominant use of pullouts today includes these basic items:

1. Stuttering, without trying to avoid or escape.
2. Realizing and analyzing what is being done incorrectly.
3. Relaxing the tension in the speech mechanism and overflow tensions.
4. Planning how to complete the word with a controlled dysfluency.
5. Slowing the involuntary spasm, extending it, and turning it into a fake spasm.
6. Converting the fake spasm into a controlled dysfluency that effectively cancels the stuttering behavior.

These points will be presented again, and expanded, during the discussions in this chapter.

History

The history of pullouts, as with cancellations, is associated with Van Riper. He certainly did not originate the basic concept, but he has made major contributions to it, structured it in the therapy sequence, and popularized it among a generation of clinicians. He did develop, or at least generate, the term *pull-out* and doesn't seem to have been totally pleased with the label. At one point, he noted (1973) that the term was invented by clients themselves, and ". . . we hold no brief for the term, 'pull-out'" (p. 328). A year later (1974a), Van Riper discussed the technique extensively and never used the popular label. Again, in 1978, he referred to the name: "This awkward term, stemming from the stutterers' own language use . . ." (p. 308). In his report on therapy experimentation, Van Riper (1958) noted that a client was taught not to fight stuttering spasms, but to slide out of them with an easy, non-struggle stutter. This was in the 1937-1938 therapy year, and he also quoted a stutterer's daily report in which progress in changing involuntary into voluntary spasms was evaluated. The relationship between these efforts and pullouts seems clear. Five years later, 1942-1943, experimentation still was in progress. In that year, Van Riper tried having stutterers use a "smooth prolongation," where the first sound of a spasm was to be prolonged until the stutterer could relax, gain control, and finish the word. He felt, however, that this method could too easily become an avoidance device, and it was dropped. Also used was the stop-go technique, where the stutterer brings the spasm to a full stop and then attempts to finish the word; but this seemed to result in too many split words. Another approach tried was "varying" or "dropping," in which the stutterer was to go ahead and stutter but, during the spasm, was to try and vary the pattern by alteration of, addition to, or subtraction from the stuttering behaviors.

The following year, 1943-1944, Van Riper made no direct reference to pullouts, by name. However, in 1945-1946, he indicated that pullouts (along with preparatory sets) had a formal identification and a significant role in his therapy program. He stated that stutterers took the modification skills learned in cancellation and transfered them to within-spasm use, or pullouts. The same year, he also reported that if a stutterer failed on a preparatory set, an attempt was to be made to turn the involuntary spasm into a pullout. Bloodstein (1969) indicated that pullouts were developed to aid the stutterer whose self-monitoring was inadequate for preparatory sets and that they worked very well in this capacity. During 1945-1946, Van Riper experimented extensively with "chewing speech" (breath chewing) in pullouts and cancellations. He did not retain this variation, but feeling that there was a basic parameter of speech production being touched in speech chewing, he suggested further investigation.

In the 1947-1948 year, Van Riper listed stutterers' assignments that routinely required pullouts (as well as cancellations) in daily efforts. A copy of one daily report listed thirteen cancellations, thirty-three or more pullouts, and forty-three preparatory sets. In that year, for the first time, his intensive therapy was organized in definite, sequential order:

Phases 1–4: Study stuttering and the stutterer; listeners and their reactions, and stutterer responses; stuttering openly, without avoidance and with good eye contact; cancellation.
Phase 5: Pullouts, getting smooth control of stuttering in process.
Phases 6–7: Preparatory sets; counseling.

In his 1947 edition of the introductory textbook, Van Riper was not discussing pullouts, and had not seemed to have evolved a clear articulation of the method, when he stated, "If his preparatory sets are still too weak, he can still bring his old blocks under voluntary control [pullouts?]. If he does not manage this, he can cancel" (p. 371). At any rate, the term *pullouts* seems to have emerged formally in 1945-1946 and been a regular part of the goals that were printed and given to stutterers at the clinic. Pullouts were also listed in 1949 as the tenth rung on the therapy ladder (Van Riper, 1949). Many clinicians experimented with having stutterers attempt to relax, gain control, and alter speech behavior during a stuttering spasm. However, Van Riper developed and refined pullouts, particularly in the linkage between cancellations and preparatory sets.

Neurological Speculations

Neurological speculations in pullouts are fascinating. As is the case with cancellations, it is appropriate to speculate on the role pullouts have in cybernetic modeling and neurological charting of inhibitory controls and timing of neuromuscular sensory and motor patterns. Compared to normal speakers, stutterers tend to become more anxious about the onset of speech and are more tense and anxious during speech (Yonovitz & Shepherd, 1977). This fact is supported by the projective findings that tension of stutterers is highest during the spasm rather than before or after (Sheehan et al., 1962). The physiological correlates of anxiety are known, and possible involvement of sensory feedback and neurological timing systems becomes potentially significant. These will make the pullouts harder to achieve, but they will make success all the more rewarding.

Research indicates that stutterers show faster jaw velocities on opening and closing cycles, suggesting a high level of muscle spindle activity (Hutchinson & Watson, 1976)—which makes it difficult to predict and time the coordination of laryngoarticulatory activity. Hutchinson and Watson suggested that pullout efficacy stems from a reduction in gamma loop activity so the afferent signals from muscle spindles are reduced, with a resulting decrement in primary alpha motoneuron stimuli to muscle motor endplates. However, Neilson et al. (1979) did not find any differences among normal persons, those with cerebral palsy, and stutterers in tonic stretch reflex responses to stretching of the jaw, lips, and tongue—although mechanical stretch may be a weak simulation of the complex afferent input of articulation and voicing actions. Early research by Van Riper (1938) showed that stutterers could, on signal, interrupt stuttering spasms and cease speech efforts. He did note that the subjects were anticipating signals to stop and that the stuttering probably invoked little anxiety, embarrassment, or other negative emotions that might be involved with real social communication. Questions and comments by other researchers (Canter, 1971; Overstake, 1979; Zimmerman, 1980b) are indicative of the interest in neurogenic aspects of stuttering in general. Pullouts represent an interesting challenge of explaining and mapping the neuromotor sequence of breaking into an habituated and emotionally conditioned different motor pattern, or slowing and relaxing of the existing motor pattern, among other variables. The explanation will not be simple, but it should be informative and valuable for therapy.

APPLICATIONS OF PULLOUTS

General Applications

General applications of pullouts have been extensive, whether the term is used or not. The publication by the Speech Foundation of America (No. 12) concerning self-therapy for stutterers does not use the label *pullouts* but, instead, refers to the technique as *in-block correction*. It is displaced out of the traditional triad sequence so that it is the third step rather than the second, following the acquisition of preparatory set (pre-block correction) skills. Stutterers are advised to use in-block correction at any time, but especially if they are inaccurate in predicting spasms or if they find themselves going into one. If they are in the middle of a spasm, stutterers are told not to stop and try again but to continue the spasm and let it run its course until it can be changed into a smooth prolongation. A repetitive spasm is to be slowed down, tremors smoothed, or fixations relaxed. While the spasm continues, the stutterer should try to analyze what is being done incorrectly and what is needed to correct or counteract it. If the correction effort (pullout) fails, the failure should be canceled. Overall, the publication does not seem to stress pullouts to any great degree, as compared to cancellations and preparatory sets (p. 125):

> It should not be necessary for you to use this in-block correction often since usually you are aware of approaching trouble and can forestall it by pre-blocking [preparatory set], but you can use this technique when needed.

Their suggestion that most stutterers are adept at predicting their stuttering spasms is open to question. Wingate (1976) feels that stutterers generally do little better than an even chance at spasm prediction. I have worked with clients who were very attuned to the subtle, prespasm indicators; but many of them, even after considerable practice, were often in the middle of a spasm before they were aware fully of it.

Earlier, Van Riper (Speech Foundation) omitted use of the label also but had pullouts following cancellation in the usual sequence. The advice he offered was similar to that provided in the previous paragraph, but it was directed to the clinician rather than to the stutterer. He suggested that the clinician show the client how to search for correct articulatory postures, demonstrate how to relax tensed muscles, and other skills. Another method (see later) is for the clinician to stutter in unison with the client, and by modeling, lead into a pullout. This method also can be reversed so that the clinician starts with a fake duplicate of the client's typical spasm pattern, and the stutterer then joins in, inserting modifications for the clinician to follow.

Shames (1978) presented pullouts as part of the operant program and had them follow the acquisition of cancellation skills. The client is reinforced each time he or she is able to stop while stuttering, pause, prolong the stuttered sound, and finish the word. This seems to be a variant combination of the smooth prolongation and stop-go approach discussed earlier. Ryan (1978) omitted pullouts entirely in his therapy sequence and moved directly from cancellations to preparatory sets. Goven and Vette (1966) followed a typical Van Riper pattern in sequencing and explaining pullouts for older children. Van Riper (1978) again suggested that the control and relaxation techniques practiced during cancellation be applied as completion techniques by speaking in unison with the clinician as the clients practice word production. These various applications of pullouts, and their placing in the triad sequence, provide some indication of how pullouts have been applied and reinforce the clinical aphorism that there may be many wrong ways to do a procedure, but there rarely is just one "right way."

Van Riper's Applications

Over time, Van Riper's organization and use of pullouts have varied, but I have made an effort to combine sources of information to represent his approach. In 1971 (p. 1,004), he noted that "In pulling out of blocks, the stutterer does not let the original blocking run its course as he does in cancellation, instead he makes a deliberate attempt to modify it before the release occurs and before the word is spoken. Basically, through all variations, this has been the form of his approach. In his 1973 (p. 328) publication on stuttering treatment methods, he discussed pullouts extensively and commented several times to the effect that they almost seem to be a semispontaneous development duringor following the cancellation process:

> One of the most intriguing observations . . . is that the modifications . . . learned through cancellations tend to move forward in time to manifest themselves *during* the period of stuttering . . . *as soon as [the stutterer] recognizes that he is in the midst of a fluency failure.*

This effect seems to result from a decision, conscious or not, by the stutterer that if a cancellation is good after a spasm, it is much better to cancel *during* a spasm. However, all clients will need modeling, evaluation, feedback, and support in developing pullouts, and some will need a great deal of help. Van Riper suggests that at the outset, you reward any attempt by the client to change the pattern while it is in motion. Then through a shaping process, in progressive, small steps, bring various elements of the total spasm under control. Your target is for the pullouts to be of the same nature and quality as achieved in cancellation practice.

The steps suggested by Van Riper are simple, but they will require considerable control and skill by both the stutterer and the clinician:

1. Prolong the abnormal posture or movement of the spasm.
2. Evaluate what you are doing in the spasm and how you are doing it.
3. Decide what elements of the stuttering spasm you want to change and how the change(s) can be achieved.
4. *Shift* into the change. Do not stop or pause and then review speech efforts.

Van Riper stated that if a stutterer makes a real attempt to pull out, and fails, it is not necessary to cancel the failure. In using pullouts, I have found early, in-clinic failures are to be expected and are useful as a teaching tool, in which stutterers can investigate the subtle aspects of their spasms more discriminatively. However, when pullouts reach the stage where they are expected generally to be successful, and one fails, I have found cancellation to be a significant reinforcement of control efforts and to uphold the client's feelings of self-efficacy.

Van Riper emphasized the wide range of possible methods leading to a pullout and suggests it is better for stutterers to find it for themselves rather than to be taught a particular pullout pattern as the only method. This statement is particularly significant as a clinician looks at programmed therapies, where it is quite common to have "one way" procedures that the client must conform to. The clinician should provide suggestions, demonstrations, criticisms, and reinforcement but be flexible in terms of what pattern the client finally develops. Personal preferences aside, part of this variability relates to the three different aspects of predominant and mixed stuttering spasms: fixations or syllable repetitions, laryngeal closures, and strong clonic behaviors.

Fixations or syllable repetitions can be dealt with by procedures previously reviewed, in which the stutterer relaxes; shifts into a slowed-down production; and terminates with a prolongation, strong movement, or similar controlled release. The strong clonic, or tremor, patterns (as distinguished from sound and syllable repetitions) concerned Van Riper a great deal. In his experimentation history (1958), he recounted a number of efforts to facilitate rhythmic patterns in his clients, efforts to vary tremor rates, and other approaches. He felt that most stuttering spasms involve a "tremor," which seems to be an oscillatory alpha motoneuron firing, possibly due to gamma sensitization. Van Riper speculated that the tremor was precipitated by a sharp increase in tension of a particular part of the speech mechanism and that this was triggered by an articulatory posture or contact not typical of nonstuttered speech (see the neurological discussion in the next chapter). It also might be a typical posture and contact made with atypical pressure or timing because of anticipatory tension. The tremor tends to be self-sustaining and will not disappear unless its amplitude and/

or frequency reduces sufficiently, or if the stutterer is able to make an abrupt, out-of-phase movement of the speech mechanism to break out. Unfortunately, such nonphase movements are difficult to time and may only result in retriggering the tremor cycle or even increasing muscle tension to the point of tetany and silent fixation (Van Riper, 1971). In the 1973 (p. 328) book on treatment techniques, Van Riper says,

> We cannot overemphasize the importance of tremor modification in the confirmed stutterer. The tremors seem to lie at the very heart of the feeling of being blocked. They seem involuntary, uncontrollable.

Several times he noted where simply simulating lip or other tremors seemed to trigger spasms in some stutterers. In pullouts, he felt the best approach is for the stutterer to decrease the amplitude of the tremors progressively, slow them down, and then shift into the pullout. This may be difficult at first, since many release devices are aimed (futilely) at tremors, and the stutterer has a history of failures to control them.

Laryngeal closure (laryngospasms) was the third trouble area Van Riper identified in pullouts. Whether the spasm was initiated at the vocal folds or whether glottal tension was an overflow phenomenon, the larynx is hard to deal with because of its visual inaccessability, lack of fine tactile awareness, and the reflexlike rapidity of its tension and aerodynamic adjustments. His recommended procedures were these:

1. Deliberately increase the silent, forced, laryngeal blocking, with any associated tremors. This is not really an attempt to phonate but is an artificial exaggeration of the laryngeal tensions.
2. Let the vocal folds relax and shift into vocal fry, as if it were bubbling between the vocal folds.
3. Continue the shift until you can ease into a steady-state vocal fry.
4. Shift easily from the continuous vocal fry into true phonation, and move to complete production of the word.

These steps can be practiced with faked spasms before it is tried with real ones. It is one method only, and others will be noted further on.

With Children

Pullouts by children are much more feasible than were cancellations. Van Riper (1973) believed that unison stuttering (with the clinician) can be used with children to "pull them into pullouts" and that more direct instructions can be used with older children. In general, he expressed the attitude that it is easier to teach the children to replace their existing patterns with new dysfluencies than to modify the old spasms.

Further consideration of using pullouts with children was given by Luper and Mulder (1964). As noted in the chapter on cancellation, their approach to children who are "confirmed stutterers" (presumably a semantic revision of Bluemel's "secondary stuttering") was very traditional. They felt that the child was ready for pullouts "When the child has become proficient in his ability to cancel and cancels the vast majority of blocks satisfactorily in difficult circumstances . . ." (p. 135). They regarded cancellation as a mandatory prerequisite and believed that the analysis and insights stemming from cancellation were needed for pullouts. Their basic instruction for pullouts was that the child, when stuttering, was to keep the spasm going voluntarily until it became a fake. As that occurred, the child was to slow down any tremors, smooth them out, and relax body tensions. The word must be finished with ". . . loose, smooth, but strong movements . . ." of the articulators. They warned that excess tension or speed in the pullout can result in recoil into an involuntary spasm, even after completion of the word.

Luper and Mulder indicated that adequacy in cancellation must be at the 75 percent level of success "at any time" before the child is ready for pullouts. There must be adequate ability in faking spasms accurately and in making a real spasm continue beyond its normal duration. In addition they recommended that the stutterer be able to attack most of the feared words directly, without substitution, circumlocution, or other devices, and that the child should be reasonably able to "avoid his avoidances." In preparation for pullouts, they recommended that the client

1. Stutter, real or faked, in the usual spasm pattern.
2. If the spasm is real, continue it until it becomes a fake.
3. Shift the locus of tension from one body part to another in order to feel tension and its opposite, relaxation.
4. Try to release oneself from the block with a sudden surge of tension, feeling the barrier to control and release.
5. Try, during the spasm, to maintain some other voluntary motor activity (hand movement, eye blink, foot tap) to realize the possibilities of pattern alteration. (This seems to have strong possibilities as a distraction-release device.)

Progress through the steps of the pullout sequence, discussed earlier, rests on the stutterer's ability to control and slow tremors before attempting the pullout. Luper and Mulder have a very useful section on phonetic factors involved in pullouts, noting that the phoneme or syllable that is the focus of struggle presents variable aspects of control and release because of its physioacoustic nature. Stop consonants, fricatives, continuants, vowels— all have their unique constriction or contact characteristics, complicated by context. The authors provide suggestions for dealing with some of these variables. In addition, they present a very useful consideration of release devices that can complicate pullouts (these will be discussed later). They suggest eliminating troubling releases by degrees; having the stutterer do the physical opposite of the release; and temporarily teaching the child competing, contrasting mechanisms to heighten awareness. One may also use penalties and reminders. Their coverage of pullouts is quite thorough, but I believe their program must rest on the assumption that the child has a sufficiently advanced stuttering pattern; awareness; the presence of, or ability to develop, good insight; and the degree of motivation necessary to move first through the prerequisite analysis, desensitization, and cancellation. This is not an easy maturation process for many adult stutterers, and it should be assessed carefully with children. In many instances, a program dedicated to fluency reinforcement may be the most appropriate approach.

Prerequisites for the Client

Overall, prerequisites depend on how you define pullouts and the uses you intend for them. I feel that pullouts are a viable interstage development in a progressing therapy, but I also think they have a continuing value in the efficacy of transfer and the stability of the maintenance program after the client is dismissed from therapy. Most of the sources discussed presumed, or stipulated, that cancellation techniques be learned prior to the development of pullout skills. Modern symptom therapy tends to retain the triad sequence referred to before and to emphasize pullouts because they do not require constant monitoring by the stutterer (Starkweather, 1980). The knowledge and abilities needed for cancellation, indeed the motor patterns used in them, are nearly 100 percent transferable to pullouts. In addition, the tolerance for stuttering and the reduction of fears that develop and increase during cancellation are significant supports to stutterers as they come to grips with a stuttering spasm while it is happening.

Nevertheless, it is possible to teach pullouts as a separate technique and not to precede them with cancellations. Very few clients will be able to start therapy and move directly into pullouts. They will lack many of the basic skills and, even more important, will not have the needed attitude. There will be a great danger that you will wind up teaching the stutterer "tricks," which after habituation has occurred, will no longer work effectively. Even worse, they may become automatic and part of the person's regular stuttering pattern. I remember a painter at my university who, as a child, had been taught the octave twist[1] as a pullout (or release) device, and it had become incorporated into his stuttering pattern. His vocal whoops were audible throughout an entire class building when he was painting there.

In listing and commenting on prerequisites, I will not assume that cancellations have been worked on previously. Pullouts will be presented as an isolated technique for application in an elective sequence of therapy.

---

[1]The octave twist was a sudden, fast increment of vocal pitch up approximately one octave and as quickly back down again. With the pitch rise, there typically was a sharp increment in loudness also.

1. There should be an acceptance of stuttering by the client, with the understanding that it is his or her problem to solve, not yours.
2. The client should have a tolerance for stuttering so that situational fears, feared words, and general speaking avoidances are reduced significantly (from pretherapy), as are specific avoidances associated with individual stuttering spasms.
3. The client should have a thorough knowledge about her or his overall stuttering spasms, behaviors during the spasms, and overall behaviors as a stutterer.
4. The client needs to be able to analyze any particular spasm that occurs, covering all aspects. This refers to postspasm analysis, and it must be feasible in real situations of any type. A reasonable criterion would be 75 percent adequacy rate.
5. In prior therapy, the stutterer should have learned to use psuedostuttering so that spasms can be faked in any situation, so that personal stuttering behaviors can be duplicated, and so that other forms of stuttering can be produced at will. If it has not been acquired, time should be taken to do so.
6. The stutterer usually needs to know or learn various forms of controlled dysfluency, such as strong movement, bounce, light consonant contact, easy onset, and prolongation. The clinician may be aiming toward one dysfluency form in particular or may want to delay them all for particular reasons. In general, the stutterer will want these control forms in pullouts and will need to practice them.
7. The stutterer must be able to pause during a stuttering spasm (or at least to stop the production effort). If this ability is not available, postspasm stoppage may have to be taught and moved temporally into the spasm.

Individual therapy programs may add or subtract prerequisites. Prerequisites that are evaluated as being absent or weak can be developed further by extra attention before starting on pullouts. The important point is that the clinician should consider why he or she is using pullouts, what they are supposed to accomplish, and where they will lead—and then make a prerequisite list to match against the client. By all means, we should avoid the therapy plan that simply lists pullouts because it is a control method and therefore can be used as soon as motivation and orientation are finished.

You will rarely need to motivate clients to use pullouts. As noted earlier, you may have to discourage them from spontaneously developing pullouts too soon. They offer the stutterer a real opportunity, perhaps the first one, to significantly reduce the duration and severity of dysfluencies. This will be of more significance to them than previously reduced secondaries, greater self-confidence, or increased tolerance. They are being given a chance to become more fluent and less frequently dysfluent, simultaneously. The clinician must not allow this enthusiasm unwisely to hasten the learning steps, basic explanations, evaluation of prerequisite skills, and transfer practice. It is important for the client to understand the basic steps and the sequence plan, and to be aware of the abuses and errors that can occur. Moving too quickly can be very costly if the rush results in failure and a loss of confidence in the method.

Clinicians will require faking skills for teaching pullouts since all modeling and demonstrating requires faking. You must be able to produce all types and severities of spasms, and especially be able to duplicate the behaviors and variations of your client. Clinicians' acceptance of pullouts usually is good, although the faking part may engender some hesitation. Compared to cancellations, clinicians enjoy pullouts, as the feedback from my classes indicated:

> This was easy compared to the ones on cancellations. Why did you wait so long? . . . I found I jerked just like the stutterers because I was trying to get the fake over and get away. . . . Do stutterers ever do cancellations after they have learned pullouts? . . . My partner says I'm the best puller-outer in the class!

It is absolutely necessary to model a good pullout, demonstrate a bad one, and show the stutterer solutions to problems. What you cannot do, the stutterer may find few reasons to learn.

TEACHING PULLOUT SKILLS

Basic pullout skills are developed in earlier steps of therapy. In teaching pullouts you should start with in-clinic exercises to probe the skills and knowledge of your client. Explain to the stutterer what skills are needed, why you are checking on them, and what you will do in the process.

1. Have the stutterers read word lists, sentences, and paragraphs aloud while you intermittently signal with a tone, bell, movements, and so forth. Mask your movements. On each signal the clients should stop during the production of the word, holding the articulatory postures of that moment. Periodically ask questions about the postures, eliciting descriptions of them and relating them to the phonemes involved. This technique is just to introduce the idea of stopping and analyzing, so make most of your signals on words that are easy to catch (early in the phrase, polysyllabic words, and so on). Discuss being aware of how the words feel as they are produced. Suggest slowing the rate down to increase awareness of tactile and kinesthetic sensations. A high percentage of stops is not needed, but be alert for the occasional persons who seem almost oblivious to what they are saying; they may need intense practice, or you may have to switch to another technique. Whether words are stuttered or fluent is irrelevant in this practice. A variant technique is to put loud, bilateral noise into the clients' ears so that reliance on tactile and kinesthetic cues will be accentuated (you can switch to visible signals for stopping exercises). Do not run the masking for more than five or so minutes at a time without stopping for auditory rest.
2. Give the stutterers a list of polysyllabic words to read aloud. On each word they should fake an easy spasm and, during the spasm, freeze it long enough to evaluate what is occurring ("freezing" is stopping all efforts to finish a word, while holding the articulators "frozen" in the production position as of the time of stopping). The clients then describe the spasm and answer questions designed to uncover any missed information. Make sure that spasm

types are varied. Model some other types of spasms and request imitation, freezing, and analysis.

3. Repeat the previous step except that when the clients freeze the spasm, they put as much tension, pressure, and effort into the speech mechanism as possible without discomfort. The "hard freeze" should be held briefly; then the clients should overtly relax and finish the word.

4. Have the clients read aloud, in unison with you, a paragraph in which you have underlined words. On the underlined words fake a spasm, continuing until the clients can blend in and catch your pattern (if necessary, back up for a retrial). When the clients can match your spasm, slow it down and move into a slow, loose, strong, deliberate movement (or some other dysfluency) on the rest of the word. If necessary, immediately repeat the word and spasm again. If you are going to use multiple dysfluencies, you can extend this practice to sample the various types and compare them. Never allow the clients to initiate any words with the dysfluencies, which always must, at this point, be used only to complete words.

The foregoing steps work mainly on the client's ability to become aware (stop) during a word or spasm. Analysis has been stressed, as has been the ability to feel tension and relax from it. You have introduced the stutterer to the idea of completing a spasm with a controlled dysfluency and practiced one or more types. In steps 3 and 4, you should insist on a performance level about 90 percent successful before moving on. I have found that if a client has been through cancellation, these five steps usually can be accomplished (in the clinic) in no more than two therapy sessions. Clients lacking the preliminary preparation may take considerably more time.

Early Misuse

Problems of early misuse with pullouts can develop. During these early stages the stutterers should be forbidden to use pullouts away from the clinic. The dangers of mislearning and failure should be stressed, and you should check regularly with the clients to see if they admit to cheating. In spite of this, probably 70 percent of the clients will cheat because of the strong attraction of pullouts. This should not discourage you from discouraging them from doing it. If they cheat and fail, they are less likely to blame the technique or you, will perhaps listen more to what you say, and will perhaps believe that it pays to follow your guidance. If they cheat and succeed because they do it relatively well, you may have a client far along the road to self-direction and self-control; you may be able to move therapy much more rapidly in this direction. The minority who listen to you and don't cheat may be paying a tribute to your forcefulness and credibility; they also may be too clinician-dependent, lacking in confidence, or anxious about pullouts themselves. Consider all alternatives. Discuss problems with the clients and make a strong effort to find out more about how they are functioning in therapy and in relationship to you. This is a critical stage where clients have to put a perspective on clinical rapport, change in speech behaviors, entertain the possibility of really developing speech control, and face other anxiety-producing developments. Listen, look, and consider all the indicators you find.

Basic Methods

Basic pullout methods can be subdivided into seven parts, which can be learned serially or practiced all at once. The options simplify teaching, depending on the client, and make it easier to concentrate on any particular aspects that are more difficult to acquire.

1. The client must be willing to stutter voluntarily without attempts to postpone, substitute use starters, or otherwise avoid the spasm.
2. The spasm's tension and abnormality must serve as a signal for the client to become highly aware of what is being done, and how, to produce the stuttering spasm. This is a reversal of the old behavior, when the spasm triggered a lack of awareness. The increased awareness is measured by analysis and ability to describe.
3. There must be a decision to relax in order to pull out of the spasm. This may be planning for the total spasm or only partial relaxation in early stages. Planning for relaxation should consider the type of spasm and associated behaviors, degree of stress felt, parts of the speech mechanism involved, physioacoustic characteristics of the phoneme(s) being stuttered on, and a decision about the most appropriate dysfluency mode.
4. The client actually must relax spasm tensions so that articulator movement, phonation, and airflow can be established properly. At first, it may be necessary to exaggerate existing tension points and then relax from the extra tension. Another method is just to continue production of the spasm until it turns into a fake from which a pullout can be made. These steps often take considerable intraspasm time at first, and yet it is important to fulfill them. If additional time is needed to accomplish all the steps, the method of continuing the spasm into a fake is used by many clinicians to provide the needed time and to ease the steps as they occur.
5. With an easy relaxation, the clients must slide into the pullout, using the selected dysfluency mode. They concentrate on the tactile and kinesthetic cues rather than on acoustic signals. Two important aspects are the relaxed movement and the dysfluency element. As will be noted later, two of the most frequent reasons for pullout failures are tense or hurried movement and attempts to complete the word without dysfluency.
6. The clients complete the word as planned. As this is done, they try to cancel any negative behaviors, such as loss of eye contact as the word is finished.
7. The clients try to carry over the feel and process of relaxation of tension into the next several words that are uttered, rather than reverting abruptly to the usual speaking pattern.

These basic steps will give the clients successive targets to work on. Some, or most, of them will be picked up with little difficulty, especially if there has been prior cancellation experience. The first two basics (stuttering openly and in-process analysis) will have had major work already if desensitization and spasm analysis stages of therapy were used. If they were not, I suggest the clinician prepare tangential therapy programs based on these areas. By the same token, clients need to be excellent pseudostutterers. If they are not, another tangential program based on the material in that chapter should be prepared.

Extension

Pullout extension follows the preceding steps. At this point, you want your client to meet the basics of stuttering openly about 90 percent of the time. The second step, analysis, should be performed satisfactorily, in all types of situations, about 75 percent of the time. Consider the basic steps:

1. Building on previous freeze and analysis formats, have clients add a description of how they would pull out of a particular faked spasm. Then have them repeat the fake, using the pullout as planned. Use mirrors and recorders for analysis and evaluation. Do not hesitate to reduplicate an effort many times to make a point or learn a move.
2. During in-clinic sessions have the clients make telephone calls and pull out of involuntary spasms (or faked ones if necessary). Analyze all pullouts, good or bad. Use role playing to rehearse telephone calls if needed. Ask the clients to self-correct errors, try different pullout modes, and generally experiment. Have them make more telephone calls. Since telephoning can be structured, rehearsed, and controlled to a great degree, don't hesitate to spend considerable time with it, and when appropriate, use it in additional solo assignments.
3. Use more aversive stimuli such as DAF, introduction of strangers, role-playing situations from real life, and sensitive topics. Let pullouts accumulate during such activities, recording them for playback and analysis.

At this point you probably should move pullouts to an out-clinic basis (the client almost certainly has anticipated you). From your knowledge of the client, look for the stutter-inducing situations, but with as low stress as possible. Many stutterers will do well at this point, but some will fall off drastically from in-clinic levels. Analyze together very carefully to find why, and then work on these problems with lower stress or in-clinic practice. Suggestions for initial out-clinic work are as follows:

1. Have the client ignore any mild spasms (less than one to two seconds) as they may pass too fast for good pullout efforts.
2. Keep situations as short as possible to reduce the number of pullouts required and to minimize cumulative stress.
3. After each situation, take time for an in-depth analysis. An unobtrusive portable recorder is a great aid (you only want to hear the stutterer) for later analysis.
4. Be sure that you go first in any situation, modeling for the client. If there is a failure, you take the next situation and try to use the word(s) the client failed

on. Then immediately have the client enter a similar situation, also trying to use the same words again (with fakes if necessary).

5. Always leave time for a posteffort analysis, instead of saving it for the next session.

ADVANCED DEVELOPMENT OF PULLOUTS

Problems

Problems with pullouts have been mentioned before. Any learning procedure generates errors, and pullouts are no exception. They can be of poor quality and hurried, with minimal dysfluency, and have other unsatisfactory elements. Primary problems usually revolve around instances when the stutterer cannot move successfully into the pullout, or the pullout slips and snaps back into an involuntary spasm. Every client you work with will have a certain number of such experiences. In those cases it is common to teach the client that the correct procedure is to cancel the failed pullout immediately, or to retrieve the failed pullout by faking immediately a stuttering spasm on the word in question and pulling out of the faked spasm. During the therapy program, errors should not only be canceled, but should be analyzed and corrected. This will be particularly important for the few clients who have a large number of unsatisfactory pullouts. In all cases, there are a number of questions that you and the client should answer.

1. Did the spasm slip by and progress so far that it was too late to pullout? This occurs frequently with short spasms, and most clients can only try to catch them, and then be consoled that any spasm so brief probably would be noticed by few auditors. Also, other techniques are more applicable to small spasms. However, if the spasms missed should have been caught, additional practice in self-monitoring, awareness, catching spasms, and stopping is needed.

2. Did it take too long to be aware of and analyze the spasm production, or was the analysis incomplete and faulty? If the answer lies in the first half of the question, sheer experience and practice should solve the problem. If analysis is incomplete or faulty, you must back up and evaluate the degree of relaxation and/or the need for further practice on analysis and evaluation.

3. Was there failure to plan getting control of the spasm and to plan the mode of pullout? Both activities have to be done deliberately at first, and both take time. As the client continues to accumulate hundreds of pullouts, a quickly available self-reference of analyses and solutions develops, easily accessed and taking little time. Anything you do frequently takes progressively less time to perform. You must determine whether the client had the capacity or the information available but did not use it, in which case a penalty may be in order, or whether there was a real weakness involved, which you need to identify and schedule activity for.

4. Was there a failure to relax? You usually can spot this visually by watching the client's face and neck, and it also can be heard on audio tapes from assign-

ments. If hypertension seems to be a problem, you want to consider the reason. If there is an inadequately developed concept of, and procedures for, relaxation, this technique will need specific work. If the reason lies in situational stress, you will need to pay attention to stress reactions and the fear hierarchy and possibly to develop activities in desensitization and relaxation. The following two points may be regarded as products and causes of relaxation problems.

5. Was there any attempt to hurry the pullout? This probably is the main reason for failure among stutterers who otherwise know how to do pullouts (although the basic cause may lie in 4). Pullouts do tend to move forward progressively in the spasm. Many clients unwisely try to pull out before they are ready, so that awareness, analysis, planning, relaxation—all become foreshortened and cannot contribute to the effectiveness of the pullout. Aside from counseling and penalty, it may help such stutterers to practice with assignments where the duration of real and/or faked spasms is preset by the clinician before the pullout can be initiated.

6. Did the stutterer "jerk" into the pullout instead of sliding easily into it? This typically accompanies a hurried effort, but it also can occur on one that is fully analyzed, planned, relaxed, and timed. It is like the sharpshooter who settles the rifle correctly, stands properly, sights carefully, and then jerks the trigger. Similar behaviors occur in pullouts because old habits and fears die hard. Moving into different articulatory sets can be difficult, and a renewal of tension results. The usual outcome is a return of the spasm on the pullout itself. You may want to concentrate on a longer period of faking, use of easy onset, self-signaling for relaxation, accentuation of tactile and kinesthetic monitoring cues, or stress resistance. Also, you may want to look closely at the acoustic characteristics of words on which these failures occur most often and determine whether or not they seem to happen with particular phonemic contexts (see next section).

7. Was the pullout dysfluency suitable to the stuttering pattern? There is relevance here also to the next section. Some stutterers may have a strong preference for one pullout mode and use it inappropriately, when another mode would be more adaptable to the acoustic environment. They also may be trying too hard for the least obvious form of dysfluency. In either case, it is useful to have clients vary the pullout modes and increase their sense of self-efficacy.

8. Was the stutterer trying too hard to be fluent or possibly anticipating preparatory sets? Just as some stutterers, during cancellations, anticipate pullouts, some clients try for an equivalent of preparatory sets during the pullout learning sequence. As before, you should not allow it. The client must understand that a viable pullout is a permanent backup for failure to anticipate and control a spasm in advance (preparatory set) or for fluency reinforcement procedures that slip because of stress or carelessness. As before, counseling, penalty, and assignment of preset spasm durations may help remind the client of proper timing.

9. Was the pullout careless, automatic, or token? Therapy requires the client to perform hundreds of pullouts, and they can become boring or motorically habituated. It is your task to provide motivation, stimulation, and different types of activities and challenges; to use rewards and penalties appropriately; and otherwise to keep the client interested and alert.

10. Are particular spasm tremor patterns or old release devices interfering with transitional movements? If so, they are likely to occur on certain phonemic

contexts and/or in particular stressful situations. The client will need to work for greater relaxation and analysis and follow some of the subsequent suggestions for stabilizing pullouts.

Overall, you will need to decide whether tangential programs are temporarily necessary to correct pullout problems, or whether just additional experience will be sufficient. Most stutterers are quite motivated toward pullouts, but they often can "see daylight" ahead and become impatient with you in the step-by-step procedures of therapy. You will want to guide this enthusiasm and not allow the client to develop a fragile pullout skill that will collapse under pressure or lose vitality over time.

Stabilization

Pullouts are stabilized to assure that they are not a temporary technique but a permanent part of the client's resources. Usually, you are trying to accomplish several goals:

1. Have the stutterer experience a large number of pullouts in a variety of speech situations.
2. Progressively reduce the duration of the stuttering spasms before the pullout becomes effective.
3. Identify and resolve special problems associated with the use of pullouts.
4. Make the client fully aware of and responsible for initiating, varying, and evaluating pullouts.
5. Direct the stutterer toward the use of preparatory sets.

You want stutterers to shift into a habitual use of pullouts and to reach the expert level of proficiency. They should develop confidence in their ability to pull out of any spasm in any situation, so that situational fears are reduced accordingly. The developing confidence should give them the feeling that when therapy dismissal occurs, they have a stable technique to apply in an ongoing maintenance program.

Reducing the length of the spasm is an attractive goal for the client. As progress occurs, severe spasms become less so because duration is reduced and many of the struggle and avoidance behaviors disappear. In addition, the temporal movement of the pullouts toward the point of spasm initiation guides the stutterer toward preparatory sets and further dysfluency reduction. Finally, individual problems with pullouts, or unique error patterns, need to be dealt with for qualitative reasons and to allow the client to have full confidence in the techniques and in the ability to use them. Some considerations or procedures in stabilization follow:

1. The client needs assignments that will generate 50 to 100 pullouts per day. This frequently means faking assignments, and few of your clients, at this stage of therapy, are going to welcome the idea of being a stutterer on purpose. You may need to use strong motivation and personal encouragement,

often. This is normal. In my experience, the degree to which the stutterer, at this advanced stage, holds back, sabotages, or refuses such assignments is a reliable indicator of the future of maintenance or relapse. Other assignments can include days when the client is to try and pull out of every involuntary spasm, keeping a record of situations, words, spasm types and severities, pullout modes, and success. Provide penalties to be self-applied for missed, unsatisfactory, and failed efforts. Try to find a variety of situations for the client, including classroom experience, talks to groups, and other situations. Assignments such as shopping for an automobile, conducting sidewalk or door-to-door interviews, talking with a stutterer just entering therapy, and participating in phone-in radio shows and items from the client's personal hierarchy of situational fears should be used.

2. In the clinic, work with the clients to fake the same spasm several times in a row, pulling out sooner each time. Repeat these exercises, having them pull out in different modes. Work to keep the pullouts unhurried, relaxed, and controlled. Use aversive stimuli (such as DAF) for practice under pressure. Fall back on the old method of prewriting telephone calls, and then repeat the same type of call several times, trying to shorten the spasms (real or faked) each time. You and the clients can agree on the optimum time for spasm-pullout balance, and then they can have all-day pullout requirements where any involuntary spasm that does not meet the time balance must be "canceled" by use of a fake-and-pullout on the same word.

3. Zero in on any special problems the client has in pullouts. As indicated earlier, there may be strong tremors, old release devices, or particular phoneme and syllable postures. Search through your and the client's memory for behaviors that have "disappeared" and bring them back for practice—because you never know when a discarded or suppressed behavior is going to return. Murray (1980) in his personal account of stuttering, recalls the resurrection of severe tremor patterns that had been absent for eleven years. In a very stressful speaking situation, the behaviors he thought dead and buried returned. You will need to determine what factors are operating and exactly what the client is doing or failing to do when the problems occur. Every stutterer will fail on some pullouts at times, but you do not want to leave any sounds, syllables, words, situations, or other variables in a state where the client is *likely* to fail or have trouble. Residual problems that remain unsolved can erode confidence and contribute to relapse. Approaches to the problem can be very individual and hard to anticipate in a general text, but the following suggestions are provided as starters:

   a. For tremors or release devices, have the clients practice isolated fakes and alterations of them to increase awareness and flexibility. Have them fake the problems you are working on, freeze them, exaggerate them, and slowly release from them. If it is feasible, they should try to perform an opposite behavior (if it is a lip tremor, to fake a lip fixation or a different lip tremor; if an upward head jerk, to try to move the head down). They also could, say, try to continue a lip tremor (or head movement) until it became a fake, allowing them to move on.

   b. For localized problems such as tongue posture or laryngospasm, concentrate on having the stutterers deliberately increase articulator or laryngeal tension to a high level and then relax. As the clients relax, have them start an easy airflow, slide phonation onto the airstream, and time articulator movements with the release of the airstream.

   c. For specific phoneme and syllable problems, identify the difficult items and then evaluate them for distinctive features. Research on stuttering

(Wells, 1983) suggests that features of +consonantal, −voicing, +continuant, and −strident are related significantly to stuttering so that it is most likely to occur when primary tension and lack of coordination are lingual and laryngeal and when the speaker must shift from no voicing to voice production. However, expect a lot of individual variation. As you locate specific points, change factors of place, sonancy, stress, and so on as little as possible in fakes or in real productions in order to facilitate movement. It may be helpful to alter a production pattern with a strong, loose, slow repetition and a progressive change on the repeated phoneme; for example a tonic spasm on the /i/ of *either* might begin with a slow and easy /ɛ/-/ɛ/-/ɛ/-/ɛ/, slowly turn into an /I/-/I/-/I/-/I/, slide into a prolonged /i/, and then slide on in to the rest of the pullout. This, or similar procedures, should be temporary, helping the client to learn the tactile and kinesthetic sensations of release and movement on the sound.

4. Emphasize to the stutterer the importance of increasing awareness of the cues that help catch the spasm and achieve the pullout. Have the client read aloud, using stronger and slower, or lighter and easier, articulatory movements in order to increase awareness. During pullout assignments, have the client keep a record of how many spasms could be anticipated (not predicted) before they began and just as they commenced. Then, probe the client about the cues that gave the advance warning. Although this will help lead into preparatory sets it also should help reduce pullout time, aid in catching the smaller spasms, and contribute to solving, or at least reducing, some of the special problems discussed in this section.

Maintenance

Transfer of skills into maintenance is the final value of pullouts. I have made several references to this already, and earlier in the chapter, I spoke of values beyond the role of an interim step in therapy. Van Riper (1971) states that many stutterers should build up self-confidence by deliberately trying to induce stuttering spasms by exaggerating trigger postures and then pulling out. Experimentation with postures and pressures that trigger spasms can be encouraged. As the stutterer receives self-reinforcement (relaxation from tension) by using pullouts, avoidances should reduce; and the client actually may start to search out feared words and troublesome situations avoided in the past, knowing that any failures can be canceled. Retaining the capacity to use pullouts (and cancellations) gives the stutterer a defense in depth against surprise spasms or sudden failures. Transfer of pullouts also should be more attractive to the client because they reduce the abnormality of any stuttering, if nothing else. Also, as a control technique it seems to be very acceptable. In a study involving 200 judges representing various age, sex, and socioeconomic divisions, pullouts were accepted at a level significantly above that of prolongation and bounce techniques. This also was true in separate judgings by stutterers and by speech clinicians (Berlin & Berlin, 1964).

It is very optimistic to talk about fluency for all stutterers, and yet it is an appropriate goal. When some clinicians define "fluency" as 0.5 stuttered words per minute, I am bemused that twenty-five stuttering spasms in a fifty minute class lecture could be called "fluent." I also am puzzled that slow, labored, monotonous, pause-filled speech patterns are labeled by some clinicians as "fluent." The tendency to separate fluent speech and normal speech is, to me, a false dichotomy; normal speech is not necessarily fluent, and fluent speech definitely can sound not normal. Whether the clinician is striving for normal and fluent speech by symptom modification or by fluency reinforcement, it seems appropriate that the client is left with some skills to utilize if slippage or crises occur. Pullouts appear to fill this need handily, and that is why I stress their value in maintenance. I think that other skills, more advanced symptom control or fluency modification, should be developed with the stutterer; but pullouts can be of significant value to the client's feelings of self-efficacy, of independence from the clinician, and for a realization that growth can continue after dismissal from therapy without the need for extensive clinical intervention or "hot lines."

ASSIGNMENTS FOR CLINICIANS

In learning pullouts, you must be good at pseudostuttering, and particularly good at faking in real situations. The mechanics of pullouts will not be especially difficult for you to master, and your biggest problem will be carelessness as you do them. However, if your spasm fakes do not appear to be real and of adequate severity, your pullouts also will be unconvincing. If you know now, or find out in practice, that your pseudostuttering abilities are weak, return to the chapter on faking, and practice until you can play the role of the stutterer convincingly.

1. Use the words provided and read them aloud, faking a moderate to severe spasm each time. Use a mirror and tape recorder. In the middle of each spasm, freeze it completely, establish eye contact in the mirror, and inspect your frozen spasm for three to five seconds. Finish the word, and then describe aloud what you did in the fake (for the recorder).

examination	plagiarism	graduate
assignment	classroom	failure
instructor	experiment	assistance

   Play the tape back, listening to your fakes and descriptions. How adequate were the latter, and how good were your fakes?
2. Use the words provided and a mirror and tape recorder. Read each word aloud five times, faking a different stuttering spasm each time. In the middle of each spasm, freeze it completely, establish eye contact in the mirror, and inspect your spasm for three to five seconds (including tactile and kinesthetic awareness). The words are *elementary, secondary, university*. Play the tape back and listen to your descriptions. How were they? Did all the spasms sound real? How did you vary the fakes? Did your fakes lose "realness" with the repetitions?

3. Repeat assignment 2, including freezes. Instead of describing your spasm after you freeze, finish the word with a pullout. On each of the five repeats of a word, use a different one of the five pullout modes that follow. You may change the list, adding other modes, or combining them differently:

   a. Strong, loose, deliberate, slow movement.
   b. Slow, easy, rhythmical bounce (five to six times).
   c. Light consonant contact.
   d. Initiation of airflow and easy onset of voice.
   e. Breath chewing.

   Play the tape back. Did each series of five fakes sound the same? Overall, which pullout mode(s) did you prefer? Did any of the pullouts feel better on particular words than on others? Did you originate any pullout modes of your own? Overall, using the criteria from earlier in the chapter, evaluate your pullout efforts.

4. Take any word list and read twenty words aloud while using the mirror. Fake a severe spasm each time, varying your spasms. In the middle of each spasm, freeze it. Holding the freeze, increase tension and pressure of production as much as you can. Hold that hard freeze about five seconds while you inspect yourself in the mirror and feel the characteristics internally. Relax the hard freeze slowly and move easily into the pullout mode(s) that you prefer. In general, describe and evaluate your fakes. What pullout mode(s) did you use, and why? Evaluate your pullouts and relaxed movement from the spasm into them.

The previous four assignments were devised to update pseudostuttering and provide experience in evaluating spasms while they were in progress. You also were asked to experiment with a variety of pullout modes to determine your preference(s) and also to relate them to different phoneme and syllable combinations. Finally, you were asked to explore the effects of relaxation by intensifying tension while withholding any attempt to move the articulators. In the next series of assignments, most of this will be repeated, with added items. You are to talk with your partner, not a mirror, and then you are to look at and listen to your partner to gain experience in evaluation.

5. Repeat designated portions (as follows) of each of the first four assignments to your partner, having her or him evaluate your efforts. Write a report of your evaluation of your partner's efforts just as if that person were a client in therapy. Briefly summarize your own efforts:

   a. From 1, on three words fake a spasm, freeze it, and describe it to your partner.
   b. From 2, pick one word and demonstrate five different spasms, freezes, and descriptions for your partner to evaluate.
   c. From 3, do the same as in b, finishing with a pullout rather than a description, and have your partner evaluate.
   d. From 4, select three words to demonstrate, for your partner to evaluate your spasm, hard freeze, relaxation, and pullouts.

6. With your partner, select five sentences and underline one word in each. Read each sentence aloud three times, faking a severe spasm on the underlined word each time, pulling out with a relaxed, strong, deliberate, continuous movement. Read the whole sentence each time. After the first and second efforts, have your partner evaluate you each time verbally, and try to improve your performance on the next effort. Write a report on your partner's problems and efforts, briefly summarize your own.

7. With your partner, underline ten words in a paragraph. Read the paragraph aloud to your partner. On each underlined word, fake a mild spasm and a pullout. Immediately repeat the same word while faking a severe spasm and pull out again, selecting your own mode(s). Continue reading. Have your partner evaluate and write a brief report on your efforts and on his or her own efforts.

8. Talk informally with your partner about any topic. Converse long enough for each of you to collect twenty fakes and pullouts. Fakes should be moderate to severe and your pullout modes varied. If any fake and/or pullout is not satisfactory, your partner is to signal you, and you must immediately cancel the poor performance.

The preceding four assignments moved faking and pullout practice into the context of semi-real situations. Your own evaluation of your efforts was compared to those of your partner, and you were asked to evaluate your partner in order to refine your criteria for judgment.

9. With your partner, make three telephone calls (each) to secure information. In each call, fake one moderate-to-severe spasm and a pullout (your choice of mode). Be sure you have a relaxation pause of two to three seconds before you pull out. Have your partner evaluate and report on them. Did you have any problems? Did you change anything on your second or third calls as a result of the evaluations? What were your feelings? Were your pauses adequate? What kind(s) of pullouts did you use? Compare your performance with that of your partner.

10. In class (if possible) or to a friend, describe your efforts to learn pullouts. During your description, fake and pull out five times, being careful to take several seconds to move into the pullout. Evaluate and report the results.

11. With your partner, stop people and ask directions or talk to people in stores. In each contact, fake two moderate-to-severe spasms and pull out. Make sure the two fakes are different. After each situation, you and your partner verbalize a thorough evaluation of the effort. Do this in three situations (each) and prepare a report that covers the situations, your feelings, the overall speech pattern, fakes (types, quality, severity), adequacy of pauses and relaxation, type(s) and quality of pullouts, and adequacy of evaluations.

12. Select a word that occurs fairly often in your daily speech (for example, *classes*). Then set a target of faking moderate-to-severe spasms and pullouts on twenty-five uses of that word. Don't forget the relaxation pause before moving into the pullouts. Collect them as rapidly as you can, but you can allow yourself up to three days. Keep a written running evaluation during the process, using the criteria discussed earlier. Also comment on the different situations, auditors' reactions, special occurrences, and so forth. Did you have

any problems? Were there any situations where you intended to pull out but avoided it?

SAMPLE ASSIGNMENTS FOR CLIENTS

The following assignments are suggestions for practice in pullouts. Although a hierarchy is attempted, the sequence is only one of many ways to approach the technique. Individual clients, the uses made of pullouts, and their place in the overall therapy sequence, as well as the effect of the clinician's preference, should alter the model assignments as they are used.

1. Go into _____ situations, and each time you stutter, let this be a signal for you to establish good eye contact with your auditor(s). After each situation, write an identification of the situation, the number and severity of stuttering spasms, and an evaluation of your eye contact each time. This assignment is to check your self-control, calmness, and ability to control parts of your behavior. In evaluating eye contact, how soon in the spasm you established eye contact and how well you were able actually to "see" your auditors are criteria. You may elect to go into two, four, or six situations, but you must collect a minimum of ten stuttering spasms.

2. Make telephone calls while watching yourself in the mirror. If possible use a tape recorder. During each call, every time you stutter, freeze the spasm totally until you have looked at the mirror and mentally analyzed everything you are doing. Then relax the freeze and finish the word. After each call, write down the words you stuttered on, the results of your analysis, and what you think you needed to do in order to finish the word. The number of calls is up to you, but collect one of the following spasm totals: ten, twenty, or thirty. If you elect either of the last two options, up to 50 percent of the spasms can be fakes.

3. Take a tape recorder and the word list provided. On each word, fake a mild spasm and a pullout. Then repeat the list, faking moderate spasms and pullouts. Finally, repeat the list a third time, faking severe spasms and pullouts. All fakes should duplicate your usual stuttering patterns. On each spasm, pull out by slowing down and exaggerating your usual pattern until it shifts into a strong, loose, slow, continuous movement. Play the tape back and rate each pullout on a 1-to-5 scale, where 1 = poor and 5 = excellent. In the following words, pay attention to the different speech sounds and whether they have any relationship to the quality of pullouts or to any tendency of some fakes to become real spasms.

parboil	ballpark	sunset	zebra
thinking	themselves	garbage	catch
telephone	dinner	father	visitor
elementary	apple	never	maybe

The first three assignments provide a recheck on willingness to stutter, situation avoidance, eye contact and the ability to control it, presence of mind during stuttering, and awareness of auditors. The basic ability to stop during a spasm without overshooting is tested, as is the client's faking ability. You also are evaluating early on the client's ability to evaluate pullouts and relate them to spasm severity and physioacoustic characteristics of the phonemes involved. The pullout evaluations should be based on practice and discussion sessions in the clinic.

4. Write a description of your typical stuttering spasm as it now exists. Be sure to consider any struggle behaviors and secondaries. Check this description with your clinician and modify it as needed. During the next _____ days collect a number of real spasms in which you continue stuttering until you can turn the real spasm into a fake. As it becomes a fake, eliminate all the secondaries and struggles so that you are left with only a slowed-down version of your basic spasm. If any spasm stays real or returns to real, note the word and other details in your report. Were you able to eliminate mannerisms and struggles on the pullouts? What were your basic spasms like? Describe your auditors' responses. Collect thirty, sixty, or ninety spasms.

5. Call a person on the telephone (your clinician will designate) and explain pullouts to her or him and answer questions. During the conversation, which should last twenty to thirty minutes, fake spasms and pullouts in which you slow the fake spasm down; turn it into a light, easy bounce; and complete the word. If any fake becomes real, stick with it until you can return it to a fake and then pull out. All fakes should be moderate to severe. Collect fifteen, twenty-five, or thirty-five fakes. Describe your results. How many fakes slipped? How many spontaneous, real spasms did you have? How did you feel?

6. Make a list of twenty words which start with sounds that seem hard to pull out on. Add to this up to twenty historically feared words you know (forty in all). Over the next _____) days fake spasms (or have real ones) three times per word (not in a row, but as they occur). Each time, use one of the pullout procedures that follow. If the pullout is not a success, put the word back on your list and try it again, using a different pullout mode:

   a. Strong, loose, deliberate, continuous movement.
   b. Slow, easy, rhythmic bounces (five to eight bounces).
   c. Easy onset of air and voice.
   d. Light consonant contact.

   How many words, in total, did you have to fake? What is your preferred pullout mode, and why? If you had problems, what were they and what seemed to be the cause(s)?

In the previous three assignments, the stutterer experiments with various types of pullouts, tinkers with the spasms to gain better control, and explores possible complications with particular phonemes or old "Jonah" words with their emotional overlays. If problems exist, a lot of them will be identified here for further work in clinic sessions.

7. Premark a selected number of words in a paragraph. Read it aloud. On each underlined word, fake a severe spasm that lasts for at least five seconds or more before you pause, start to relax, slow down, and pull out. Do this on 60, 90, or 120 words. What pullout modes did you use, and why? Did any fakes slip? Evaluate the quality of your pullouts.

8. Read a paragraph aloud under DAF, with the machine set at 200-msec delay. As you read, pull out of every spasm that occurs. Read until you have forty, sixty, or eighty pullouts. If you find that you are not stuttering, speed up your

rate until you do have a problem. How long did it take to reach your goal? Overall, what was your speech like? Evaluate the pullouts.

9. Record yourself as you make telephone calls. Each call should continue until you pull out of a real spasm or fake a severe spasm that lasts five to ten seconds before you relax and pull out. Play back the results as you have done during in-clinic sessions. How many times did you have to fake? What were your real spasms like, and how were the pullouts? What pullout mode(s) did you use, and why? Collect pullouts on ten, fifteen, or twenty-five telephone calls.

The previous three assignments are designed to increase pressure on the stutterer, demand more speech and pullout activity, and give the stutterer more responsibility for selecting and evaluating pullout methods. The final three assignments are designed to continue the increase in pressure, expand verbalization, encourage pullouts to occur sooner in the spasm, and sharpen analysis. Also, some attention is paid to pullouts on small spasms.

10. Over the next _____ days collect the selected number of spasms and pullouts *each* day. If you cannot collect them, the clinician will help by arranging outside assignments in which she or he can be with you and assist. If any pullout is not adequate, immediately repeat the word with a faked spasm and pull out from the fake. Describe your efforts to collect the pullout, the results, and your evaluations. Collect 60, 90, or 120 pullouts per day.

11. Arrange with your clinician to talk to a class or group. Talk for about thirty minutes, describing your stuttering, explaining and demonstrating pullouts, and answering questions. Use pullouts on every spasm. If you miss or if a pullout is poor, stop and explain what happened; then fake a spasm and pullout on that word. How many times did you stutter? How did you feel? How many times did you have to fake, and why? Evaluate the audience's reactions and your own reactions.

12. Enter a number of speech situations and pull out on all spasms you can catch. Do your best to pull out as soon as possible on each spasm. If a spasm gives you trouble, immediately fake stuttering on that word again, and pull out as you had planned to do in the first try. What spasms were hardest to control quickly? Why? How many pullouts were unsatisfactory, and why? If you had any fakes, how did the repeats go? Talk until you collect 50, 100, or 150 pullouts.

This final section emphasized pressure, with a significant increment in the number of pullouts to be collected. The client must pull out a great deal, in all situations, and come to think of pullouts as being possible anywhere, anytime, under any conditions. Self-responsibility was increased, but some samples were to be brought back for checking. Additional assignments will be needed, based on the individual characteristics of your clients.

9

Preparatory Sets

OVERVIEW

A definition and description of preparatory sets have been implied in previous chapters, in a misleading way. Strictly speaking, preparatory sets are not a technique of therapy. It is an incorrect physioanatomical pattern to be corrected in therapy, but the condition became associated with the treatment, and the label was transfered.[1] Behaviorally speaking, *preparatory set* is voluntary and/or a reflex preparation by the organism to respond in a certain way to anticipated stimuli. I include both voluntary and reflex preparation since different conditions can create different sets. You can organize your body systems into a general set so that you are ready to respond to any stimulus, but not necessarily in a specific pattern. However, if I instruct you to shout "stop!" when you hear a particular stimulus, you will prepare a set to perform a very specific action. Similarly, you might "generally set" for a demanding speech situation (reflex level) or specifically be prepared to say certain words when the proper question is asked. Most people tend to adopt a preparatory set prior to initial utterance,

[1]Preparatory set, as will be shown, is neither a technique nor an incorrect pattern. It is a process we all use. The therapy technique we call "preparatory sets" actually is prespasm correction of an *abnormal* preparatory set. However, as with DAF and DAS cited earlier, I will continue the traditional use of the term.

particular phrases, or stressed words or in other aspects of special concern over delivery.

The preparatory set tends to include the combined respiratory, phonatory, and articulatory systems. Frequently, after a major inhalation for speech, we will set the respiratory and phonatory combination with a slight exhalation as the vocal folds adduct to the desired tension and shaping configuration. Some people, speaking normally for them, tend to use a pronounced preparatory set, even to the extent of silently moving the articulators in and out of the appropriate initial position.

During most of speech, normal speakers do not use a static preparatory set but move from one sound to the next. Sounds may be anticipated more than one unit in advance, and articulation postures and movements are delicately altered because of that anticipation. This so-called context effect helps explain the variability of articulation errors and is the rationale for articulation tests that evaluate repeated recombinations of the same phoneme. In stutterers, however, several things occur with preparatory sets:

1. They occur more frequently and inappropriately than in fluent speech.
2. They occur with greater tension and duration than is normal.
3. They may occur with postures or distortions so that proper production of the desired phoneme or syllable is not possible.
4. They may become triggers to set off major tremors that oscillate into involuntary stuttering spasms.

Not all stutterers conform to these possibilities, and probably none of them conform on all occasions. Nevertheless, they are major problems and are the focus of much of our therapy, fluency or symptom.

History

The history and development of preparatory sets, as a concept, is very long, covering centuries. Many stuttering techniques referred to at the beginning of this book had the secondary, or even the main, effect of altering the speaker's preparatory set pattern. Even the use of anesthetic or blistering applications to the tongue (Gottlober, 1953) resulted in either changed tactile cues or altered articulatory postures. Many teachers who concentrated on the proper elocution of speech with "round, pear-shaped tones" actually were altering preparatory sets. However, the European clinician, Freund, claims that he hypothesized the preparatory set in 1932 (1966). As with cancellations and pullouts, Van Riper is associated with preparatory sets in stuttering therapy. Nearly fifty years ago, he defined a preparatory set as a neuromuscular adjustment that precedes the stimulus and selects, determines, and controls the response to the anticipated stimulus. He hypothesized that the preparatory set pattern of a stutterer could be as variable and unique as the different spasm patterns presented by different stutterers. The preparatory set could be respiratory, phonatory, articulatory, or a combination of these. At this time, Van Riper favored the stop-go technique to break up the ongoing preparatory set, a technique he subsequently abandoned (see later). The recommended therapy (including a shift of handedness, if necessary) involved elimination of the overlaid avoidance and struggle behaviors in order to bare the primary or basic spasm and its preparatory sets. The basic symptoms were then attacked with the stop-go to change the preparatory set and complete the stuttering in an altered pattern. As you will remember from the previous chapter, this development probably was part of the pullout evolution (Van Riper, 1937).

Previous therapy (Van Riper, 1958) had involved large amounts of simultaneous talking and writing, group psychotherapy, and voluntary stuttering.[2] Preparatory sets were not mentioned that year (1936-1937) or for several years after. However, the 1942-1943 report indicated concern over their function. During the intervening years therapy had moved closer to dealing with the preparatory set phenomenon. Spasms were faked on nonfeared words, and it was noted that many fakes would turn into involuntary spasms, especially when stutterers attempted to duplicate their typical stuttering spasm. These duplications seemed to trigger tremors far more rapid than usual, leading into the real spasm. Some clients triggered spasms just by adopting a certain articulatory posture. In working with planned variations of the fakes, Van Riper (1958) found that an unaltered number of phonemes, rather than sound and syllable repetitions, seemed to be most desirable (that is, prolong, don't repeat). Also, it was better to use a normal, relaxed, slow production pattern. Van Riper, searching for something to approximate normal utterance more closely, dropped the old form of voluntary stuttering and experimented with "varying" and "dropping," where the client either changed or shaped the stuttering spasm in progress or totally dropped certain behaviors—aspects found across cancellations, pullouts, and preparatory sets.

In the same year (1942-1943) Van Riper reported experimentation with speaking while inhaling helium gas and the effects of dental anesthesia on articulation. The stuttering reduction effects were attributed to the alteration of sensory feedback, shift of focal tension and pressure points, and alteration of motor patterns. They were regarded as support for the concept of altering speech preparatory set patterns to eliminate stuttering triggers. The therapy reports of the next two years (1943-1945) contained no general discussion of preparatory sets, but reference to them occurred in clients' daily self-therapy reports. In 1945 through 1947 there were several references to the use of preparatory sets with cancellations and

---

[2]At this time, "voluntary stuttering" meant the substitution of a highly voluntary and deliberate repetition of the first syllable or sound (not the "easy Iowa bounce") without any of the usual struggle and avoidance behaviors.

pullouts, revision of the habituated preparatory set, and other comments. These included a brief experience with motokinesthetic therapy, which produced no startling results but seemed to emphasize the importance of tactile and kinesthetic cues, both in the monitoring of speech and in the triggering of stuttering spasms. The 1947-1948 summary contained the first definite, sequenced ordering of intensive therapy, including preparatory sets, where Van Riper reported "efforts to vary stutterers' preparatory sets, changing tense, abnormal postures into easy, slow movements." At that time, a client's daily report summarized thirteen cancellations, more than thirty-three pullouts, and forty-three preparatory sets.

Preparatory sets clearly had matured as part of the regular therapy program, and the therapy process had acquired the label from the condition. In 1948-1949, they were the eleventh of fourteen steps, and the clients practiced different ways to initiate feared words with controlled dysfluencies. In the following year, one client's report showed seventeen plans to initiate words with a timed release of air and/or sound, thirty-two plans to start with loose or light contacts, twenty-eight plans to begin with slow and easy movement, and twelve plans to initiate words with the sound following the initial sound as the production target. In following years concern was indicated over increased monitoring of speech through increases in (and greater attention to) tactile and kinesthetic cues. This "high-stimulus speech monitoring" was used as a replacement for preparatory sets, briefly, but clients found it fatiguing and irritating (it will be discussed separately in a subsequent chapter). Incidentally, Van Riper tried having clients monitor emotional feelings (rather than tactile or kinesthetic feedback) as cues but found that too many stutterers became engrossed with their feelings and neglected the stuttering symptoms.

In the last two years of the therapy experiment reports, Van Riper tried the deliberate triggering of stuttering tremors. The clients attempted to study them and then learn to control them by deliberately altering the frequency and amplitude of the tremors. He felt that a major pattern in the stuttering syndrome had been identified for therapy, in which therapy had to attack fears and articulatory triggers of stuttering at the same time. His therapy reflected this philosophy, and preparatory set development was just one aspect of the overall therapy plan. It should be emphasized that the work on preparatory set formation did not occur until the stutterer was advanced in therapy, and Van Riper did not allow the development of artificial speaking patterns as an avoidance of stuttering. These artificial devices did provide awareness and feedback, but why not emphasize feedback from *normal* speech production?

In the 1947 edition of his introductory text, Van Riper briefly described a sequence for preparatory sets in which the stutterer, first, was to rehearse the old spasm pattern, rejecting it and the associated fears.

Then, he or she was to assume a new preparatory set to start the feared word from a position of rest, to look forward to the second sound of the word, and to relax the articulators so that initial sounds were a movement rather than a contact. The major factors were to start the speech attempt with relaxed articulators, synchronizing airflow and voicing, and producing the feared sound as a movement rather than as a posture. Seven years later (Van Riper, 1954), the procedural description for preparatory sets was nearly verbatim to the first. Emphasis was placed on using the controlled utterance to hunt diligently for feared words and situations, and experience them over and over again, while habituating the new motor patterns, extinguishing the old avoidances, and reducing the accumulated reactions of anxiety and fear to communicative stimuli. Bloodstein (1969) summarized Van Riper's prior work on preparatory sets, noting that they attack the characteristics where many stutterers have a tendency to develop muscle tensions in the speech mechanism before an utterance, to adopt fixed articulator positions on the initial sound, and to rehearse or preform the first sound. He felt that changing preparatory sets was a way to help the client toward the goal of ". . . learning to stutter with a minimum of abnormality" (p. 251). This statement basically is true, but I believe the ultimate goal of preparatory sets is to allow the stutterer to initiate speech with normal relaxation, timing, and movement.

Current Applications

Current applications of preparatory sets have not departed too far from the Van Riper developments just discussed. In the latest edition of the introductory text (Van Riper & Emerick, 1984), they are basically unchanged from descriptions provided nearly forty years ago. In another source (Van Riper, 1971) there is extended coverage of cancellations and pullouts, but preparatory set discussion is limited to approximately one paragraph, with no procedural explanations other than ". . . new competitive responses [of pullouts] . . . have moved forward in time so that they now exist as *preparatory sets*" (p. 1,005). The client finds that pullouts can be moved forward in the word to smooth out and slow down, in advance, the tremors of stuttering. In this way the stutterer can control the existence or duration of any spasm, reduce auditors' penalty to minimal or null levels, and alter the abnormal approach-avoidance and avoidance-avoidance conflicts into approach-approach behaviors. Preparatory sets are seen as a logical extension of cancellation and pullouts, the latter being inadequate for "lifetime use" if therapy stopped at that point (Van Riper, 1974a).

Other clinicians have used preparatory sets widely. Luper and Mulder (1964), however, despite their extensive discussion of cancellations and pullouts, only refer to preparatory sets without amplification. Ryan (1971a), omitting pullouts, moves from pseudocancellations to "preparatory sets." In his application the client is told to ". . . prolong any word on which he anticipates stuttering," either on the vowel or the initial consonants. It is taught by the clinician, who models initiation of prolongation, and the client repeats the example ten times. Correct prolongations are reinforced verbally or tangibly, and a success level of 90 percent is the goal. This approach is so different from the so-called traditional approach that it might be more appropriate not to call it preparatory set.

Shames' treatment of preparatory sets (Shames & Egolf, 1976) also lacks some features of the historical model. Following a programmed sequence of cancellations and pullouts, preparatory sets are taught in the following pattern:

1. Instead of stuttering on a word, the client is to repeat the first syllable three times and then say the word fluently. Positive reinforcement is provided for each correct performance.
2. The client performs, and is reinforced, as before—except that the repetitions are reduced to two on the initial syllable.
3. The client performs, and is reinforced, as before—but only a single repetition of the initial syllable is used.
4. Words must be produced without stuttering. Positive reinforcement is provided for fluency and punishment for any stutterings.

This approach would depend heavily on attitude and desensitization to provide any feelings of efficacy for transfer and maintenance. Many other clinicians have applied preparatory sets in therapy. A Speech Foundation of American publication (No. 9) reports the advice of twenty-four stuttering clinicians (in both senses of the term, since all twenty-four stutter). Many of them use and/or recommend the use of preparatory sets. Starkweather (1980) commented that pullouts could be moved forward in time until the stutterer can reduce tension before stuttering. He stated that ". . . this happens only with clients who anticipate their stuttering most of the time, and many do not" (p. 335). This observation is contradicted somewhat in a study in which thirty stutterers read passages wherein they previously had marked words on which they anticipated stuttering. There was a higher percentage of stuttering on predicted words than on those not predicted, and in repeated readings, there was greater consistency of stuttering on those words that had been predicted initially (Martin & Haroldson, 1967).

A current application of preparatory sets in the traditional mode can be found in *Self-Therapy for the Stutterer* (Speech Foundation, No. 12). The label was changed to "pre-block correction," and it is taught *before* pullouts. There is, perhaps, a rationale in self-therapy for reversing the sequence, but I would not recommend it for clinical therapy sequences. It assumes a complete mastery of cancellation (post-block correction) prior to this procedure. The stutterer is told to

1. Anticipate stuttering. (There is an assumption that the stutterer is a pretty good anticipator, but as we have noted, there is disagreement about this view.)
2. Pause before attempting the word, slowing the rate down to a complete stop. As you stop, identify tense areas and completely relax them.
3. Estimate the probable spasm pattern and the nature of the anticipated stuttering, based on past study of and experience with the stuttering, particular words, and specific levels of stress.
4. Plan how to correct or modify the usual initiation of the first sound or syllable.
5. Rehearse mentally, or actually pantomime, how the initiation effort will be performed. Most auditors will recognize that an effort is being made to overcome an obstacle.
6. When breathing is normal, and not before, utter the word with a sliding, resonant, prolonged manner—exaggerating the effort without tension and paying more attention to how it feels than to how it sounds.
7. Complete the rest of the word in the same fashion as in 6, and let the production mode carry over to the next few words, if it feels natural. However, do *not* adopt the mode as a habitual speaking pattern.

The stutterer is advised to practice on words that frequently cause fluency problems. If trouble is anticipated in a speaking situation, the stutterer should spontaneously use some preparatory sets to boost self-confidence and promote relaxation. Also, it is suggested that the stutterer develop a repertoire of different preparatory set patterns for different needs. As skill and confidence develop, the pause-stop aspect can be eliminated because anticipation and prediction will allow the stutterer to slow down and start planning before a particular word is reached.

The previous paragraphs have defined the preparatory set, described its recent history, and provided several examples of current applications. Before moving to therapy applications, it should be worthwhile to examine certain aspects of the neurological control of the speech mechanism and some of the physiological factors involved in speech production.

PREPARATORY SETS IN SPEECH

Neurological Considerations

Neurological considerations relative to pullouts and cancellations (or to any speech controls) were omitted in previous chapters to avoid redundancy and because of the speculative nature of much of our information. However, preparatory sets may be an appropriate point at which to consider briefly some aspects of neuromotor control. The central nervous system (CNS) reflects faithfully the state of the body musculature. To many this sounds contrary to the idea that the CNS "controls" the body's muscles, yet it is the basic concept underlying such functions as the Bobath therapy for cerebral palsy, Jacobson's progressive relaxation, and many other therapies. The body's sensory input determines the functional levels and responses of a normal nervous system. Changing the location, degree, and timing of muscle tension changes the functional pattern of the regulating system. From that point of view, it should be valuable to look briefly at the controlling system and its functions.

Starting "at the top," we deal with the cerebral cortex, and immediately run into confusion, disagreement, and lack of information. Localization, nonlocalization, and association theorists disagree and overlap in a bewildering array of beliefs. Without falling into the dispute, I will propose that our accumulated information suggests that motor speech and speech perception are anatomically related in the precentral gyrus, superior temporal gyrus, insula, somatosensory area, frontal lobe, and premotor areas (Larson & Pfingst, 1982). The old concept of Broca's area controlling motor speech and Wernicke's area decoding and interpreting input, solo, is no longer accepted. How we produce utterances depends on our perceptions and sensory inputs, and our decoding and interpretation are affected by the stored patterns of motor sequences. When the stutterer (or any speaker) organizes a sequence of motor impulses and emits them via the pyramidal fibers to the brain stem nuclei responsible for control of the speech mechanism, they are modified by the basal ganglia and related subcortical areas because of their own feedback loops to those areas and the extensive sensory inputs and relays from the thalamic divisions. Similar modifications, timing, smoothing, and coordinating influences are exerted by the cerebellum with its sensory inputs from exteroceptive and proprioceptive neurons and its motor relays. Part of this system, and more than the parts that comprise it, the reticular formation (or system) functions as a core or hub receiving information from all areas and influencing all structures. ". . . It organizes sensory information through facilitation, inhibition, organization, and synthesis" (Heiniger & Randolph, 1981, p. 189).

The activities of the RAS and RIS (reticular activating and inhibiting systems) components of the complex largely determine our willingness to "notice" certain stimuli and our responses to them. Van Riper (1973) speculated that the abnormal speech postures or sets of stutterers might be linked to reticular activity. Similarly, it may be that his emphasis on practicing preparatory sets under stress relates to applications of reticular activity; that is, learning is facilitated because of RAS stimulation due to stress. What we do with speech behaviors, as we learn them, also is part of the neurological complex. Remembering, extinction, and relapse depend in part on memory, and memory is a neurological phenomenon. In teaching any skill we stimulate sensory areas of the cortex that provide input for retention. Research indicates that the complex of hippocampus, fornix of the corpus callosum, and the mamillary bodies form a facilitating mechanism for the storage (memory) of newly learned data or skills. However, long-term retention of this learning seems to depend on a different mechanism maintained by spontaneous activity of neurons (Espir & Rose, 1970). In short, the methods we teach must be learned for immediate recall and practice and then shifted to "permanent hold."

Thus far, we have seen that motor speech production depends on speech perception (and vice versa) and that neurological control of speech is not a clear, hierarchical pattern. Neuronal units at all levels act on, and are acted on by, centers at other levels. Abnormal movements or positions of the speech mechanism provide a sensory input to the control centers that is stored in immediate and, possibly, in long-term memory functions so that appropriate sensory stimuli can call up these patterns as needed. In addition is the previously unmentioned aspect of emotions. Lamendella (1977) notes that as speech functions shift from sophisticated propositional levels (cortical) down to simpler communications at lower levels, the limbic system becomes progressively involved and speech more and more becomes subject to behavioral imperatives. Where emotion (for example, fear or anxiety) becomes overwhelming, limbic influence could disrupt the neopallial control of propositional speech. His review of research that suggests the left hemisphere acts to inhibit limbic expressions through the right hemisphere raises interesting questions about the studies proposing hemispheric differences between stutterers and nonstutterers. Overall, the performance or learning of motor behaviors is affected by the emotional levels involved, and therapy may deal with this by reducing the physiological correlates through relaxation or desensitization, by removing stimuli from the emotion, or by changing the productive behavior linked to the emotion.

The final step in looking at neurological factors relative to speech production is to consider the high level of automaticity in many of its aspects. The rate of production is too great for step-by-step decisions at subcortical, much less at cortical, levels. Heiniger and Randolph (1981) state that we develop a response sequence by chaining certain simple reflex movements into a series, and we then integrate responses to where a single stimulus sets off two or more reflexes. These grouped responses are sorted and recombined into schema so that they can operate more or less automatically without constant attention—as in our reduced monitoring of speech as we mature. The repetitive performance of motor acts may even affect the synaptic patterns of the columnar neurons of the cerebral cortex, increasing the probability that a particular stimulus (or class of stimuli) will elicit an automatic response (Edelman, 1981). The volitional behaviors of childhood ultimately become mature mandates that dictate adult responses because of neurological presets. There has been a tendency to think in terms of voluntary and reflex motor behaviors, as an exclusive dichotomy, when this is not the case (Kennedy & Abbs, 1982):

> Intermediate between reflex and voluntary motor behaviors are *triggered actions* that comprise complex motor behaviors released by the applications of external sensory stimuli and shaped by previous instruction or intention (rather than stimulus parameters).

Our motor speech behavior involves a range of nervous system functions. These seem to vary from sensory-response servomechanisms for some movements to preprogrammed patterns for others, with an infinite variety of subtle, task-dependent patterns in between.

Neurological control of speech is a complex process. The apparently simple utterance, "My name is John Smith," is an incredibly sophisticated series of separate and combined neurological actions of the respiratory, phonatory, and articulatory systems. These actions combine voluntary motor and spinal reflex motor patterns and variations between those extremes. For stuttering, we would have to add the distortion and interference of emotional reactions to situational and word variables. To ask clients to slow down or start on an easy release of the airflow, when they are habituated to rapid attack or a laryngospasm, is to try to reroute the sequence and timing of millions of neuron synapses away from long- established routes and patterns, and to do so despite emotional interference from the limbic system. However, the point to be made is that emotions can be reduced, and the motor patterns can be altered, and these changes will be reflected in the central nervous system.

Physiological Factors

Physiological factors in production follow neurological considerations. There are many excellent references on this subject in our profession, and I do not need to review it extensively here. Reference has been made to the nervous system's coordination and timing of respiratory, phonatory, and articulatory mechanisms. This coordination and timing is achieved through a mixture of voluntary, reflex, and intermediate sequences already mentioned. Prior to the utterance, respiratory inspiration occurs to a degree required to satisfy the anticipated length of phrase utterance, to be released in ballistic pulses appropriate to the myoelastic-aerodynamic resistance of the vocal folds. The emitted air and/or sound will be modified by resonance shaping and the constriction and interruption effects of the articulators.

Research concerning respiration and laryngeal activity in stuttering will be discussed in the chapter on airflow therapy. For respiration, I refer the reader to Hixon's chapter on the basic aspects of the respiratory system

(Hixon, 1973) and to Zemlin's text (1980) for an excellent review of the respiratory system and physiology. The phonatory aspects of stuttering are of more immediate interest in preparatory sets. Under control of the superior and recurrent branches of the Vagus cranial nerve and its brain stem nuclei, the larynx has been of growing interest to researchers in stuttering. The reader is referred again to Zemlin for overall coverage and to Starkweather's monograph (1982) concerning stuttering and laryngeal behavior. Freeman (1982) summarized a large number of research studies and indicated that their findings support the following statements:

1. The larynx is involved in stuttering to varying degrees.
2. Stutterers appear to have difficulty in both initiating and terminating phonation.
3. Fluency-evoking conditions appear to be accompanied by changes in the manner or timing of phonation or both.
4. In stuttering adaptation, the practice or rehearsal of phonation along with respiratory and articulatory efforts seem critical.

As stated, the larynx is involved to a variable degree in stuttering. Freeman and Ushijima (1978) reported that during stuttering, there was a significant occurrence of cocontraction of the antagonist laryngeal muscles, instead of typical relaxation. They did note, however, instances of the opposite occurring. On fluent utterances, antagonists generally relaxed as expected. Possibly some stutterers, or many stutterers part of the time, are characterized by atypical laryngeal muscle contractions. Starkweather (1982) differentiated between predominantly oral and predominantly laryngeal stutterers and suggested that certain therapy choices can be inappropriate, depending on the predominance presented.

Most attention in stuttering has been focused on the articulators, probably because the tension, tremors, grimaces, and other distortions are either visible or can be related audibly to particular sounds or both. The articulators are limited by their speed, physical constraints, and influences of adjacent sounds and coarticulation effects. If speech efforts are too rapid, there is probability of error. If articulators are preformed into atypical postures, other (proper) contacts are impossible or distorted as they follow. Also, if following sounds are anticipated too soon, the articulator muscles may receive shaping and movement signals too soon from the previously discussed control system, so that production is disturbed. Even the apparently simple condition of verbal environment will affect sound production:

1. Vowels are shortened at the beginning of words and sentences, compared to other locations.
2. Vowels and consonants, both, are shorter in long than in brief utterances. As we speak longer, we tend to speak faster and clip our phonemes.

3. After a pause, phonemes tend to be shortened.
4. Consonants initiating a word generally are longer than middle or final consonants.
5. Consonants and vowels generally are longer in stressed than in unstressed syllables.
6. Consonants are longer in shorter words than in longer words.

The foregoing refer to normal production and omit considerations of information, situational complexity, speaker's stress, or other effects. As the studies indicate, we err when we look at a speech sound as "a sound," as an isolated production posture or contact (Daniloff et al., 1980, p. 334):

> Indeed, the sounds of speech are not separate entities, free to be changed at will. Individual sounds occur within a sound pattern for a given language. The sound pattern is like a fishnet. Each sound within the net stands connected to and in opposition to all other sounds in the pattern. Change of one sound tends to release compensatory shifts for many of the other sounds in the pattern.

It seems clear that we cannot separate respiration, phonation, and articulation; that is, an effect on one produces changes in the others. Small wonder that it takes children years to establish accurate, coordinated patterns; that there is such diversity in the so-called normal range; and that we often have trouble defining the limits between normal and abnormal. In stuttering, the presumption is that the near-infinite combinations of sound movement sequences become arrested and then deformed by the speaker's efforts to cope with an anticipated fluency disruption. The limbic system may override the cortical (or lower) systems and result in the abnormal preparatory sets, or the reverse may be true. Whether high levels of muscle tension upset coordination and timing of respiration, phonation, and articulation, or whether the system's efforts to overcome disrupted coordination and timing result in high levels of muscle tension, is debatable (Freeman and Rosenfield, 1982). In preparatory sets, and many other control techniques, a deliberate effort is made to break into the previously closed loop of abnormal production and feedback. By interfering through relaxation of peripheral tension, an effort is made to create a "stuttering r.i.p.,"[3] whereby muscle spindles stop sending hyperstimulus messages to alpha motoneurons and spinocerebellar tracts. Similarly, rate is slowed down to provide a more reasonable duration for timing and coordinating movement series and giving proper place to the prosodic or suprasegmental elements. This slowdown, it is hoped, is facilitated by voluntary (cortical) intervention in the release of air through the vocal folds where antagonistic muscles have been inhibited (basal ganglia?) so that phonation has a gentle onset and an on-off cycle appropriate to the beginning and ending of

[3]A borrowing from Bobath's "reflex inhibiting posture," used to establish normal muscle tone and sensory feedback in cerebral palsy therapy.

voicing sounds. Finally, emphasis on monitoring, at least temporarily, increases that capacity overall, and particularly stresses tactile and kinesthetic cues over the mature, habituated auditory routes and makes even more difficult the interposition of reflexive or semireflexive responses to partial sensory signals stimulating habituated, abnormal responses.

Whether these limited events occur or function as described is completely arguable. However, while the preceding statements are hypotheses and not necessarily accurate, none appear to be contradictory to what we know about neurological control and speech production. They do not support or invalidate any theory (even neo-Freudian) and are compatible with fluency reinforcement or symptom control approaches to therapy. They suggest a rationale and, it is hoped, invite experimentation with techniques so that revisions, combinations, and differing applications to different stutterers are encouraged.

Applications to Therapy

The applications to therapy of preparatory sets are somewhat confusing. It is one thing to speculate about the neurological control systems and their function and dysfunction in speech control. However, it is quite another thing to move from speculation to application and attempt to describe how the system breaks down, exactly where the circuit malfunctions, and the particular factor or factors that precipitate the breakdown. I do not want to return to the theory thicket discussed in Chapter 1, yet that confusion ultimately must be resolved if our therapy is to be relevant and adequate. Studies by the thousands have poked and probed at "factors that influence" every aspect we can think of—many of the studies investigating a molecular aspect of an undefined whole. However, at some time, all the points must come together and give us a structure we now lack.

Reference has been made previously to the finding that stuttering (and presumably preparatory sets) is more likely to occur when a speaker must shift from a −voice to a +voice phoneme (Wells, 1983). However, it may be that the problem is focused on the initial consonant and that the apparent deviant formant transitions to a following vowel are the result of initial faulty formation of the consonant and not errors in transition dynamics (Montgomery & Cooke, 1976); that is, the incorrect formation of the first phoneme is responsible for following distortions. This hypothesis may or may not be supported by research suggesting that stutterers, in general, are inferior to nonstutterers in sound-making abilities (Wingate, 1971b). Adams (1978) indicated that there are three types of phonetic transition, two within and one between words. He suggested that these are related to instances of stuttering, which could result from initial incorrect preparatory set patterns on either side of the transition points. At any rate, this suggestion reinforces the significance of the preparatory set.

Another area of application has been in attempting to identify *when* stutterings (or preparatory sets) are likely to occur, since therapy can then focus on such points. The chapter on evaluation extensively discussed anticipation and predictability of stuttering. Many early studies, cited previously, on word position, grammatical function, information level, and so on. As indicated in the previous paragraph, this development often resulted in exploration of very finite possibilities without development of an overall context. However, many researchers have worked at combining factors and collating results. Quarrington (1965) correlated word predictability (high-prediction words seem more probable for stuttering) and sentence position (initial position is more probable), finding that sentence position related more to stuttering occurrences. Another study combined word predictability with word frequency, finding that words with low predictability and low frequency of use were most likely to trigger stuttering (Schlesinger et al., 1965). Tornick and Bloodstein (1976) reported that the simple factor of sentence length affected stuttering occurrences, and longer sentences generated more stuttering, as possibly there was increased demand of motor-planning capacities. Frick (1965) reported similar length-related problems and directly involved motor planning. Wingate (1979b, 1979a, 1982) generated a number of studies concerning position, grammar, meaning, and so forth in stuttering occurrences. He suggested that these various factors are not isolated, ranked factors but are linked and driven by the overriding features of prosody, particularly that of stress.

Other approaches to prediction have been based on anticipation of difficulty. Many clinicians have assumed a "law of audience size" in terms of stuttering produced, but Young (1965) reported that advance knowledge and time for anticipation by the stutterer was necessary for there to be a consistent relationship between stuttering and the size of the audience. This finding concurred with a very early anticipation study (Johnson et al., 1963), which reported that definite, or even doubtful, expectation of stuttering was more likely to be followed by stuttering. This conclusion has been confirmed with children, where expectation of being called on in school was found to be a factor in stuttering occurrences. Peins (1961) suggested that expectancy of stuttering (over a period of four days) does not adapt, with reference to reading. In a reverse finding, James and Ingham (1974) reported that reducing the expectancy of stuttering did *not* reduce stuttering. However, their presumption that they actually did reduce the expectancy of stuttering (by verbally assuring the subjects and by using a placebo "tranquilizer") cannot be verified and probably is unwarranted.

Some clinicians have suggested that stutterers are good at predicting spasms, whereas other clinicians disagree. Wingate (1976, p. 27) suggested that prediction operates at no better rate of success than does chance. This is a misleading judgment, however, since it also can mean that any one stutterer is as likely to be accurate in predicting spasms as to be inaccurate in that ability. Avari and Bloodstein (1974) found that about half their subjects did not predict (at all) whether nor not they would stutter, but those who predicted tended to stutter on those words. Similar findings occurred in another study (F.H. Silverman & Williams, 1972), in which eighty-four stuttering children were evaluated. About half the subjects were able to predict 50 percent or more of their spasms. The authors suggested that children good at prediction might be most responsive to therapy involving recognition of anticipatory feelings and then changing behaviors on the basis of that anticipation. Children who are poor predictors probably would respond better to "expectancy task" types of therapy, where anticipation is not a critical factor. This varied ability may have been involved in Lanyon's suggestion that high adaptation and low consistency (that is, weak prediction) may correlate with improvement in therapy (Lanyon, 1965).

Whether anticipation is a genuine function in which the speaker assimilates sensory and situational cues to make a genuine prediction, or whether prediction is self-serving and predisposes the subsequent occurrence of stuttering, is not important for therapy. The important factor is whether or not it exists. The clinician's error will lie in making an a priori assumption that a client does or does not predict stuttering spasms with any accuracy. The generation of critical, erroneous assumptions about a client's capacities, fears, patterns, needs, or goals can be a major factor in failures in evaluation, establishment, transfer, or maintenance in therapy (Adams, 1983). Not only with reference to preparatory sets should each client be viewed as an individual. Further, whereas behavior such as prediction may be reduced by initial stress and unfamiliarity of clinical exposure and/or enhanced by self-analysis and discussion later in therapy, the actual prediction capacities of a client may not be apparent until hours of therapy have elapsed (Andrews et al., 1983). Therapy dealing with preparatory sets can be facilitated by skill at prediction, since it will zero in on trouble words. However, the previously cited studies on loci of stuttering indicate that the clinician will be reasonably accurate in predicting for the clients, and as the clients learn, will encourage awareness and development of prediction by them.

TEACHING PREPARATORY SETS

Learning by the Clinician

Learning of preparatory sets by the clinician is, for a change, not too different from the learning by the stutterer, except that the clinician does not have to deal with negative feelings or conditioned avoidances. In order to understand preparatory sets and teach them effectively, you should be familiar with the phonetics of production, covered by courses in phonetics, speech science, and/or anatomy of the speech mechanism. Although it has been emphasized that articulation is a continuous movement and not isolated contacts, you should be familiar with the usual postures and movements involved in sound production. The more that is known concerning normal variations in sound production, effects of context, and so on, the better prepared you will be. Advanced study in phonology, experimental phonetics, and similar courses will help. In addition, every client with articulation or phonation problems can help build your information, awareness, and judgment. The lateral lisp, uvular /r/, omitted fricative, vocal nodule, and so on will improve your eye and ear in detecting and evaluating production efforts.

The next significant area is knowledge about stuttering itself, which can be divided into two categories: general information about the characteristics of stuttering spasms, and specific information about when and where stuttering is most likely to occur. This information does not help *you* learn preparatory sets, but it is an important aspect in teaching the client. General knowledge covers material discussed in Chapters 2 and 3—types of spasms, severity, adaptation, concomitants, associated behaviors, and so on. Since preparatory sets are a "subtle" aspect of stuttering, you need to be very familiar with the more overt or major components of involuntary dysfluency. Specific information includes accumulated data from the many studies cited thus far, data that suggest stuttering is more likely to occur

1. At the beginning, usually among the first three words, of sentences or of phrases following a pause.
2. When preceding production has been nonvoiced (surd) and the following production is voiced (sonant).
3. On consonants rather than on vowels.
4. On longer, rather than on shorter words.
5. On content rather than on function words.
6. On words occurring less frequently in our language.
7. On initial syllables, and more on the initial consonant than on the following vowel.
8. When the following word is less predictable by context, grammar, or other factors.
9. On words with greater informational importance.
10. On longer, rather than on shorter, utterances.
11. When the number of auditors is increased.
12. When the stutterer anticipates greater difficulty, overall.
13. When the stutterer anticipates or fears difficulty with a particular word or sound.
14. When a particular word was stuttered on previously, particularly among severe stutterers.

Since you will be modeling and demonstrating preparatory sets to clients, you should have a thorough knowledge of your own speech patterns. Further, you need to enhance any skills you have in self-monitoring by auditory and oral sensory feedback channels. For some of you this will be a problem. As I have noted earlier, people vary in their ability to self-monitor. Some are able to catch small variations in their use of words and modes of production, whereas others are capable of what seem to be incredible spoonerisms, malapropisms, and production errors, with little awareness. Practice can markedly improve your abilities in self-monitoring, but be prepared to accept variation. As a particular point of self-analysis, and this involves the following suggestions, learn the similarities and differences of how you exactly produce different sounds. You will want to note the following items:

1. How do you produce the general phonemes of the English language in terms of structures used, placement, and degrees of pressure and tension involved. Use a mirror and a recorder to help in analysis.
2. Without being exhaustive, how does your production pattern on different phonemes vary with context, stress, following pauses, rate variations, and other factors?
3. Pick several phonemes and listen to and watch other people in their productions of the same sounds. Note variations in position, formation, timing, pressure, and other factors.

Most of these areas are included in the assignments for clinicians, as well as other suggestions to increase awareness and information.

Learning by the Client

This discussion will be more specific than the description in the preceding section, and the sample assignments at the end of the chapter will be reduced correspondingly. As noted before, stutterers vary in their capacities to predict stuttering spasms, yet they can be sufficiently consistent that rereading a passage in which previously stuttered-on words were removed still resulted in significantly more stuttering in the areas adjacent to the words that had been eliminated (Avari & Bloodstein, 1974). This consistency factor, which can vary from stutterer to stutterer, needs to be raised to a level of functional awareness. With some degree of anticipation, stutterers can attempt to change the abnormal preparatory set, but they will not be at all the same in their abilities to predict or to anticipate. In order to alter preparatory set patterns, a stutterer must do one of two things: predict and/or anticipate spasms with sufficient accuracy to control significant spasms, or adopt an altered overall speech pattern so that all motor speech patterns are altered. This latter approach was used by generations of therapists, both well-meaning and dishonest ones, as clients tapped, sighed, waved batons, chanted, swung Indian clubs, and did other things to slow, stereotype, and prolong speech production. After a period of disrepute, these techniques have been resurrected and refurbished in many variations of "speak fluently" programs. The label, of course, is a misnomer for the techniques and refers to the ultimate, laudable goal. However, many clients find that transfer and maintenance of the revivified techniques are, at worst, difficult under stress and with adaptation and, at best, tiring or irritating for months and years of postdismissal life. It is probable that the altered speech patterns will become habituated without controlling the anxiety avoidance behaviors, so that stuttering reappears with the new patterns incorporated into it.

Similar relapses can occur with symptom modification techniques, such as preparatory sets. Criticism of "speak fluently" approaches stems from the lure they have extended to some clinicians to automate clients in rapid, intensive programs without concern for anything but the mechanical procedures taught on a limited, in-clinic basis. Preparatory sets also can be taught inappropriately and misused so they lose effectiveness over time. For best preparation, learning, and transfer of preparatory sets, the following criteria should be considered:

1. Is the stutterer thoroughly familiar with every aspect of the stuttering spasm? This is mandatory, in fine detail, and not just in identifying spasm types and severities.
2. Can the stutterer go ahead and stutter without preliminary avoidance and with a minimum of struggle and associated behaviors during the spasm? Avoidance elimination must include mutism and situational withdrawal and extend to subtler postponements, starters, substitutions, and circumlocutions.
3. Is the stutterer aware of the overall speech patterns of articulation, pronunciation, rate, stress, and other characteristics? It is important to know how one talks when *not* stuttering.
4. Can the stutterer have both the presence of mind and the tactile and kinesthetic awareness to monitor speech as it occurs? This requirement implies a combination of information, anxiety control, and awareness.
5. Prior to this time, has the stutterer developed an ability to control stuttering spasms? It is important to eliminate the avoidances, releases, exaggerated struggle, and other excess dysfluency baggage; but stutterers also need the ability to regain control of their speech through cancellation, pullouts, or other procedures.

The foregoing criteria will be applied in the following procedural steps on preparatory set development. If your client meets some of the criteria, skip the appropriate steps and utilize the ones on which the client needs to work. The steps are not in unchangeable sequence, and you may want to arrange them differently for different clients. Also, many of them will be worked on simultaneously, with emphases shifting as progress is made.

The first step is *clinician analysis* of the stutterer and the stuttering pattern. This step is begun in Chapter 2 with the usual diagnostic assessment, but it continues as therapy goes on. How many of you have said, "I never knew that about you!" to friends and relatives, sometimes after years of close association? Some clinicians tend to regard a diagnostic report as the final, definitive statement about the speech patterns and behaviors of a client. It is useful to reread periodically the initial report to see how many alterations (and corrections) can be made after therapy sessions. Continue to refine the data so that you know more about the history of the client's stuttering pattern, its changes over the years, and its basic variations in different phonemic contexts. After awhile, you should be able to construct a hundred ways in which the client might stutter, given changing variables, and know the shifts in attitude, avoidance, self-confidence, accuracy, and cooperation. There is, of course, no end to this study. You will be continuing it up to the minute of dismissal, and beyond, in maintenance efforts.

The second step is *client self-analysis*, discussed in Chapter 3. As argued there, clients must learn to know themselves and their speech pattern, regardless of the therapy used. The information referred to in Chapter 3, and in the preceding paragraph, is vital for the performance of preparatory sets. The self-confidence and desensitization that come with self-analysis are equally important. As the client progresses through the therapy program, self-analysis should continue as an ongoing study of three areas:

1. The traditional analysis of stuttering and speech behavior, attitudes, and adjustments—continually refining and specifying information.
2. Changes in stuttering behaviors as a result of ongoing therapy, noting things omitted, those altered, and behaviors resistant to change.
3. The characteristics of speech when it is fluent.

You want to inculcate a habituated pattern of self-study and awareness that, in addition to the values cited, will help stabilize maintenance and foster continued growth.

The third step is to *avoid avoidance*. Clients, in progressive steps, must stop avoidance in their speech behavior and stutter in an open, voluntary fashion, maintaining eye contact with auditors. Until speech avoidances are eliminated, preparatory sets cannot be used effectively because the avoidance behaviors prevent, distort, nullify, or mistime during preparatory set rehearsals and productions. Indeed, the first elimination of, say, postponements, actually is an initial modification of abnormal preparatory set behavior.

The fourth step is modification of *behavioral avoidance* in communication. You will note that I suggested modification rather than elimination. Overall elimination, after years of habituation and personality set, cannot be achieved reliably. The development of fluency should stimulate social interactions that were previously avoided and enhance those that were previously minimal, but you are not likely to change the basic social personality of the individual. It will help if you work with the stutterer to develop a triplex fear hierarchy along the lines suggested in the chapter on desensitization. One hierarchy would be traditionally situational and build on a mix of progressive complexity, stress, and prior conditioning. The second list would be of people, combining specific persons and categories such as wife, Aunt Emily, police officer, clerks, my boss, and so on. The third list would be based on speech production and would arrange avoidance stimuli on the basis of "Jonah words" (my name, any numbers, "hello," questions, and so on), particular phonemes or combinations, the first three words of initial utterances, and other factors. These hierarchies should be reviewed consistently and updated as therapy simultaneously reduces and refines them (see the second step).

The fifth step is an ability to *alter stuttering* by some form of symptom control or fluency-inducing speech pattern. As indicated before, preparatory sets are not an initial technique. They are used to make symptom control more total or to apply fluency modes when they are needed (rather than continuous overuse). Clients need the self-confidence of having used cancellations and pullouts successfully, knowing they are there as a fail-safe technique, and they also need the motor pattern modification experiences such techniques generate. Similarly, in fluency control, prior success with rate control or airflow procedures is important so the clients know they can fall back to a homebase slow rate or exaggerated control of air release and phonation onset, if needed.

The sixth step, subsumed by several of the previous steps, is that the client must be able to *relax* as a feared word is approached. The stimuli that once precipitated tension must convert to a signal for overt relaxation. This can be accomplished through other techniques in this book, aimed directly at relaxation, and/or as part of other procedures of which relaxation is a part. It is vital, and it is impossible to develop and use a stable preparatory set program in the absence of consistency in relaxation.

The final step is for clients to develop correct information about how they speak when not stuttering and to *self-monitor* the speech-production process. Speech monitoring involves a heightened awareness of the tactile and kinesthetic processes; it is a compound of the sensory nerve ending distributions and dorsal pathways of the spinal cord and the RAS[4] gating (perhaps) that allows attention to the incoming stimuli. Any monitoring is tiring when carried on consistently, and few people will do so for more than brief periods of time. However, oral sensory monitoring is very helpful in alerting clients to the need for preparatory sets and, paradoxically, in reducing the occasions on which they will have to be used on specific words.

In the sequence for teaching preparatory sets to stutterers, we will assume that most of the procedural steps outlined previously have been met, at least in part, and proceed with more specific steps in the acquisition

[4]Reticular activating system.

of preparatory sets. Because of the triad sequence discussed before, I will assume that the client has had prior therapy with cancellations and pullouts, although other techniques for formats will be referred to at particular points:

1. Review the analysis proficiency levels in the first two procedural steps and assign in-clinic and out-clinic practice work, where needed. This is best done with cancellation and (especially) pullouts. Seek out situations, people, and words from the fourth procedural step to precipitate stuttering, while garnering the added values of desensitization and increase in self-confidence. Concentrate on finer analysis, focusing on prespasm tremors, phoneme variations, and other affecting factors. Concentrate particularly on the immediate prespasm period to uncover clues, such as slight changes in rate, short inhalations, shifts in eye contact, lip tremors or postures, laryngeal strap muscle tightening, that will warn of a probable spasm and its possible form. Your goal here is near 100 percent accuracy in analysis. Even small spasms that fly by should be estimated accurately on the basis of past performance. Use every available method, from in-clinic mirror work to progressive levels of complexity and stress outside the therapy room.

2. Revive, or institute, the previously discussed techniques of stop-go and stop-freeze for spasms. However, the thrust now will be, ". . . as soon as possible, and try to react faster and faster." The client should practice stopping the instant stuttering occurs, even to the point where an auditor would be unaware there was any difficulty. The just-cited prespasm cues should be used extensively. The goal is for the client to utilize stops so that the clinician is caught by surprise. Signal practice can be used, but be careful not to build higher tension levels. If pullouts have been learned previously, continue to work on them, pulling out as soon as possible without losing the qualities of a good pullout. In every case, the stop or the pullout should be followed by a relaxed, slow, normal production of the word.

3. For as long as is necessary, have the client repeat a stop-go or a pullout in a pseudocancellation, where the entire word is reuttered in the same production mode as would be used for a pullout. All negative behaviors should be canceled, and production should be in the slowed-down, relaxed, easy mode. During in-clinic practice, you may want the client to cancel a single spasm three or four times, stop and discuss it, cancel again, and then proceed.

4. Now that analysis, relaxation, stopping, and slow-normal production patterns have been practiced, move the client to out-clinic efforts by using hierarchy situations or people—high enough to secure some stuttering but not high enough to overload the system. With the use of role play, aversive stimuli, and faking, tell the client to practice as follows:
   a. Upon anticipation, slightly slow the speech rate on the syllables or words preceding the probable spasm word. In practice, you can generate a signal that signals the next "appropriate" word for the use of preparatory set.
   b. Prior to the word utterance, mime an abnormal preparatory set, as if it was going to lead into a spasm. Use tension, preformation, and if typical, start a tremor. Do not actually attempt to utter the word.
   c. Pause, review the abnormal preparatory set, and deliberately relax from it. Check to see if there is adequate air supply for the coming production. If there is not, inhale and then recheck relaxation.

    d. Initiate an easy airflow. Once there is a flow of air (not a gasp or gusty sigh), gently add phonation if the initial phoneme is voiced. If desirable, use a slight /h/ sound to start the folds vibrating easily.

    e. With airflow running smoothly and a gentle phonation onset in process, move the articulators *through* the movements needed to produce the sound and lead to the following sound. Do not adopt a set posture.

    f. Complete the entire word with the same slow, easy, light, continuous movement. Do not deliberately prolong any particular sound, but just keep the movement going.

    g. You may let the easy production mode spill over to the next two or three words, but don't attempt to adopt this method of utterance for the general run of speech.[5]

5. Have the client apply the procedures listed in 4 in some controlled situations where the steps are all practice. Utilize persons you bring to the clinic, telephone calls from the client to you or to persons you select, and conversations between the client and family members or selected friends. Evaluate behaviors closely and, if necessary, refer to the next section on preparatory set problems. Have the client keep a record of preparatory set efforts, rating performance with reference to a matrix (see p. 241). Instruct the client to tally as "successful" any preparatory set that observes each of the steps in 4 and *remains under control*, whether it is a really good production sequence or not. For each effort in which control fails and a spasm results, the client is to put an X by each performance area that was omitted or inadequate, entering it under the *Problem Variables* that most applied. In theory, there could be an X for one production in every row and column, but most occurrences result in only a few; for example, Anticipation Prediction may have an X under Situation, Relaxation the same, and Phonation Onset an X under Phoneme. For some clients you may need a column headed J.P.F. (Just Plain Forgot). Use this matrix, or a simpler version, to measure successes against failures, comparing sheer numbers. Also, discuss the results to determine how many failures were due to mild spasms slipping by too fast. Then review, accumulate, and keep reviewing the rest of the matrix to see what part(s) of the preparatory sets fall down and what variables seem to be involved most often. At this point, you want your attempt-success ratio to be 100 percent to 75 percent on severe spasms, about 75 percent to 60 percent on moderate ones, and 30 percent to 90 percent on mild spasms. The last 90 percent is set high because quite a few mild spasms may be missed totally, but when they are caught they rarely should fail.

6. Using the procedures outlined in step 4, and eliminating the mimed rehearsal unless it becomes necessary as a problem solver, practice reducing the time spent on relaxation, review, and airflow initiation. This can be done in the terminal stages of step 5 and then shifted to broader transfer in this step. Using the hierarchy lists discussed before, start the client on the items; be sure you accompany her or him on the initial ones and periodically afterwards. Note: In an intensive program, steps 4 through 6 could be achieved in as little time as one day; in a conventionally paced program, the three steps probably would take about 6 to 10 weeks. Use the matrix idea, suitably modified, from step 5 and, as before, analyze it with the client (see Chart 9-1). On a progressive basis, work for 100 percent performance of severe spasms, 75 per-

---

[5]Certain fluency reinforcement methods do have the clients use their mode entirely, but their target usually is to work for "normally fluent speech" and to return to the high-control mode only when under pressure or need. Preparatory sets in this case would be quite applicable, and the warnings would still apply.

CHART 9-1   *Preparatory Sets Report Matrix*

NUMBER OF SUCCESSES
(make a slash mark for
each one)

PERFORMANCE AREA	PROBLEM VARIABLES				
	Spasm Mildness	Word/ Phoneme	Person	Situation	Other*
Anticipation/Prediction					
Initial rate reduction					
Awareness of tensions					
Pause					
Relaxation					
Adequate air supply					
Airflow initiation					
Phonation onset					
Easy movement					
Slow movement					
Continuous movement					
Following words					

*For example, general emotional and physical state, overall rate of speech, significance of communication.

cent on moderate spasms, and 30 percent to 40 percent on mild spasms, with cancellations setting the last figure back up to 60 percent to 70 percent. (In fluency reinforcement modes, you can "cancel" misses by deliberately uttering the next five to ten words in the base-level modes of earlier establishment levels.)

7. This step is to consolidate a final form of preparatory sets that is smooth and continuous, to search out highly feared words and situations, and to solve specific difficulties that develop. Van Riper (1973, p. 338) states that a "surge of fluency" is typical at this time, where the client may go on talking binges just to experience fluency control and self-acceptance. He warns that stabilization has not been attained yet, and early dismissal would result in operation of Jost's Law: In two learned responses that are competitive, the older response will, over time, tend to replace the newer response. Would that more "package programs" and some clinicians would observe this law! At this point the stutterer's pullouts are

. . . pretty largely a slowed version of the standard utterance. Some writers have misunderstood this and have asked the stutterer to prolong the first sound or the vowel of the feared word. . . . We reject this as being very unwise. We do not want the stutterer to distort the motor sequence by such prolongations; we want the whole sequence to be slowed down, all sounds and transitions proportionally.

The client frequently will resist drudgery of assignments, or even of clinic sessions, at this point, if preparatory sets are operating at or above an averagely successful level. The clinician may need to adopt more of a counseling mode, motivating the client, searching for interesting and stimulating activities, generating stress against the preparatory sets, and generally helping the client. High performance targets should be set, and the client asked to equal or go beyond those cited in step 6. In final stages, mild spasms (one second or less) may be the major problem, and two approaches can be used, in addition to reductions through increasing practice, self-confidence, and relaxation:

a. Use high-stimulus speech monitoring, discussed briefly in Chapter 11, to help in overall speech awareness and in catching minor dysfluencies.
b. Work on general aspects of language, voice, articulation, and prosodic elements. Remember that the majority of stuttering children may have other communication deficits, as well as stuttering (Blood & Seider, 1981). This is discussed further in the next section.

Another focus in this prolonged final step is also discussed in the next section—fears of and adjustment to controlled fluency. Additional counseling and/or referral may be necessary.

Problems

Problems with preparatory sets extend from the very first efforts to the final stages. Although it is a highly motivating target, its complexity and adjacency to fluent utterance can create difficulties. Also, since it is a near-terminal technique, the individual and social characteristics of each client become more significant and can create special problems. In discussing each problem, I will divide it into the early practice and learning stages of steps 1 through 3 (initial), the application stages in steps 4 and 5 (interim), and the refining and transfer stages in steps 6 and 7 (final).

1. An overall mild pattern of stuttering will make it difficult to achieve consistency and adequacy in preparatory sets because of lack of motivation; difficulty in catching spasms; and trouble in effecting a properly timed, patterned preparatory set. If the client is a "mild stutterer," preparatory sets may not be indicated. You may wish to try as far as the interim stages, but do not hesitate to switch to a fluency-reinforcement technique.
2. Mild or not, the existence of a covert-predominant stuttering pattern is bad for preparatory sets, from initial to final stages. Even if covert stutterers learn preparatory set procedures, their camouflage of stuttering behaviors is liable to undermine maintenance and stability. Most stutterers mix covert and overt behaviors and are likely to show some variation in different situations. In general, a covert-predominant stutterer has at least several of the following characteristics:
    a. Extensive, skilled use of substitutions and circumlocutions.

   b. Development of surface-logical postponements that seem to be careful pauses for thought, requests for restatement by the first speaker, searching for the "right word," and so on.
   c. Carefully timed, apparently appropriate gestures and body movements and similarly appropriate words or sounds—used as starters and/or release devices.
   d. Mutism, refusal to speak, "I don't know" answers, and extreme avoidance of speaking situations.
   e. Internal struggle that may be invisible or noticeable only after thorough familiarization. One stutterer, after ten weeks, still had to tell us when she had stuttered.

   Other devices are possible, and you will run into them. It is almost certain this type of stutterer would not survive cancellation efforts, would probably not find pullouts much of an improvement over the present speech pattern, and would be unwilling or unable to open up sufficiently for the proper use of preparatory sets.

3. Reduced talking was a possible aspect of the covert stutterer, but it can be a problem in any syndrome. It often can be compensated for in the initial step because the client, by this time, usually is willing or even eager to talk with the clinician. However, out-clinic speech avoidances may have changed little. Such cases can be dealt with if the interim stages stress motivation, clinician support, and situations carefully selected to generate successes. This pushing-supporting practice will have to be continued in the final stages and planned for in maintenance schedules, or Jost's Law will operate.

4. Dependence on auditory feedback is characteristic of most speakers, although we tend to use it minimally except under special circumstances. There is no clear evidence to support hypotheses that stutterers are more, or less, dependent on auditory feedback. However, sufficient data have accumulated to suggest that, at least, stuttering subgroups differ in certain areas of auditory perception and processing. In most instances, therapy programs in awareness, high-stimulus speech monitoring, masking, and speech chewing will improve monitoring abilities.

5. Occasionally a stutterer will be unable to slow down, relax, and move easily into the preparatory set. Except for the problem source in 7, this failure usually is attributable to anxiety levels that inhibit desired behaviors. In most instances, this is due to the clinician's failure to deal adequately with desensitization, self-confidence, and confidence in the technique and with the clinician's credibility. It may be desirable to plan a program of desensitization or switch to a fluency-reinforcement program.

6. Preparatory sets can fail, or be erratic, because the client is not prepared well in self-analysis of stuttering. This is the clinician's fault and is inexcusable. A temporary tangential program in analysis should correct the problem. However, the clinician must not blame the clients for this problem and must not let them feel they have failed.

7. Rapid rate is counterproductive to preparatory set control; it can catch the clinician by surprise since so many in-clinic exercises occurred at slower practice rates. Excessive rate may be anxiety-linked, an avoidance pattern, a symptom of aggression, or environmentally habituated. It may be possible to use suggestion, monitoring emphasis, and practice to slow down. However, in some cases you may have to go to a rate-control program, such as those suggested in the DAF chapter.

8. As noted before, many stutterers have had other communication problems in the past. Even though most of these problems have been corrected or out-

grown, there may be a residuum. In addition, adjustments to and avoidances of stuttering may have habituated patterns of loudness, pitch, rhythm, inflection, and stress. They usually do not interfere with initial preparatory set work, but they can become a growing problem in interim and final stages, as the client becomes more aware of overall speech patterns. In such instances, preparatory sets will be facilitated, general speech patterns improved, and self-confidence increased by standard voice and articulation improvement or correction procedures.

9. Rarely, in initial stages, somewhat more during interim steps, and often in final activities, the client becomes aware of and concerned about the dysfluencies that are typical of so-called fluent speech. These include hesitations, interjections, postponements, starters, repetitions, mispronunciations, and other breaks. Many of these, of course, have occurred in the speech of the client as part of the stuttering pattern. Clients may become overly concerned about eradicating these normal dysfluencies, fear that they mask returning losses of control, or puzzle about differentiating them from the stutter-associated dysfluencies. Some counseling may be needed to reassure the client, plus assignments to listen (again) to the "fluency" of nonstutterers. In general, clients can be advised to tolerate dysfluencies but to use preparatory set methods on words around the dysfluencies if they want to. They usually stop doing this after a short time.

10. Fear of fluency can be a problem, especially among stutterers who think of themselves as victims. Despite all its negative effects, stuttering can provide a ready excuse for any failure or omission. "Why apply for a certain job? They won't hire a stutterer." Now, a rejection would be for reasons *other* than stuttering. Spouses may become negative as the person they married changes into a fluent or a controlled speaker. Such problems tend to surface during the interim and final steps, if they occur at all. They should not be ignored, but carry them only as far as your skills can be applied. When necessary, refer the client to the appropriate resource for further help.

I have not covered all the problems that can occur or cited all the aids to correct them. In general, at this point in therapy, it is wise to think of your client in whole terms and not just in a stuttering frame of reference. What does he or she need *as a person* to function effectively with preparatory sets?

ASSIGNMENTS FOR CLINICIANS

The first series of assignments are to check your general awareness of how words are spoken and your ability to spot differences. If you have trouble noting differences, you might want to check your hearing acuity; otherwise, keep repeating the practice series until you improve.

1. For a period of at least one week, carry several 3-by-5 cards with you and (unobtrusively) make phonetic notes on how people pronounce various words. Look for obvious utterances such as *liberry* for *library* and *nucular* for *nuclear*, but also listen for smaller differences, such as *pin* for *pen* and *wen* instead of *when*.

2. With your partner, and various friends, alternate recording readings of the

same sentences. Play back several times and note variations in pronunciation, articulation, stress, inflection, and other suprasegmentals.

3. Administer ten to twenty articulation tests, preferably to preschool children. If children or persons with articulation problems are not available, use a dictionary to prepare a list of unfamiliar words and "test" your friends.

4. Ask at least five persons to read aloud the following ten words. As they read, note variations in pronunciation and stress:

deciduous	universal	emissary
obsolete	meritorious	philanthropic
statistical	centennial	reservoir

The next assignment series is intended to focus on how phoneme variations occur. You want to become more aware of your own production patterns but also to pay attention to articulation differences by other people.

5. Using a tape recorder, utter the following word pairs. Listen to the playback and note differences in the transition phonemes and/or differences because of phonetic context. Repeat the list, slowing down your production and trying to feel the transitional effects. In the slowed version, concentrate on continuous movement of the articulators as if each word pair was one word and you were uttering it in slow motion.

got to	want to	he ran	pass tray	walk in
got some	have to	dog ran	pass some	walk on
got a	you to	sun ran	pass bulb	walk good
got it	drop to	fish ran	pass it	walk proud
got free	leaf to	cliff ran	pass on	walk early

6. Repeat assignment 5, only have three other people read the list to you while you record them. Play back and compare their productions to your own and among themselves.

7. Select five words, two syllables or more, that you use fairly often (for example, telephone, breakfast, upstairs, weather, father) and listen to yourself for three days, trying to catch each time you use those five words. Listen for those same words from other persons. Compare their productions to your own.

8. Use the following words in everyday speech. On each use, on the initial phoneme and syllable, apply one of the techniques listed until you have used all of them on every word. Take _____ days to complete this assignment. If need, check the Index in order to review particular techniques.

How did different techniques affect production of the same phoneme? Which technique, overall, did you prefer? What technique(s) did not work too well on what phoneme(s)?

WORDS	TECHNIQUES
hello	Bounce
give	Light consonant contact
I	Easy onset
some	Prolongation
really	
please	
at	

How did different techniques affect production of the same phoneme? Which technique, overall, did you prefer? What technique(s) did not work too well on what phoneme(s)?

The final series of assignments is aimed primarily at increasing your awareness of tactile and kinesthetic stimuli. They also provide experience in self-monitoring. Further practice can be gained by selecting activities from the assignments for clients that follow.

9. Using the audio circuit on a tape recorder or audiometer or an auditory trainer, turn up the volume until your own voice through the earphones is just below the discomfort level. Read material in paragraphs aloud for about three minutes while you record your reading. What happened to your pitch, loudness, inflection, and rate? Play back a few more times. Then read the same material aloud, without earphones, while you try to imitate "exactly" your speech pattern of the first time (amplified). What did you have to do the second time to duplicate the first effort, and how difficult was it?

10. Repeat the procedure in 9. However, mask your voice with white noise, taped music, or other sounds. Be sure it is just below the discomfort level of loudness. Answer the same questions as before.

11. Repeat 10, on your partner, and observe her or his adjustments. If any were different from yours, attempt to imitate them.

12. Set a DAF unit at 200-msec delay, with loudness just below the level of discomfort. Read a paragraph aloud for five minutes. As you read, slow your rate and restrict your phrase length to five syllables or fewer per phrase. Use an easy, strong, continuously moving production. Deliberately exaggerate movements so that plosives "drag" slightly, fricatives "scrape" through articulator positions, and vowels are elongated. Concentrate on feeling the touch and position of articulators as you continuously move through an easy, slow production.

13. In ten situations, utter the first three words of each sentence with a slow, continuous, strong articulatory pattern. Make sure you start the first word each time with an airflow followed by a gentle voicing onset. Report on your efforts.

SAMPLE ASSIGNMENTS FOR CLIENTS

If there is a need to check on, or update, awareness by the client of what is happening during stuttering spasms, draw on the assignments in the self-analysis chapter. Similarly, reviews and reminders of "avoiding avoidance" and relaxation patterns can be drawn from the activities in the chapters on pseudostuttering and desensitization and relaxation. The following assignments will relate more directly to preparatory sets, but the foregoing comments are important; the stutterer must be excellent in knowledge and analysis, good at stuttering openly without avoidance, and at least aware of and able (in easy situations) to relax.

1. Put several 3-by-5 file cards in your pocket. On each card, draw a line dividing it in half. Label one box "Yes!" and the other box "Oops!" For the next _____

days, after every verbal interchange, count the stuttering spasms you were aware of before they happened, and enter that number under "Yes!" Count the spasms that surprised you and enter the number under "Oops!" Write a brief report on the "Oops" factor—situations, words, feelings, and so on that made it hard to anticipate.

2. Repeat the first assignment for ＿＿＿ days, but divide each 3-by-5 card into three boxes. "Yes!" now means you anticipated soon enough to do something to change the spasm, "Barely!" means you caught the spasm just an instant before it happened (too late to change it), and "Oops!" is a total miss. Report as before. What do you think you can do to shift "Barely!" items into the "Yes!" category?

3. Make ten telephone calls to secure information or services. Before each call, review what you are likely to say, and try to predict what words you will be most likely to stutter on. Make the calls and note stutterings. How accurate were your predictions? Why do you think you missed on the words you did not predict, and what can you do to improve your accuracy?

4. Telephone a person your clinician designates and talk for fifteen to twenty minutes, doing most of the talking yourself. During the call, try to anticipate each stuttering. Do nothing if your anticipation is right or wrong. However, for each unanticipated stuttering, pause immediately afterward to relax, and then repeat the word with initiation of airflow, easy onset of voice, and a slow, continuous movement of the articulators.

The preceding assignments can be varied in many ways. Their purposes are to secure practice in anticipation, search for cues that will aid prediction, emphasize simple monitoring, check on factors reducing anticipation accuracy, and introduce (or reintroduce) control patterns that can be used in subsequent preparatory set work. The following assignments concentrate more on situational variables.

5. Bring in your old hierarchy list of situational fears and, with your clinician, review and update it. Don't accept in-clinic evaluations, but check on the situations you feel are not a problem or that you think have shifted lower in the hierarchy (checking can be done while performing the first assignment series). When finished, you should have an as-of-now ranking of your fear hierarchy in communication. How has it changed over time?

6. Complete the Erickson S-24 scale and compare its results to your earlier scores. If possible, ask a person close to you (parent, spouse, sibling, roommate) to fill out one on you (as that person sees you) and compare it to your own evaluation. Discuss the results with your clinician and decide whether special work is needed in any areas.

7. From the first four assignments, and using the fear hierarchy and attitude evaluations, construct a list entitled "Factors Reducing My Ability to Anticipate Stuttering." Review these with your clinician and use or avoid them appropriately as you go through the preparatory set practice stages.

The next assignments sample activities during the initial, interim, and final stages of preparatory sets. They are designed to foster transfer and refinement of preparatory set skills in the clinic and to reduce future problems uncovered in assignments listed previously.

8. In _____ speech situations, *stop* after each stuttering spasm and pause. During the pause, silently mime the articulatory postures you used in the stuttering spasm. Then, relax your speech mechanism tensions and continue talking.

9. While alone, underline thirty "possible stutter" words in a paragraph, and record the passage as you read aloud. As you approach each underlined word, slow your rate by 30 percent to 50 percent on the two or three preceding words. Then produce the word with the preparatory set movements we have been practicing in the clinic. Play back the recording and evaluate your efforts.

10. Without the recorder, repeat 9, but read the paragraph to a friend after explaining what you are trying to do (or call your clinician and read over the telephone). Afterward, ask the auditor for an evaluation of your efforts, and compare that to your own evaluation.

11. You are now at or in stage 6 of preparatory set activity. Take your hierarchy list of situational fears and work on preparatory sets according to the following options. If you fail on *any* severe spasm, on more than 20 percent of the moderate spasms, or on more than 60 percent of the mild spasms, repeat the entire assignment.

    a. In twenty instances (total) of your three or four easiest types of situations.
    b. In ten "easy" and five "medium" situations.
    c. In five "easy" and three "hard" situations that your clinician has approved.

12. With your clinician, discuss and analyze particular words and/or phonemes that have given you trouble in achieving smooth, controlled preparatory sets. Draw up a list of ten troublesome words (or ten words with the troublesome phoneme). If necessary, make several lists. Practice on these in the clinic and at home. Then use each word with successful preparatory set patterns, three times, in real situations. As you eliminate each word, pull in another word from the extra lists.

These final assignments are to improve monitoring skills and to stabilize preparatory sets. The important factors of self-confidence and flexibility are stressed.

13. In _____ situations you are to use preparatory set patterns on the entire first sentence each time it is your turn to speak. Do this to evaluate your rate, tension, and speech pattern. You may use preparatory sets elsewhere in the situation, as you wish or need to. Do this in

    a. Fifteen "easy" and ten "medium" situations.
    b. Ten "easy," five "medium," and five "hard" situations.
    c. Ten "medium" and five "hard" situations.

14. Call a friend or a person the clinician designates. Make sure you talk for at least five minutes. Use preparatory set patterns on every word you utter. What were the effects and how difficult was it?

15. Enter five situations where you will talk for at least one minute each time. Use the preparatory sets as you need to. In each situation, fake one deliberate spasm, pause afterward, say "Let me try that again," and repeat the word with a proper preparatory set pattern.

10

Respiration and Phonation

Organization of this chapter will differ somewhat from previous chapters in that two functional therapy areas are being covered. Some research and therapy have been concentrated on the abnormality of stuttering respiratory habits and have ignored phonation or assumed that corrected airflow errors would be accompanied by improved phonation. Similarly, there is research and therapy concerning phonation that ignore respiration or regard adequate airflow and other respiratory habits as being available for proper use while attention focuses on the laryngeal area. Since the primary biological purpose of the larynx is to function as a valving complex for the respiratory system (protective and regulative), it is not surprising that many studies and therapies combine attention to both areas. This chapter will follow both approaches, separating and mingling the two areas to reflect both aspects.

History

The background and history in respiration and phonation reflect the mixed approaches just mentioned, with respiration perhaps receiving greater historical stress. In the pre-Renaissance period (about second century A.D.), Abu Ali Hussain of Avicenna advised taking deep inspirations before speaking. In general, the tongue (rather than the larynx) was blamed more often in stuttering. In the nineteenth century, there was notable interest in respiration. Thomà, in 1867, cited respiratory malfunction, and de l'Isére, in 1831, recognized two types of stuttering—what we now call "oral stuttering" and stuttering caused by spasms of the laryngeal and respiratory muscles. He recommended, among other things, breathing exercises and work on vocal rhythms. The great European surgeon Dieffenbach, in 1841 assumed that stuttering was caused by glottal spasms, but his treatment of excising a wedge of tissue from the base of the tongue was dropped after a year or so. Gregorie used a mixture of peppermint oil and chloroform to regularize movement of the diaphragm, which is only one example of the many substances applied topically or swallowed by the suffering clients. For laryngeal spasms, part of Bates' complex apparatus, in 1854, included a leather collar for the neck, fitted with a metal plate and set-screw over the thyroid cartilage. The screw, set against a spring, could be turned to increase pressure on and deform the cartilage until the muscle spasms in the larynx stopped (or breathing did). Of tremendous influence in European speech therapy and, by transfer, in America, the great German specialist Hermann Gutzmann (and his son, Albert) stressed breathing exercises among their methods. Into the twentieth century, there was increasing emphasis on breathing, singing, and other regulatory exercises. Scripture, who studied with Gutzmann, opened a clinic at Columbia University, prior to World War I. He used the "octave twist" to impart variety to phonation. Subsequently, a rapid growth of psychotherapy emphases tended to replace some of the phonatory and respiratory approaches, except in many private "schools" where secret techniques were guarded jealously. However, in the 1930s, Froescehls experimented with "breath chewing" as an approach to laryngeal and respiratory coordination with the articulation process (Eldridge & Rank, 1968). A fascinating account of laryngeal release and breath control therapy was provided by Judd (1983) in his writing about the Australian specialist Logue, who in 1926 began work with England's King George VI (then the Duke of York), work that extended over a period of years. He initiated breathing exercises, gargling, intoning vowels at fifteen-second duration, and many other exercises (along with strong suggestion, charisma, and encouragement) to greatly improve his royal majesty's fluency.

By this time, none of the techniques were new. The Schwartz system of the passive sigh is at least 200 years old (Jonas, 1977). Richter (1976) provided a history of breathing exercises and concluded that they are still significant in therapy today. People were, and are, divided in their opinions about breathing emphasis in therapy. Pellman (1947) condemned breathstream therapies, arguing that the techniques were inconsistent and contradictory. He felt that the stutterer had enough problems without worrying about breathing, and he felt improvements that might result would only be temporary. Falck (1969) combined respiration and intonation methods, suggesting that breath control was better applied (if needed at all) after fluency had been established completely. He felt it was better to develop adequate breathing ". . . indirectly as a by-product of improved speech fluency than to try to achieve speech fluency through direct breathing exercises" (p. 91). Proponents of breathing therapy could be found in Robbins (1931) and other early clinicians. Boome and Richardson (1931) recommended that the stutterer learn ". . . to relax his muscles, and to *allow* his breathing mechanism to work of itself, instead of *forcing* it to do so" (p. 86), so that breathing would drop to its desired automatic status. Berry and Eisenson (1945) instructed the stutterer to inhale quickly, on signal, and then exhale and phonate on a set temporal pattern while counting, naming, and so on. Practice in different modes of speech breathing was used to build up monitoring of air use and reserve. Therapy then moved to phasing, choral reading, solo reading, and on into conversation. Muirden (1968) stated that almost all stutterers breathe inefficiently, usually because of upper chest overemphasis and excessive inspiration. Proper breathing patterns were to be learned (diaphragmatic) with ". . . a slight intake of breath which must always precede correct vocalization . . . [if this is not done, the vocal folds are] . . . caught in a stiff, static position from which they must jump suddenly and hurriedly . . ." (p. 34).

Currently, breath control and/or phonation coordination are frequently applied in Europe (Lennon, 1962; Richter, 1976), although Russian speech therapy (Vlasova, 1962) in residential treatment centers does not include breathing exercises for children on the grounds that it disturbs their concentration and makes them self-conscious. Van Riper (1974b) borrowed Fernan-Howe's term, *ablauf*, which is a Germanic combination indicating synchrony problems between respiration and phonation and coordinated articulation. He suggested that this is a third stuttering pattern (in addition to repetitions and prolongations) and noted that it can be a stimulus (preformations?) as well as a response. Therapy procedures are recommended (see later), but they do not involve respiration per se. Van Riper discussed breathing exercises extensively, noting their popularity with such early clinicians as Gifford (1940) and their appearance in Hahn's (1943) classic summary of theories and therapies. He noted current applications around the world and special techniques such as breath chewing and ventriloquism. In general, he feels that most respiratory anomalies are the habituated residual components of naive efforts by stutterers to time the release of speech and will respond better to therapy focused directly on stuttering (Van Riper, 1973, p.75).

> In our opinion most of these [breath training] techniques are at best mere vehicles of suggestion, self-discipline, or distraction.

In his view (p. 75), some of the breathing exercises may aid in breaking laryngospasms and help time the coordination of respiration, phonation, and articulation.

> . . . some of the minor effectiveness of this breath training may be explained in this way. Yet there are dangers in the deliberate control of the breath for speaking.

Van Riper worried that the therapy efforts might further disrupt the automatic respiratory sequence or even turn them into "gross abnormalities."

Some of the current practitioners of respiratory and/or phonatory therapies will be summarized later. Many of the approaches cited in the previous paragraphs involved "breathing," but a major effect of their use was the timed, relaxed initiation of phonation. By the same token, therapy emphasizing phonatory aspects assumes or stipulates an adequate air supply and a normal breathing cycle. Although they have a variable history, respiratory and phonatory therapies are frequent today and deserve inclusion among the techniques available to clinicians.

Preparation of Clinician

Preparation for therapy in respiration and phonation involves both the normal and abnormal aspects of these areas. As in many techniques, it is possible to apply them in rote fashion, with some success. Unfortunately, stutterers do not cooperate by having identical respiratory and vocal fold habits. Indeed, beyond basic similarities, nonstutterers also differ (which will be discussed in the brief sections on normal respiration and phonation). We need to understand the structural, mechanical, and neurological information that underlie both functions. Academic courses in phonetics and speech science acoustics are important, as is study of the normal anatomy, neurology, and physiology of respiration and phonation. Knowing that "most people" are diaphragmatic breathers does not explain those who seem to use upper chest musculature in apparently normal breathing. In addition to the normative bases, you will want to understand the anatomy involved in opposition breathing, reversed breathing, clavicular breathing, vocal fry, adductor spasms, and other abnormalities. If it is possible, you should work with instruments that measure quantity or patterns of respiration (spirometer, pneumopolygraph, pneumotactograph) and evaluate the various phonatory functions (pitch analyzer, sound spectrograph, stress analyzer) and instruments (electromyographs) to detect and record muscle activity. The availability of such instruments can be limited, but you can learn a great deal simply by *observing* the normal breathing and phonation patterns of friends and the abnormal patterns of different clients in speech clinics. You should observe the breathing patterns of stutterers during fluent and stuttered speech. It is important to know what stutterers do and how they vary. Finally, you should practice every technique you are going to use, and if possible, practice on friends. Some of the procedures are hard to explain or demonstrate because so much of respiration and phonation is invisible, involuntary, does not involve high level tactile cues, and can be rapidly variable.

RESEARCH IN PHONATION AND RESPIRATION

Discussion of research in the two areas will become mixed, as in the previous section. However, since stutterers vary in the degree to which one system or the other is involved, some separation will be attempted. After the review, an effort will be made to tie the two areas together before going on to therapy.

Respiration

Respiration research and observation have been conducted for many years in stuttering, consistently reporting anomalies. Murray (1932) stated that stutterers had more variable breathing patterns, identifying six, as compared to two for the nonstuttering group. Weller (1941), in studying over 100 stutterers, found disturbances such as rapid, shallow, and irregular breathing and a predominance of abdominal breathing patterns. In a comparison of stutterers and nonstutterers, Starbuck and Steer (1954) found that the stutterers showed significant reductions in the number of complete abdominal and thoracic cycles but (unlike the nonstutterers) did not show a significant increase in the depth of thoracic inhalation or in the depth of abdominal inhalation or exhalation. Schilling (1960) indicated that the quiet, nonspeech breathing of some stutterers may show short, spastic muscle contractions in the respiratory area. Interestingly, on short CVC words, Adams et al. (1975) reported that airflow, duration, and respiratory volume scores for stutterers (during fluent speech) were the same as, or greater than, the scores of nonstutterers. Hutchinson and Navarre (1977) evaluated stutterers during metronome-paced speech, finding that they (like their controls) showed lower pressures and greater pressure durations during metronome pacing at sixty bpm. However, whereas the airflow rate increased for nonstutterers during pacing, it decreased for stutterers. Intraoral air pressure onsets were much more rapid on dysfluent productions than when the same sounds were uttered fluently elsewhere. Sheehan (1970) summarized a great many observations and research on respiration and seemed to accumulate the following information:

1.   There is greater variability (compared to normal), from moment to moment, in stuttering respiration.
2.   There is no coordination between thoracic and abdominal movements.

3. There is shallower breathing during troubled speech.
4. There is fixation of respiratory muscles during moments of stuttering.
5. There tend to be sharp, rapid initial respirations.
6. There are stereotyped, prolonged inspiratory and expiratory patterns with shorter cycles superimposed as brief interruptions.
7. Stutterers vary among themselves, and there is no "typical" pattern, universal to all.

In brief, then, we are likely to find respiratory problems associated with stuttering, but not in all cases. Further, among those who do have problems, there is no set pattern to the respiratory anomalies. It would seem reasonable to say that airflow therapy will not be the best approach for some clients and that "one way" systems will be undesirable unless the clinician can adapt them to shifting patterns.

Phonation

Phonation research ties into respiratory function because of the linked functional relationship. However, extensive study has been limited to the laryngeal area. Phonatory research has been complicated by the relative inaccessability of the larynx, which limits measurements and confuses interpretations. It has also been complicated by persons who want to believe that the larynx is the key to stuttering (Schwartz, 1974), who argue that the stuttering spasm is centered in the larynx and that therapy should focus on the larynx (Shapiro & Decicco, 1982). Van Riper (1982) on the other hand, agrees that there may be abnormal tension, ventricular adduction, discoordination of reciprocal muscle groups, and other phenomena, but he states, " . . . it seems unwise to attribute the core discoordination in stuttering to laryngeal functioning alone . . ." (p. 403). This reminder should be kept in mind as further research is reviewed.

Use of instruments, such as fiberoptic laryngoscopes (Wolk, 1981) has resulted in reports of vocal fold asymmetry and abduction-adduction conflict. The tendency to abduction on repetitions, adduction on sound prolongations, and abduction on broken words has been reported (Conture et al., 1977), although Revdi (1976) did not find a consistent relationship between external stuttering behavior and internal laryngeal patterns. Using electromyography, some researchers (Bar et al., 1969; Freeman, 1978; Freeman & Ushijima, 1975) have reported that stutterers show, before speaking, increased and prolonged laryngeal muscle activity compared to normal talkers. Also, they have reported reciprocal contraction of antagonists during stuttering (not present during fluent speech). However, not all stutterers showed this reciprocal antagonist conflict. In other research it has been stated that stutterers *and* nonstutterers, when speaking under metronome pacing, lower their fundamental frequency, reduce variability of the first formant, speak more softly, and show fewer variations in loudness. In other words, stutterers and nonstutterers show similar laryngeal behaviors while under the influence of a strong rhythm. With another alteration, singing, it was found that stutterers increased voicing duration without significant changes in their peak or average SPL. Nonstutterers showed significant shifts in the last two measures (Colcord & Adams, 1979). In general, it seems that direct observation or measurement of muscle activity indicates possible abnormalities among stutterers, but not a consistent pattern, and some of the behaviors are similar to (and others different from) those of nonstutterers.

Some clinicians have suggested that the absence of stuttering among laryngectomies is proof of the crucial role of the larynx in stuttering. Other clinicians have reported on stuttering in laryngectomized patients, some of whom stuttered and some of whom were fluent before surgery (Freeman & Rosenfield, 1982; Rosenfield & Freeman, 1983). The significance of the larynx relates directly to points of involvement with the articulatory system in producing voiced sounds. Wells (1983) stated that stuttering was most likely when the primary tension and discoordination are lingual and laryngeal, as the speaker shifts from nonvoice to voiced production. Manning and Coufal (1976) had reported earlier that the fewest stutterings occurred on voiced-to-voiced transitions compared to the other three possible combinations. Adams and Reis (1971) used two reading passages, one of which required 400 percent greater occurrence of no-voice transitions; they found fewer dysfluencies and significantly higher adaptation rates with the "on-voice" passage. In contrast, another study compared mixed qualitative, not quantitative, differences in stuttering factors on the two passages (Runyan & Bonifant, 1981).

It was reported that compared to clutterers, stutterers have greater mean pause times and lower mean phonation times, reinforcing the idea that stutterers have problems with laryngeal initiation (Rieber et al., 1972). This could be explained by the hypothesis that the speaker presets the tension and position of the vocal folds so that vibration starts to occur when constriction and airflow reach mutually critical levels (Gautheron et al., 1972). Stutterers seem to start with too high a vocal fold tension level, so that a stronger than normal airflow is required. This, in turn, tends to create a hard glottal attack and cause, or contribute to, stuttering spasms. Webster (1978) felt that the larynx functions in a distorted pattern and, therefore, disturbs other speech movements. In his view the other abnormalities of stuttering may be learned responses to the basic laryngeal struggle. Wingate (1981) felt it was inappropriate to regard the larynx as a source of stuttering. However, this does not eliminate its involvement in the development and maintenance of stuttering. Jones (1969) recounted a personal contact with Russian radiographic research personnel. Their position was that each articulate sound has a characteristic shaping and volume size of the pharynx. This preset is related to, but distinct from, those of the oral articulators. Since according to the Russian researcher, articulator control is cortical (?), and pharyngeal function is controlled by lower centers, intrusive emotions of anxiety, fear, and so forth can distort the pharyngeal presets. Presumably, this distortion could trigger a stuttering spasm. Adams (1983) argued strongly in favor of applying differentially the evaluation of causation or major involvement of the larynx in stuttering. He felt that it is significant in our understanding of stuttering, but he rejected efforts to make stuttering a laryngeal phenomenon only.

A laryngeal research area that has drawn much attention in recent years is that of planning, timing, and onset-termination phases of vocal functions. Do stutterers respond at a slower pace in initiating and stopping phonation? Wyke (1974) answered in the affirmative, suggesting that some stammering may be a variety of phonatory ataxia. Disruptions could occur because of incorrect phonatory preparatory sets prior to phonation and/or a breakdown in the coordination of reflex adjustments during ongoing phonation. Research has indicated that stutterers are slower in voice initiation time (VIT) on vowels and, with practice, can significantly reduce their VIT measures (Adams & Hayden, 1976). The adaptation effect had been observed earlier when stutterers read passages that involved different requirements for rapid VIT efforts. The poorest adaptation occurred on the passages with the most rapid VIT requirements (Adams et al., 1974). Ciambrone et al. (1983) also found a relationship between VIT values and adaptation, and the correlation was quite low—possibly indicating strong individual variations. Starkweather et al. (1976) tested stutterers and controls on the production of twenty-six different syllables. Overall, the stutterers were about sixty-five msec slower than were normal speakers on a range of syllable types. When particular phonological conditions delayed syllable production by a time equivalent to the delay just cited, the significance factor between the two groups disappeared.

Other timing studies have cited the existence of longer VIT values in stutterers (Hillman & Gilbert, 1977; McFarlane & Shipley, 1981; Metz et al., 1979; Reich & Goldsmith, 1981). One study suggested that stutterers exhibited delayed glottal closure in their respiratory adjustments for speech (Baken et al., 1983). Disagreement on prolonged VIT values for stuttering can be found in the research that indicates no differences between stutterers and nonstutterers on a vocalized and a whispered vowel, although the difference between voiced and voiceless production was significant for the stutterers. In a related study, stutterers as a group did not take longer in production of /z/ and /s/ phonemes, but the severe stutterers *did* take a significantly longer time. The mild stutterers resembled the normal speakers (Venkatagiri, 1981; Venkatagiri, 1982b). Also, Watson and Alfonso (1982) failed to find longer reaction or initiation times among stutterers. However, it was noted that subjects were given a preliminary signal before a response was required, and also, the stutterers tended toward the mild end of the severity continuum. This mild-severe dichotomy was reinforced in a subsequent study (Watson & Alfonso, 1983) in which it was determined that both the period prior to voice initiation efforts and the severity of the stuttering syndrome significantly affected laryngeal reaction time. Janssen et al. (1983) attempted to combine onset measures for phonation and articulation, failing to find a difference between stuttering and nonstuttering groups. However, nearly all the stutterers were at the high end of variability measures, and the authors suggested that patterns, not speed, of activity might be more important.

Comparisons of children to adults have shown different results than those discussed previously. Murphy and Baumgartner (1981) evaluated children aged 4.5 to 6.8 years and found no VIT differences between stutterers and nonstutterers (on vowel initiation) relationship to severity. In disagreement with this finding, Cross and Luper (1979, 1983) evaluated subjects in small age groups of 5, 9, and 18 years or adult, who produced a vowel or pressed a signal key in response to a stimulus. Reaction times for both functions (laryngeal and manual) were significantly slower for stutterers than for nonstutterers, and all groups reduced their reaction times with increasing age. McGee et al. (1981) evaluated stuttering children who read high and low "on-off" characteristic passages (in passage A, 71 percent of the syllables began with stops; in passage B, 77 percent began with continuants). They found more dysfluencies on the first passage, but not significantly so, and they reflected lack of support for the earlier Adams and Reis (1971) study, which stated such a relationship. Finally, Cullinan and Springer (1980) evaluated twenty children who either stuttered or stuttered and had other speech, language, and/or learning disabilities. Using a warning signal, they reported that stuttering children were slower, overall, on both VIT and VTT (voice termination time) values—although the "stuttering +" children showed the greatest time values.

As so often happens, the variety of research procedures, the unwise mix of levels of stuttering severity, and the lack of uniformity in other variables result in incomplete and, to an extent, incompatible findings. However, Freeman (1979) reviewed a large number of laryngeal studies and concluded that the larynx is important in stuttering. He doubted the imputation of cause by some clinicians, but agreed that abnormal or mistimed laryngeal behaviors are important in evaluation and therapy.

In a major contribution, the ASLHA monograph (Starkweather, 1982) on laryngeal behavior and stuttering summarized 125 studies or expositions on the subject. Starkweather examined laryngeal muscle activity in stuttering and concluded that although laryngeal stuttering does exist, it is no more (or less) important than oral stuttering, and there is no proof of causation. He felt that the adaptation studies have done little to assist us in studying laryngeal behavior and stuttering, and that research into vocal reaction time is questionable because of the possible existence of unobserved and unmeasured abnormal muscle activity in other laryngeal or related areas. After a careful review of voice onset and termination time studies, Starkweather felt generally that they have been valuable but have not settled any particular questions about the role of the larynx in stuttering. He pointed out that VIT and VTT also are affected by articulatory and respiratory factors, not just laryngeal ones. Also, the questions of anxiety level, arousal level, and unmeasured (subacoustic) muscle dysfunctions further complicate the picture. After further review and discussion of related areas, Starkweather made several points:

1. During stuttering, the larynx shows abnormal function and timing of muscles.
2. We cannot say that laryngeal behaviors are "primary" in either the causative or in the physiological syndrome senses.
3. In comparing stutterers and nonstutterers, laryngeal abnormalities seem to be of the same nature and significance as the oral anomalies when they are compared.

Through clinical observation over the years, it is obvious that there are "laryngeal stutterers," just as there are also "oral stutterers." Starkweather made a useful point in suggesting that the former type are harder to work with and probably have a poorer prognosis. In another study (Starkweather, 1980) he noted that you cannot work on just laryngeal stuttering (or just avoidances or just anything else). Some of the techniques that propose or encourage such a course do not serve the client well. Just as we cannot untangle phonation from respiration (or from articulation), we cannot separate therapy from the past experiences, learning, needs, and personal goals of the stutterer.

Summary

A summary and review of the preceding research can be done fairly briefly. It is evident that wide separation of the overt events of stuttering is, at best, unwise. Stutterers often show disruptions of respiratory timing, pattern, and control during dysfluencies. They also may show deviations during fluent utterances and in quiet breathing. There can be an extreme range, where at one end, respiratory anomalies appear to be a logical result of stuttering struggle and anxiety arousal, and at the other end, disturbed respiratory patterns seem to be a major component of the stuttering spasms and the overall syndrome. Similarly, laryngeal abnormalities are common in stuttering and show evidence of being present during what we ordinarily perceive as fluent speech. Some stutterers present laryngeal disruptions as a major aspect of their stuttering, whereas others are predominantly oral (or respiratory). Timely initiation, duration, and termination of phonation can be disturbed so that the intricate timing patterns of connected syllable strings are thrown into disarray. Again, whether this is cause or effect is less significant than the predominance, the severity, and the associated struggles. Tying respiration and phonation together simply illustrates the fallacy of trying to categorize stuttering as belonging to only one area of physiology. To say that stuttering is caused by discoordination of the posterior cricoarytenoid muscle is as superficial and untenable as blaming stuttering on malfunction of diaphragm timing (and dosing it with chloroform and oil of peppermint)!

THERAPIES STRESSING PHONATION

Normal Process

The normal process of phonation is not well understood. Anatomists disagree on muscle divisions, structural characteristics, and possible combinations of functions. Physiologists are not clear on all of the sequences and interacting variables involved in phonation. Generally, we accept the theory that phonation is a combination of tension adjustments in the myoelastic (muscle) structures and shaping of the aerodynamic contours of the same structures in the vocal folds. The added factors of air pressure, velocity, and resonator complete a complicated picture. For phonation to occur, the vocal folds adduct as subglottal air pressure increases. As a critical point of closure, or near closure, occurs, the folds are forced apart by subglottal air. Relaxation and muscle elasticity, antagonist muscle contraction, supraglottal air pressure, and the Bernoulli effect help explain closure. We must also add, first, the subtleties of vocal fold vibration to produce a precisely desired pitch, loudness, and duration. Complexity is increased as we consider that each cycle of vibration is affected by the cycle pattern preceding and by the pattern following. Finally, the larynx is affected extensively by the state of the body's limbic system; dry throat, nervous swallowing, faulty phonation, and other laryngeal disruptions—all can accompany anxiety, fear, anger, and other emotional states. Variation in production is normal, and we rely on a complex of sensory receptors responsive to stretch, position, and air pressure to provide reflexive and semireflexive modulations toward whatever is the norm for us. In stuttering, the normal process (possibly including monitoring) is disrupted, either by limbic interruption, faulty learning, neurofunctional insufficiency, or some combination thereof.

Phonation Therapy

Phonation therapy will be covered primarily in the discussion on respiratory therapy. As stated before, many phonatory procedures either build on the basis of airflow control or assume its adequacy. Van Riper (1973) pointed out that Arnot, in the nineteenth century, recommended using a set vowel to precede all phonation efforts in order to secure a timely onset of phonation. Gifford (1940) used a vocalized sigh to initiate phonation, and some of our present-day therapies do the same, or near to it. Van Riper felt that such methods function basically as rhythm techniques, and he rejected them because they can become habituated and may acquire exaggerated and distorted characteristics as time passes. This also can be said about certain stages of preparatory sets if they are not preceded by adequate preparation and followed by further progression in technique. Singing also has been used in many forms, including chanting and intoning. These various methods may allow the stutterer to break a laryngospasm (clonic or tonic) by superimposing a rhythm on which the stutterer may "ride out of" the spasm or perhaps slide into a prolongation and complete the utterance.

Earlier reference in this chapter was made to the *ablauf* problem in stuttering (Van Riper, 1974b), or the asynchrony between respiration and phonation and articulation. Van Riper suggested that many of these stutterers seem to produce a jerky, fragmented, vocal fry phonation, and he offered suggestions:

1. Deliberately adopt the laryngeal block posture typical of the usual stuttering.
2. Produce the tense, irregular, brief vocal fry efforts associated with the usual spasm.
3. Consciously relax the laryngeal tensions and let the abnormal vocal fry smooth out and settle into an easy, relaxed, "bubbling" fry.
4. Without interrupting vibration, and without sudden increases in tension, turn the vocal fry into a soft, easy, continuing phonation.
5. Finish the word.

Vocal fry should be a temporary expedient, just as is the use of speaking on inhalation in some therapies for functional aphonia. Vocal fry also has been called *vocal creak* and *glottal roll*. Breath noises usually are lacking, there is no loudness effect, frequency is extremely low, and there is a distinctive popping or ticking sound because of the slow vibration rate (Greene, 1972; Moore, 1971). I would be reluctant to use the technique unless the stutterer already has an exaggerated vocal fry with tension and fragmentation, or unless I was stymied for something to get phonation started out of a laryngospasm pattern.

After the client becomes proficient in the vocal fry shift to phonation and can perform it on an out-clinic basis (the duration will not be particularly longer or the quality more noticeable than that of laryngeal stuttering), the client can eliminate steps 2 and 3, retaining the relaxation and easy phonation concepts. It may be necessary, first, to drop step 2, retaining a relaxed vocal fry, before eliminating both steps. Van Riper also suggested that the client be assisted in not shaping any articulator preformations or postures until he or she actually is in step 4, the emission of a relaxed, easy tone with a steady airflow.

A different approach to phonatory therapy is the use of biofeedback cues, or EMG signals, to train laryngeal relaxation. Its use in stuttering therapy has not been limited to the larynx. Guitar (1975) taught several stutterers to relax, using analog EMG feedback from different muscle groups. Concentration areas varied among clients (oral, laryngeal, oral-laryngeal). Results were positive, in terms of fluency, but clients varied in terms of their relaxation areas. Another study evaluated the effect of truthful and false signals of tension increases and false decrease signals of EMG feedback from the tension levels of stutterers' laryngeal muscles. Truthful and false increase signals were accompanied by subject manipulation that resulted in a reduction in stuttering frequency. However, false decrease signals did not result in a decrement in stuttering spasms; that is, people can be persuaded that they are more tense than they are but not that they are less tense (Cross, 1977). This raises a perennial question: Does actual biofeedback "do" anything, or is it simply a useful attention-focusing method for symptom modification?

In another approach to phonation control, effects of masking and of rhythm pacing were evaluated (Hayden et al., 1982b). Stutterers were compared on vowel VIT in a controlled condition in which intervals between signal tones varied under masking noise with varied intervals between signals, and under a timing condition in which the intersignal interval was constant and matched the duration of the signal itself. Results indicated that VIT was significantly faster under masking than under the control condition, and significantly faster under pacing than during either masking or normal conditions. In a related study (Hayden et al., 1982a), it was reported that SIT (speech initiation time) values for stutterers and for nonstutterers increased during masking and decreased under pacing conditions. Under all conditions, stutterers' SIT values were longer than those of normal speakers. The significance of timing the onset of phonation is reaffirmed in these studies, but this does not raise timing, per se, to a value above that of techniques that result in a regularization of phonatory timing patterns as an aspect of the therapy procedure.

Perkins et al. (1979) discussed the linkage of phonation to respiration and articulation, emphasizing the mutual interaction effect. They felt that phonatory changes in therapies where whispering or "lipping" occurred (articulation without producing any airflow) were not really dealing with the presence or absence of phonation but with progressive reduction in the complexity of physiological adjustments required (plus a significant rate reduction). They considered the effects of possible reduction of subglottal air pressure affecting the larynx but retained their original points (simplification and rate reduction) because the so-called slow-rate speech therapy results in a stuttering decrease without an appreciable drop in subglottal air pressure. An additional factor may be the increased duration that also tends to occur in slow-rate speech. Also, familiarity of the material and the mode of expression used could simplify motor planning (Healey et al., 1976). Further application of these and related phonatory techniques will be found in the subsequent section on airflow procedures.

THERAPIES STRESSING RESPIRATION

Normal Function

Respiration in normal function is the power source on which phonation depends. The laryngeal valving mechanism abducts to allow inspiration of air into the lungs, adducts to provide the buildup of subglottal air pressure for phonation or physical effort, and reflexively protects the lungs from environmental dangers such as the accidental ingestion of solid or liquid material. Internal thoracic air pressure also depends on a complex of thoracic and abdominal muscles that coordinate agonist, synergist, and antagonist balances as we breathe. Inhalation typically will be through contraction of the upper thoracic muscles, supported by the shoulder girdle and/or by lowering of the diaphragm. The latter action appears to be the more common one. During speech, the rapid changes in air pressure seem to be related to rib cage changes rather than to significant alterations in the abdominal and thoracic relationship. It may be that ballistic pulses of the intercostals are involved. The speaker normally inhales an amount of air that is appropriate for the anticipated duration, intensity, and other characteristics of an utterance. If we are going to say "No, thanks," our inhalation will be short and shallow; if we are planning a long answer, the inhalation usually would be slower and deeper. As we speak, air is exhaled at a (usually) steady rate. In slower, softer speech, air pulses corresponding to syllable releases can be detected, perhaps because of internal intercostal contraction, but these tend to smooth into "ripples" for faster, louder speech. On these ripples, we superimpose the variations in irregular pressure associated with stress, inflection, and other factors.

Following inspiration, especially if it is extensive, there will be a checking action of the respiratory muscles against elastic recoil and relaxation pressures of the thorax. As we will see, this checking action will figure variably in some of the therapies discussed subsequently. Expiration for speech is prolonged greatly, compared to normal breathing for life. As we talk, we must interrupt production for additional inspirations of air, and we tend to minimize this effect by adopting a "thoracic posture" of abdomen in, chest out that facilitates diaphragm movements for rapid inspiratory action. The maintenance and release of air pressure is a complex process involving voluntary effort, blood chemistry, and baroreceptors and muscle spindle receptors of the thorax and pharyngeal tract. Most of the function operates on reflex levels and is particularly susceptible to physiological states associated with stress and anxiety. In the following section we will consider some of the breathing characteristics associated with stuttering (Daniloff et al., 1980; Dickson & Maue-Dickson, 1982; Hixon et al., 1976; Zemlin, 1980).

Respiration Therapy

Respiration therapy has had a long history. Application varies when airflow and control are secondary to a major technique or when the technique takes for granted the preliminary establishment of good breathing habits. Airflow is also found in application, where it is the significant factor and other variables are secondary to it, or apparently so. As a generalization, our experience leads to several conclusions:

1. Many stutterers show major disturbances or distortions of breathstream function, but some clients show it only to the degree where amelioration of the spasm pattern will improve or correct the airflow pattern.
2. The more severe the stuttering, the greater the likelihood that there will be serious airflow problems.
3. Some stutterers display airflow abnormalities as a predominant part of the stuttering syndrome, including use of airflow in postponement, starter, release, and other associated behaviors for avoidance and/or struggle.
4. Some stutterers will display disturbed vegetative respiration, but "variability is standard" in breathing, and we should be cautious in labeling different breathing patterns defective.
5. Therapy based only, or with extreme emphasis, on respiration very likely will be of minimal benefit to many stutterers. Some of them will not present major airflow problems in the first place. Also, too much focus on one approach to therapy leaves the client with unresolved problems in other areas. This criticism can apply to any therapy approach that is too monolithic in its orientation.

Earlier discussion categorized some of the possible respiratory abnormalities of stuttering and the stutterer. Fiedler and Standop (1983) particularly cited speaking on inhalation, speaking on residual air,[1] and reverse and opposition breathing during speech efforts. In evaluating stutterers, the *Disfluency Descriptor Digest* (Cooper, 1982) lists predominance of clavicular or upper chest breathing, asynchronous and disruptive breathing patterns during speech, abnormally rapid or insufficient or abnormally prolonged inspiration prior to speech, and occurrence of dysfluencies near the end of speech exhalation cycles. He also lists additional descriptors concerning pitch, loudness, pausing, and stoppage that involve

---

[1]Residual air, averaging 100 to 1,500 cu cm in young adult males, is retained by the constant intrathoracic negative air pressure. Many persons mention "speaking on residual air," which is not possible. "We cannot speak on residual air, of course, and it is unfortunate that reference to 'residual breathers' or 'residual speakers' continues. Confusion between the terms *residual volume* and *functional residual capacity* . . . may account for misuse of terms" (Zemlin, 1980, pp. 92-93).

or affect the respiratory pattern. Brankel (1961) urges the use of a pneu-motactograph to provide a printout of breathing and diaphragm movements, to effectively evaluate and treat stuttering. Unfortunately, few clinicians have access to such devices. Overstake (1979) states that a "majority" of stutterers have nonsynchronized, quiet breathing patterns in which the even balance between duration and depth of inspiration and expiration is disturbed. He relates timing to normal cardiac rhythms where each cycle lasts two to three pulse beats in normal respiration. According to Overstake, there may be short inspirations and long exhalations, with several rapid cycles being followed by a period of apnea, and then a deep inhalation, and so on. He also cites other irregularities previously discussed, plus stutterers' attempts to initiate phonation during the "set" or transition period between inspiration and expiration. In general terms, there are a number of characteristics that can be evaluated in assessing the client's respiratory pattern:

1. Record vital capacity, or the maximum amount of air that can be exhaled following the deepest inhalation possible, by a volume measurement device, such as a wet or dry spirometer. If no equipment is available, use two very rule-of-thumb measures. For both measures clients should first inhale the maximum amount of air possible.
   a. The clients hold their breath for a minimum of fifteen seconds; most people can hold much longer.
   b. After a second peak inhalation, the clients gently blow air out (it helps to have a candle flame or feather) as long as possible. At least ten seconds is desirable. Guard against too forceful a use of air.
   Vital capacity will rarely be a significant factor, since we typically use only a small portion of our volume potential for speech.
2. Check the phonation relationship by having the client inhale deeply, set, and phonate (any vowel) for at least ten seconds. This will indicate sufficient respiratory support of phonation for most speaking demands.
3. Either specifically, or as part of other diagnostic procedures, observe the nonspeech breathing patterns. Watch for a long enough period of time to "average out" what you see. A number of Overstake's characterizations (irregular pattern, apnea, and so on) can be found in normal breathers intermittently, in reactions to stress and anxiety, or even in the absence of any concomitant speech problem. Patterns to watch for include
   a. Consistently erratic patterns.
   b. Frequent occurrence of apnea.
   c. Particularly rapid (shallow) or slow (deep) breathing.
   d. Upper chest, clavicular breathing, particularly if there are visible signs of excess tension in the strap muscles of the neck.
   e. Reverse breathing, where the thorax is seen to drop and/or the abdomen to contract on inhalation.
   f. Opposition breathing, where abdominal contraction and thoracic expansion occur at the same time.
   If you feel the need, have the client remove outer garments that are masking torso movements. Generally, however, try to avoid any reference to your interest in respiration, since awareness by the client tends to create an artificial pattern.

4. Specifically observe respiration as you evaluate reading, monologue, and spontaneous speech. These observations apply to nonstuttered and to stuttered speech, and it might be useful to record them separately:
   a. Prior to the speech attempt, especially on initial utterances, is there an unusually prolonged inspiration?
   b. Prior to the speech attempt, especially on initial utterances, is there a noticeable pause, or "set," before exhalation and phonation begin?
   c. Are there speech attempts during inhalation?
   d. Is there noticeable release of air before phonation begins?
   e. Is there a breathy, gasping quality to phonation?
   f. Are there noticeable glottal (hard) attacks?
   g. Is ongoing speech interrupted by inappropriate glottal stops?
5. In addition, observe respiratory actions during moments of stuttering, to determine if abnormalities are there:
   a. Are inhalations or exhalations apparently used as postponing, starting, or releasing behaviors?
   b. Does the spasm type, severity, locus, or other spasm variable relate to any particular respiratory acts?
   c. Is there a predominance of laryngospasms in the stuttering?
   d. Is there evidence to indicate that spasms start as oral and then spread to laryngeal, or vice versa?

Other questions of respiratory and phonatory examination are discussed in the chapters on evaluation and self-analysis.

Schwartz's Therapy

Schwartz's airflow therapy, or passive airflow, has received a disproportionate amount of attention for a procedure that involves very little that has not been practiced for several centuries. Were it not for his insistence that stuttering is caused by and centered in the larynx and that the posterior cricoarytenoid muscle and an inhibited airway dilation reflex explain moments of stuttering, and the book's title, *Stuttering Solved* (Schwartz, 1976), the therapy would not have received nearly so much attention.

Schwartz (1974) suggested that stuttering basically is a strong, ill-timed contraction of the posterior cricoarytenoid muscle (PCA) as a result of subglottal air pressure stimulus. Observations of nostril flaring in some children prior to stuttering spasms, and of his dog flaring its nostrils before every inhalation, caused Schwartz (1976) to examine the phenomenon further. He noted similar nostril flaring in adults preceding such reflex actions as yawning, coughing, and sneezing. Ultimately he concluded that there is an airway dilation reflex (ADR) along the length of the respiratory passage. In stuttering, there is an inappropriate reflex response to stress where the ADR triggers a strong adduction response (laryngospasm). These stress reactions depend on seven categories of anxiety or stress stimuli—situation, sound or word, authority figures, uncertainty, physical factors, external influences, and rapid rate (probably the most important). In his therapy, Schwartz recommended five days of work (eight hours per day). The client practices daily for the next year in four fifteen-minute periods. One minute of each solo session (twenty-eight minutes per week) is recorded on a cassette and mailed to the clinic for evaluation and feedback. A telephone "hotline" number is provided, and recommendations for maintenance are discussed with the client.

In therapy, the client seems to be asked to emit a prolonged, relaxed, audible sigh (passive sigh). This is produced immediately following inhalation so there is no intervening "set" or transition period between inhalation and exhalation. Then the client, midway in the passive sigh, "releases" a one-syllable word without any interruption, change in tension, or other alterations in the passive ongoing flow of air. Articulators are not preset and should move into position during the airflow. The number of one-syllable words is increased progressively on each breath and then turned into sentences. Syllables should be slowed (prolonged). Acquisition, then, is practice, error correction, and private sessions described earlier.

Gregory (1978) referred to the controversies about Schwartz's presumptions and generalizations. Sheehan (1980) was more specific in objecting to the theory and the assumptions, asking why we are still talking about stuttering if Schwartz "solved" it. Lee (1976) applied the Schwartz system to thirty-one adult stutterers for the recommended forty-hour, intensive period. At the end of that time it was reported that 90 percent of the clients were symptom-free in a wide variety of structured, stress-inducing situations. The interpretation of "symptom-free" was not clear. A second phase of therapy was a weekly group meeting and daily home assignments, both of which the authors felt were of significance to the continuance of fluency. In another study (Falkowski et al., 1982), two stutterers received the Schwartz-type program, omitting the elongation phase. One client dropped from a stuttering baseline of 30 percent SW to 1 percent SW and, on follow-up, was at 5 percent SW. The second client went from 40 percent SW to 16 percent SW and, on follow-up, was at 12 percent SW. The authors commented that overall the spontaneous speech improvement was erratic and seemed unrelated to elongation, airflow, or a combination of both. Andrews and Tanner (1982) applied Lee's modification of Schwartz's therapy, wherein eight-hour sessions were conducted on three consecutive days, and on the eighth and thirtieth days. After the first trial, all six stutterers showed positive results, but only two were reliably stutter-free. After the complete program, follow-up indicated that after one year all clients experienced regression, and the authors concluded that the approach is not superior in the short term, or any more effective over time, when compared to precision fluency shaping or to prolonged speech. Ingham (1984) pointed out that Schwartz's data are not specific or adequately substantiated, and he did not view them favorably.

Regulated Breathing

At about the same time there was another therapy system called the *regulated breathing approach* (Azrin & Nunn, 1974) based on earlier work with nervous habit elimination. Azrin and Nunn reported on a program with fourteen stutterers. In one two-hour session, stutterers were brought through an extensive sequence. They are asked to remember and discuss the history and development of their stuttering, recalling and verbalizing unpleasent experiences. Stuttering behaviors are analyzed, and an effort is made to develop awareness of stuttering. Also, a fear hierarchy that includes words and persons, as well as situations, is developed to clarify precipitating factors in stuttering. Basic relaxation training is covered, in various postures and including self-instruction. In speech control, the stutterer is taught, when stuttering occurs or is anticipated, to stop, exhale deeply and slowly, inhale while consciously relaxing, and consciously formulate the word that is to be spoken. The word should be uttered as soon as inhalation is complete, with an emphatic delivery on the first syllable that carries over into the next few words. Initial efforts should be brief, expanding as practice improves ability. Desensitization is attempted through symbolic rehearsal and visualization of unpleasant situations while attempting relaxation. The new breathing pattern starts with reading, where the client is to pause, relax, and breathe after every word. When this can be done consistently, the pause is shifted to every other word, then to every third word, and so on. When necessary, "cancellation" can be used by saying the word a second time. The clinician works with the client to set up a careful plan for transfer and maintenance. Reminders, environmental familiars, finding new situations for speaking, seeking out feared situations, and reports to the clinician are among methods used, along with telephone checks.

Azrin and Nunn reported stuttering decrements in the 90 percent to 99 percent range for a period of four months following the in-clinic procedures just described; they stated that the treatment, requiring a great deal of effort from and motivation by the client, was effective either for severe or for mild stutterers. They felt their approach would be more effective clinically than the programs in use at that time. Another comparison study (Poppen et al., 1977) involved one subject who previously had received many types of therapy. In serial order he was given metronome therapy, which dropped his stuttering frequency to 5.5 percent SW but did not carry over; use of a portable metronome resulted in 4 percent SW (at 100 bpm) but did not hold up. Poppen stated that the "regulated breathing" included elements of prolongation, rate reduction, semipreparatory sets, pullouts, cancellation, anticipation training, and social support. Fiedler and Standop (1983) evaluated the Azrin and Nunn system, criticizing the design and evaluation of the methods, as well as what they thought were very vague descriptions of the clinician's activity. "Before we share the optimism of both authors it seems that controlled replication of the investigation is called for" (p. 123). Ladoucer et al. (1982) applied the Azrin system to twelve stutterers, dividing them into four groups. Each group received the procedure described earlier, but three of the groups received special training in awareness, in biofeedback on respiration, or in biofeedback on muscle tension. They found no significant differences among the four groups and could not confidently report stuttering decrements nearly as good as those claimed in the original study.

Early on, Weller (1941) reported on 100 stutterers who had been trained to establish rhythmic breathing patterns. Number counting was used, and results indicated that new, slower, deeper inspiration patterns could be established with good permanency. Gronhovd (1977) approached stuttering control through the management of breathing, rate, airflow, and tension (BRAT). The client first was taught deep muscle relaxation while supine. Therapy went on to a voiceless sigh, a vocalized sigh, and counting progressively. During counting progress the client concentrated on maintaining

1. A smooth, moderately deep inhalation and a smooth, easy exhalation.
2. Slow rate.
3. Uninterrupted airflow.
4. Relaxed state without excess tension.
5. An easy glottal attack with a breathy voice.
6. Easy, automatic production.

The client then would move from counting to short responses and finally progress to monologues. Physical position now became semireclining, and the cycle was repeated. The cycle was repeated again in the sitting position. Rate was increased from one to two syllables per second, and work on quality, intonation, stress, and so on was added.

Overstake's System

Overstake's system of respiration management was introduced partially in the chapter covering relaxation, since he includes that as a first step of the treatment program (1979). He feels that most stutterers have non-synchronized respiratory patterns but, unlike Schwartz, states that "Stuttering is not caused by the irregular breathing patterns. These deviant patterns are the symptom of the problem" (p. 53). Following a complete Jacobson-style program of progressive relaxation, the stutterer (who has been evaluated previously for breathing abnormalities) is introduced to "block breathing." In this set, clients sit, or lie supine, and relax. Their cardiac pulse is located and allowed to settle from any initial fast rate. Then they are instructed to

1. Inhale, as rapidly as possible, what feels like a normal inhalation, holding the breath at the stopping point until signaled by the clinician to exhale.
2. Exhalation follows the previous step, as quickly as possible; then stop-hold until the clinician signals the next inhalation.

The clinician calculates both stop-hold times from the client's pulse rate, with approximately four beats being typical. Overstake suggests that the clinician audibly count at first in an ". . . in, hold, 3, 4 . . ." type pattern. This should be repeated eight to ten times before having the clients relax (they usually will relax to brief apnea, deep breath, and sinusoidal quiet breathing). If available, a pneumograph tracing should be made, and the clinician should check for blocklike inhalation and exhalation (see the following), where each phase and the hold periods are equal. Also, thoracic and abdominal tracings should be as synchronous as possible.

The foregoing steps are repeated in patterns of eight to ten cycles, followed by a rest. The block pattern and thoracic-abdominal synchrony tend to carry over into the rest period, but clients will vary in how soon they revert to the old pattern. Overstake reports that most clients permanently change their cycle pattern after a few sessions, but some take months to achieve stability. The clinician continues practice until satisfied with the client's pattern. Home practice can be assigned when the clients are able to monitor and control their own breathing patterns. Pneumograph tracings can be replaced with observation andd hands-on contact by the clinician, but Overstake warns that this requires "years of experience" to supply equivalent information.

Vital capacity for speech should be checked, but it is quite variable and each client must be judged in terms of his or her own breathing pattern. Overstake describes a normal respiratory speech pattern as consisting of a rapid inhalation, slight exhalation during a transition or set period, and then a slower exhalation as speech occurs. Just prior to the next inhalation, there usually will be a final, small release of air during the transition or set period. In describing respiratory anomalies of stutterers, Overstake cites the usual problems previously described. However, he also points out an error wherein stutterers try to start talking without the transition set between inhalation and exhalation. This may occur at the end of the exhalation, too, and can result in abdominal reversal and gasping in opposition to thoracic movement. Overstake says that this error is "quite common," and it is an interesting conflict with some of the therapies described previously in which the transition-set period deliberately is eliminated.

In progressing to the correction of respiratory patterns for speech, Overstake's first step is to coordinate the inhalation and exhalation cycles of the abdomen and thorax, and the block breathing for quiet respiration will serve as the foundation. Progressive steps that follow are these:

1. Clients take a full, normal inhalation, concentrating on simultaneous elevation of the thorax and protrusion of the abdomen. They practice until both occur in synchrony.

2. On exhalation, clients produce an easy, prolonged, breathy-whispered but loud vowel. They prolong the phonation until
    a. The exhaled breath stream becomes forced, or
    b. The abdomen begins to move outward, typical if there is pressure against the lower rib cage.
    The clinician, carefully, can press down on the abdomen and/or put a "marker" on it for the client to monitor. Breathy vowel production is practiced until consistency of balanced movement, breath release, and easy phonation are obtained.

3. The previous step is repeated completely, except a clearly phonated, non-breathy vowel production is used. At first, it may be necessary to alternate productions of breathy and clear production.

4. Clients produce a clear, stable vowel and let it form smoothly into the word *one*. They repeat until the production is smooth and balanced and then increase to *one, two* and stabilize. They continue to add numbers until the limits of a normal exhalation duration are reached.

5. Clients repeat step 4 but omit the preliminary vowel. Have the clients take a normal breath and start counting. Apply the same criteria as before.

6. Prior to the onset of production (vowels or numbers) have the clients practice releasing a small amount of air that blends smoothly into the onset of phonation. If needed, to start, an unstressed /h/ sound can be used. Monitor to assure that there is no stop between the air release and phonation onset. Counsel the clients against using this technique out of the clinic as a starter device or concentrating on breathing as a distraction from possible stuttering.

7. Transfer the stabilized breathing pattern to production of automatic phrases, nursery rhymes, or any material having strong patterns of rhyme or rhythm. Begin with short phrases and increase the length, but not to the point where two respiratory cycles are needed. The clients should inhale, utter the phrase, finish exhalation, inhale, and so on.

8. Work with the client to use a single exhalation more efficiently so that it lasts longer and more than one phrase can be uttered on a single exhalation. Monitor for signs of forcing and for reversion to old patterns. Add more phrases.

9. Start switching from rote, memorized, low propositional material to productions that are more spontaneous and propositional. Ask questions that tend to require brief, stock answers. As the clients are able to formulate the answer and maintain the new breathing pattern, ask questions requiring longer answers and increase the rate at which you ask the questions (stay below stress levels).

10. Shift propositional speech and practice until the clients can ask questions, use monologue responses, and generally converse while maintaining the stable respiratory pattern. Stuttering, which typically disappeared during in-clinic practice on earlier stages, may come back, although adaptation and other factors usually make it minimal. However, the clinical goal is a stable respiratory pattern, not control of stuttering.

Overstake continues therapy, primarily in aspects of rate control, with emphasis on timing and other prosodic elements. This technique will be discussed briefly in the chapter following.

Froeschels' Approach

Froeschels' approaches to therapy were always interesting and frequently unconventional. Although his basic orientation was psychotherapy, the so-called "breath chewing" method was one of his preparatory techniques. Some have regarded it as a semimotokinesthetic method; others felt it operated as a timing and motor coordination variation. Hollingsworth (1939) regarded it as a relaxation procedure, and Van Riper (1973) thought it basically was a persuasion and suggestion (of fluency) therapy. He also felt its apparent simplicity might disguise sophistication. It has been used for nonstuttering communication disorders. It has been taught in various sequences, and I will present it as I have learned it and used it. Other sources are available for those who wish to learn about the technique in its original form and about other applications of it (Froeschels, 1952a, 1952b; Froeschels & Jellinek, 1941; Kastein, 1974). As background, the biological mechanism interacts complexly in its primary oral, laryngeal, and thoracic functions of chewing, swallowing, and respiration. Oral and laryngeal systems protect and valve the respiratory area. In chewing and swallowing, they coordinate to bypass the respiratory system and to allow simultaneous functions to occur without choking. Normal speech, an overlaid function, continues the coordination symmetry. Stuttering disrupts that coordination and makes the stutterer feel that speech is difficult to produce. Breath chewing, on the other hand, reestablishes coordination of the parts and the system and demonstrates that normal speech, built on primitive biological coordinations, is quite feasible (Froeschels, 1952a, 1952b).

1. Clients are instructed to chew "nothing," with the mouth closed, concentrating on feeling the movements of the lips, jaw, and tongue. At first, the clients may be allowed to chew "something" and observe in the mirror, but then they should move to chewing with an empty mouth. The clinician demonstrates, informs, instructs, and corrects.
2. Next, clients are instructed to chew "savagely" on nothing, with an open mouth, while observing in the mirror and feeling the tactile and kinesthetic sensations.
3. Breathstream is added so that the clients are now "chewing air," or breath.

Attention is paid to regular respiration and not pressing or forcing the air out. Often, there will be some aperiodic vibration that increases the savage quality of the production, but this is a side effect.

4. Voicing is added to the airstream, after chewing begins. Initially, or after brief practice, the clinician might have the clients phonate a steady /n/ and then manipulate the clients' jaws and lips, directing them to listen to the different "vowels" that are produced. These are compared to the "vowels" produced by chewing the voiced tone. Moncur and Brackett (1974) note that the purpose here is to provide a variety of nonsense syllables instead of a continuous, monotonous sound.

5. As the clients become able to relax and chew sound with variation, begin adding words, phrases, and sentences. The clinician participates and models.

6. Progress to "conversation," reducing the strength of the chewing but falling back to more basic levels if dysfluencies develop. Home assignments are given, and the clients are instructed to visualize chewing motions and concentrate on movements of the articulator system.

I have found few stutterers (or student clinicians) who respond well to the technique, and many persons resist it. When it is accepted, however, it seems to work surprisingly well and is of value for a number of speech problems.

> . . . the success of the method seems to depend not only on the personality of the patient, but also that of the clinician. . . . Those who use procedure interlace it with a great variety of vocal psychotherapeutic techniques. (Murphy, 1964, p. 120).

Other Approaches

Other clinicians use breathing therapy in different ways. Fiedler and Standop (1983) have a complex system of two levels and subdivisions within levels, but they provide for relaxation work and practice on easy breathing. Similarly, significant combinations of airflow control, easy onset of phonation, continuous airflow or phonation, and coordinating articulation with phonation can be found in various programs (Ingham, 1984; Perkins, 1973b; Ryan, 1974; Shames and Florance, 1980; Van Riper, 1973; Webster, 1974).

The overall significance of airflow as a major technique is disputed. Sheehan (1980, p. 184) blasts the whole concept.

> We hear of stutterers cured in half an hour through "discovery" of an airflow technique or an operant program that turns out to be an elaboration on or variation on discredited breathing exercises. After all, the stutterer has been breathing a long time without programmed instruction.

Van Riper (1973, p. 21), recalling his own experiences, is not charitable toward airflow as a major component of therapy.

> . . . interminable breathing exercises: lying down, sitting, standing up, chest breathing rituals, "costal breathing" exercises, diaphragmatic ones,

abdominal ones. (Our chests were measured each week to see if they were benefitting from the practice).

He argues that, at best, most breathing therapy techniques are ". . . mere vechicles of suggestion, self-discipline, or distraction" (p. 75). He does not deny some "minor effectiveness" in helping to break up laryngospasms or aid in timing respiration, phonation, and articulation. However, he feels there is danger of habituation and losing control of respiratory efforts, which could add "gross abnormalities" to the old pattern.

Falck (1969) seems to agree that direct respiratory work is not necessary and that normal breathing patterns are achieved more appropriately as byproducts of ". . . improved speech fluency than trying to achieve speech fluency through direct breathing exercises" (p. 91). Perkins (1983) stipulates his own use of breath management as part of a seven-skill therapy complex but feels it (breath control) is not a universally effective technique. Miller (1982) provides what probably is the best current overview of comments concerning airflow therapy. She states that in its various forms, it is an aid to stuttering therapy and its value ranges from none to complete elimination of stuttering symptoms and to support of fluent speech. Miller states that, typically, the average stutterer will experience a noticeable reduction in stuttering, but that it should be recognized that other variables (for example rate) are being manipulated at the same time. Finally, she cautions that the existing 90 percent improvement claims well may be exaggerations of a generally positive fluency picture, and that some of the "fluent" speech is noticeably different from normal speech.

This chapter does not lead to one particular method or sequence of breathstream management, airflow, breathing exercises, and so on. The range of emphasis, integration, and significance is too great. The best orientation may be one between Overstake and Perkins, where all the steps of the former are not followed, but there is more emphasis than by the latter. Perhaps, dividing stutterers into therapy-need categories, we might use a shifting concentration of airflow and breathstream in therapy:

1. Those stutterers for whom respiratory anomalies are characteristic in non-fluent and fluent speech and non-speech breathing. A predominance of laryngospasm dysfluencies may characterize these persons. For them, a therapy program emphasizing breathstream management could follow self-analysis and preliminary relaxation and desensitization and precede either fluency reinforcement or symptom control procedures.

2. Those stutterers for whom respiratory anomalies are strongly evident during stuttering but are minimal or absent at other times. For these, breathstream management usually can be a substep of an overall program, or breathing adequacy may be achieved as a byproduct of other therapy management techniques.

3. Those stutterers for whom respiratory anomalies are not strongly evident and who probably have an oral predominance in their stuttering spasms. Any needed breathstream improvements could be byproducts of other techniques.

4. Those who present a variable mix from the preceding three types. Further evaluation, queries about previous therapy, and flexibility in planning are indicated.

ASSIGNMENTS FOR CLINICIANS

The following assignments are a mixture to help acquaint you with aspects of phonation and respiration and then to provide practice in certain breathstream management steps. For this reason, the assignment section will be considerably longer than the usual ones at the ends of chapters. It surely would be unwieldy to cover the entire section for a class, and individual users probably will find parts of it not relevant to their needs. More than usual, it is suggested that the reader select those sections where information and experience are needed and skip the remainder.

General warning: In many of the assignments, do not breathe so frequently and/or deeply that you become dizzy or feel faint. If you or your instructor has access to a pneumograph or other respiratory measurement devices for volume and pattern, they can be used in many of the following assignments and will improve your information. Since such instruments are often not available, the tasks have been structured on a "make-do" basis as far as equipment is concerned.

Because the text of this chapter provides a number of step-by-step procedures to follow, the assignments are only approximate in the sequence followed and tend to sample from the different procedures rather than develop just one method. Because of this, and because of the extensive previous discussions, sample assignments for clients (usually following this subsection) will be omitted.

The first four assignments are intended to increase awareness of respiratory capacity and the uses of air. Comparisons are implied between simple exhalation, breathy and economical phonation, and the amounts of air required by different types of speech sounds. Most of you will be able to monitor your productions without difficulty, but a few may need the help of your partner to supplement self-awareness. Be careful to avoid hyperventilation or oxygen starvation; rest briefly between each series of exercises.

1. Exhale all the air you can, and then inhale to the maximum. Hold the inhalation briefly, and then exhale at a slow, steady rate by blowing air against your finger (held an inch or two from your lips). Try to make the airstream last for about fifteen seconds. Try this five times, and average the times of airflow duration. What was your average? How did it compare to your partner's or to that of other persons?

2. Exhale and inhale as in 1. Then produce a continuous /a/ vowel, recording it on tape, until you run out of air. Do this three times. Play back the recordings and answer the following questions, comparing results with your partner.

    a. How long did phonation last, on the average?

    b. How long did phonation last before strain, quaver, noise, or other indications of stress appeared?

3. Repeat 2, but on the three productions of sounds, generate one with a continuous /s/, the second with a /z/, and the third with an /n/. Answer the questions as before, comparing the different sounds.

4. Exhale and inhale as in 1. Record consecutive productions (no more than two per second) at a normal voice level of /pʌ/, /kʌ/, /dʌ/, /tʌ/, and /bʌ/. Play back and count the number of productions for each syllable. Compare with your partner on

    a. The number of productions of each syllable.

    b. The difference, if any, on voiced and voiceless sounds.

    c. The difference, if any, between bilabial /pʌ/ and /bʌ/.

    d. The difference, if any, between /pʌ/, /tʌ/, and /kʌ/.

The next four assignments are designed to stimulate your awareness of how you breathe and the pattern of regional predominance. As before, do not overbreathe and become dizzy. The last two assignments provide practice sessions in speaking while monitoring and controlling respiratory patterns. It may be necessary to repeat the four assignments in several different sessions until you are able to achieve the control and pacing desired.

5. Loosen restrictive clothing—belts, straps, and buttons. Lie supine on the floor. Place a styrofoam cup, open end down (any lightweight, visible object can be used) on your sternum (adjust placement for variations in physical geography) and another cup over your navel. Close your eyes and relax while your partner observes. The observer may speak, but you are to remain silent. Continue for several minutes. What was observed in terms of thoracic-abdominal movement during respiration? Compare to your partner.

6. Repeat the arrangement for 6 for about one mintue. This time make an effort deliberately to expand your thorax and protrude the abdomen on every inhaltion; do the reverse on exhalation. Compare and report as before.

7. Repeat the arrangement for 6 but for one to two mintues. Count aloud to 100 at a steady, normal pace, breathing whenever it feels appropriate, while your partner observes. Compare and report as before.

8. Repeat the arrangement for 6, but for about three minutes of conversation with your partner, while he or she observes the movement of the markers. Look for long respirations, phrase interruptions, laughter effects, and so on. Compare and report as before.

Assignments 9 and 10 are inserted to suggest that people vary in their respiratory patterns and that the system we take for granted can be used in different ways. You will notice shifts in predominance among persons, and you may note a particular individual varying what is his or her common pattern. Posture, duration of speech effort, intensity of effort, and other factors may affect predominance and pattern. Notice as much as you can.

9. Observe at least twenty different people to notice their breathing predominance (abdominal or thoracic). Consider whether they are standing, sitting, or reclining. What did you find out? Note: Seasonal weather variations and/or costume can facilitate or hinder this assignment. If circumstances warrant, reduce the number of required observations.

10. Observe five different persons as they are talking. Try to sample about three minutes' talking time per person. In approximate fashion, answer the following:

	SUBJECT NO.				
OBSERVATION/QUESTION	1	2	3	4	5
1. Breathing was mainly thoracic, abdominal, or mixed.					
2. Major respirations were frequent, moderate, infrequent while talking.					
3. Phrase breaths were frequent, moderate, infrequent while talking.					
4. Voice was breathy frequently, some, not at all.					
5. Hard glottal attacks were frequent, moderate, rare.					

The following four assignments are a series related to Overstake's procedures for breath management. The first two can stand separately and are to be used with any client who would profit from awareness and regularization of vegetative respiratory patterns. They can be a preliminary to other therapy techniques or to the two assignments following—in which Overstake's procedures are provided for speech production. These four assignments, particulary 14, can be quite lengthy and time-consuming. Unless in-depth practice is desired, revision to a sampling exercise might be desirable.

11. Find a quiet place where you can either lie down (supine) or sit back and relax. Sitting or lying, let yourself relax until you can sense your cardiac pulse. If it seems difficult, use your fingers to find the carotid pulse in your neck (anterolateral area at the level of the thyroid cartilage; don't press too hard). Once you have located the pulse, count the number of beats in ten seconds. Do this five or six times over a period of several minutes. What was your rate and variability, and how did they compare to those of your partner?

12. Practice "block breathing" as in Overstake's description on page 269. It might help at first if you can set a metronome to signal almost at the same rate as your pulse rate (from 11). You can make a cassette signal tape if you lack a metronome. Inhale for three beats, hold the air for the same period of time, and exhale for three beats (you may change the beat rate to one that is more comfortable). Practice until you can evenly pace your respiratory cycle. Concentrate on simultaneous action of the thoracic and abdominal muscles. Compare notes with your partner about how easy or hard it was to establish a

respiratory cycle where your inhalation, hold, and exhalation each lasted the same amount of time.

13. Practice the "block breathing" you learned in 12 in a variety of situations. Continue until you are able to maintain the equality of the three divisions. Remember to time your pulse rate. If situational conditions create the need, you may change the duration, but continue to keep all three divisions equal. Use the following situations:

    a. Sitting and reading or watching television.
    b. Sitting in a class, a meeting, a car, and so on.
    c. Standing in privacy.
    d. Standing in a line or listening to another person.
    e. Walking on a level surface, not carrying a weight.
    f. Lying in bed, supine.

14. With your partner, proceed through the ten stages of the summary from Overstake's procedures, starting on page 270. When you are the "clinician," explain each step as if your partner knew nothing of the procedure. Watch for retained shifts in rate, stress, inflection, loudness, and so forth as you progress toward more typical speech production. If it will help, use thoracic and abdominal markers to monitor respiratory movements (adhesive labels, masking tape, and so on can serve). Write a brief summary of your experience, and evaluate your partner.

The last six assignments combine sampling release procedures and breath control. The continuous flow methods of Azrin and of Schwartz are suggested, but you could substitute Overstake's methods if you wish. The important point is that you carry over and habituate new respiratory patterns in real speaking situations. You will find it is easy to slip back into your old patterns—which emphasizes the need for heavy doses of in-clinic practice, coupled with daily out-clinic practice assignments. If you have used, or plan to use, relaxation exercises, by all means relate them to controlled, correct respiratory patterns. They will reinforce and cue each other. Similar linkages can be made between respiration and pullouts, preparatory sets, rate control, easy onset, and other control or fluency methods.

15. With your partner, practice production of a vocal fry. After inhalation, adduct the vocal folds and concentrate on "bubbling" a low-pitched /a/ at the vocal folds. Once you obtain it, move articulator around to modify the sound. Another initiation method is to "gargle" the sound. Be careful to avoid excessive production and irritation of the vocal folds.

16. Record the following list of words. Before each word inhale. As you end an inhalation, immediately switch to a gentle exhalation, easily start phonation, and then move articulators to form the sounds. Have your partner watch you closely to make sure there are no anticipatory movements of postures of the articulators before phonation. Each word should be produced with extra breathstream but not with a gasp or with effort. Remember: Inhale normally, immediately exhale with a steady flow, easily slide phonation onto the airstream, and move the articulators to form the word. Produce the entire word in the gentle mode.

A	B	C
alone	about	baggage
zero	zebra	exaggerate
newsman	newspaper	pandemonium
sure fire	sure to	cerebral palsy

Did you notice any differences in producing the words in A, B, and C? Could your partner clearly identify your inhale, exhale, and phonate shaping stages? What sounds or syllables were harder to do?

17. Read a paragraph of 300 to 500 words to your partner. On the first word of every sentence, follow the breathing-production sequence set forth in assignment 16. Have your partner, on a copy of the passage, mark each respiration other than those on the first word of each sentence. Swap passages. Read the paragraph aloud a second time, performing as before, and add the word following each of your partner's marks (to the production sequence method). Evaluate your respective performances.

18. Converse with your partner on any topic. On the first word of each sentence, or after each inhalation, use the technique described in 16. If you miss any break, your partner should stop you at once; you should relax, inhale, start phonation, say the missed word, and then proceed. Talk until each one of you has accumulated about three minutes' talking time without error (time each other). If you are stopped more than five times in any one three-minute accumulation, add another minute to your requirement.

19. Select five words you commonly use. During the next twenty-four to forty-eight hours, use each word in speech with other people, with the production pattern described in 16. The words should be produced five times each. Report on the situations, success, any responses from auditor, and your feelings.

20. Prewrite three telephone calls for information, service, or products. For each call, underline five words on which you will use the technique described in 16. Have your partner observe and evaluate. Report on the results, any reactions from auditors and your own reactions.

11

MASKING

OVERVIEW

General applications of masking in stuttering therapy have been varied. Silverman and Trotter (1973) listed forty-seven references concerning masking noise and stuttering, indicating a lively interest in the subject. In preparing this chapter, I reviewed quite a few additional references, many being eliminated to avoid redundancy or because they otherwise were not applicable directly to therapy. In a somewhat contrary view of masking's significance, Andrews et al. (1983), in a cursory review of treatment, cited only a few references and appeared to confuse the concepts of therapy with those of programs that utilize masking as a part or step. We are concerned here not with the overall programs of therapy, which can be comprised of one or many techniques and used in many different ways.

Therapy programs have utilized masking in several ways. Peins et al. (1970) described a tape-recorded therapy program for self-administration by the client. The program, in eight steps, mixes progressive levels of speech production and masking, with masking operating in decrements at each stage. MacCulloch et al. (1970) reported on a program of low-frequency (300 Hz) masking used over a period of twenty-four therapy sessions. They obtained a significant increase in fluency, with an average of 41 pretreatment dysfluencies dropping to 15.5 after twelve therapy sessions.

However, further treatments did not result in additional significant improvement. Nevertheless, the authors felt that the results were preferable to those obtained by DAF or rhythm techniques, and they recommended the development and use of portable masking devices (see later). Zsilavecz (1981) suggested that 150 Hz noise can be used to demand an increased use of and attention to somesthetic feedback. Van Riper (1973) made a similar suggestion, using masking as a diagnostic instrument to assess the degree to which the stutterer was aware of tactile and kinesthetic cues. Although he generally did not favor the use of masking (see later) in therapy, he did suggest that its use could be scheduled in a sequence of loudness decrements and increasing "off" periods. It was not to be used in early stages of therapy (Van Riper suggested using it in the final stabilization phase of his MIDVAS sequence) and never to be used to suppress spasms through induced fluency.

Variable applications of masking have shown that it can be used as an aversive stimulus, where a reduction in stuttering is followed by a cessation of noise (Flanagan et al., 1958). Sutton and Chase (1961) reported that continuous masking, masking only during speech, and masking only during silence, all reduced the frequency of stuttering. In a study comparing the fluency effects of TO, DAF, metronome, "wrong" after every stuttering, and masking (100-dB SPL in a five-minute on and five-minute off cycle), the masking resulted in only a 40 percent reduction in stuttering frequency and a 12 percent reduction in spasm duration. This was compared to a 70 percent and 90 percent reduction in spasm frequency and a 74 percent and 46 percent reduction in duration for TO and metronome conditions, respectively (Martin & Haroldson, 1979). However, the data indicate that a number of stutterers actually increased duration under masking; it may be that their noise design (on/off cycle) was inappropriate or that they had condition-subject interaction on a subgroup basis. Andrews et al. (1982) compared fifteen fluency-inducing conditions, including masking. All conditions improved fluency, but masking was not one of the most effective. As in other studies, stutterers varied in their responses to different conditions.

In spite of varied reports of masking's effectiveness, a number of clinicians have developed portable masking devices so that the stutterers can carry noise with them in order to block their auditory monitoring of speech signals. Battery-powered units that fed masking through hearing-aid-type receivers were mounted either in spectacle frames or in larger pocket-belt units. Van Riper (1965) reported on the use of a portable unit with twenty-five stutterers, who used intermittent (speech-only) masking. He stated that there was only a moderate reduction in the frequency of stuttering, although the severity was reduced markedly. Trotter reported on thirty months of using a portable masker, manually controlling the masking (if he felt he was going to stutter or was surprised by a stutter). He wore the device about 50 percent of the time and actually used it about fifteen minutes per day. He stated that, generally, the portable masker reduced his stuttering by about 75 percent or more in frequency, and usually reduced spasm duration to one second or less (typically, without masking, 40 percent of his spasms would have been longer than one second). He found that the ear inserts caused a mild hearing loss for outside sound, and prolonged use of the masker (more than ten to fifteen minutes) disturbed mental concentration and tended to make his speech louder, faster, and less precise than normal (Trotter & Lesch, 1967).

Subsequently, Trotter and Silverman (1973) reported on four studies of a "stutter-aid." This was a 7/8"-by-2 1/4"-by-1/8" noise generator with manual controls for loudness (97 to 120-dB SPL) and pitch (35 to 770 Hz) and fitted with standard hearing-aid receivers. In the four studies, it appeared that masking did reduce frequency and severity of stuttering on some occasions but not on others. The authors also reported problems persuading clients to use the device outside the clinic, and when they were wearing it, to turn it on when caught by a stuttering spasm.

Perkins and Curlee (1969) discussed use of a portable masking unit, and Donovan (1971) reported on a portable unit that could generate a metronome beat, a continuous masking noise, or a rhythmic beat masking tone. Intensity and duration of tones could be preset, and the stutterers could select which of the three signals they wanted with controlled on-off time. Gruber (1971) reported using a portable masker at a summer speech camp, to help clients gain control after (not before) a stuttering spasm had started. It was used to increase tactile and kinesthetic awareness as the stutterers worked on pullouts for symptom control.

In 1976 it was reported (Dewar et al., 1976b) that AFM (auditory feedback masking) eliminated accessory eye muscle movement associated with stuttering spasms and caused similar effects in "ex-stammerers." The researchers noted that using a voice-activated (laryngeal vibration triggering) noise generator eliminated the tendency of clients not to trigger manually the masking switch after they had been talking for awhile. They also reported (Dewar et al., 1976a) on using a voice-activated masker with fifty-three stutterers. In reading, automatic speech, and picture description there was a 93 percent to 95 percent reduction in stuttering frequency and a 40 percent to 60 percent reduction in the duration of spasms. They noted that five clutterers who used the device improved significantly, but much less than did the stutterers. In a very thorough study (Dewar et al., 1979) results of using a portable masker with 195 stutterers were reported. The clients first were started with a stationary, in-clinic masker to establish the best loudness (just above normal conversational level) and frequency range (up to 500 Hz). After practice in trying not to talk louder than the machine, using the throat microphone, and so on, the clients were switched to the portable unit, which was built to vary the frequency of the masking tone as the speaker's fundamental frequency varied (within its 500-Hz ceiling) and set at the preferred loudness level. The clinicians reported that only 11 percent (twenty-one) of the clients did not respond well. Overall, sixty-seven clients used the portable AFM for six to twenty-eight months; 82 percent reported "considerable" to "great" benefits, and eighteen percent reported "slight" benefits. About half reported a decreasing need to use the unit. Wearing time averaged about 200 minutes a day, although the range was 5 minutes to 8 hours, and the estimated exposure to noise was about 26 minutes per day.

The previously described research led to the marketing of a unit known as the Edinburgh Masker (University of Edinburgh Bulletin, 1979). At that time, it was claimed that over 500 stutterers in twenty-three countries had used the portable masker and that 90 percent of the stutterers who tried it could speak more fluently with it. This device is a set-frequency, variable volume, voice-activated (by laryngeal contact microphone) masker, which also can be controlled manually (separately or along with automatic control). It is about 3-1/2" by 1-1/8" by 2-1/4" and is powered by a standard nine-volt battery. It has a 0.5 second turn-off lag, so it usually continues masking during production of voiceless sounds or during very brief pauses. The manual control allows the speaker to initiate masking prior to an utterance attempt if desired. There is a precaution that some "mild-to-moderate" stutterers will reject the device as being more obvious and distracting than their own stuttering and that some clients find the noise too objectionable (Williams, 1984). Walle (1980) reported effective use of the device with severe stutterers as part of an overall program of intensive therapy. Ingham (1981) reported on using the Edinburgh unit with four stutterers. One client exhibited almost 100 percent reduction of stuttering on every use, two clients had marginal or temporary reductions on either reading or open speech (but not on both), and the fourth person was helped on spontaneous speech. Ingham noted (see later discussion about masking effects) that no reduction in stuttering was associated with a reduction in rate.

Wingate (1970) also discussed masking studies. In an exhange with another clinician (Conture, 1973; Wingate 1973), he reviewed the effects of masking on increasing loudness, pitch, and syllable duration and on decreasing rate. Ingham (1975a) reviewed a number of masking studies and suggested that simple masking of the voice signal is not an adequate explanation of the resultant reduction in stuttering. He felt it probable that individual changes in rate, syllable duration, vocal intensity, and pitch may be significant. Wingate (1976) and Van Riper (1973) both presented excellent summaries of masking research and application. Van Riper traced the use of masking in Europe from 1920 to 1930 and to its "rediscovery" at the University of Iowa (Shane, 1955). He indicated that the Russians first used portable maskers, followed by a number of the satellite countries. Wingate suggested that the induced changes in manner of speaking, not the blocked auditory feedback, per se, caused by masking are responsible for changes in stuttering (slowed rate, increased syllable duration, articulatory alteration, changes in stress, and changes in pitch).

Bloodstein (1972) suggested that . . . almost any form of novel auditory feedback . . . can reduce stuttering, but this seems to fall short of being an adequate explanation. He rejected anxiety reduction by masking, finding only partial support for any theory involving an inherent abnormality of auditory feedback in stutterers that masking would suppress. Distraction effect was supported because of the novelty and the simplification of motor planning. Another clinician (Dijk, 1973) substantiated the nondistraction factors in masking. Many studies report little or no adaptation to the effects of masking, which would not be the case if masking simply was distraction. Intermittent masking is not more effective (that is, distracting) than continuous masking. Also, masking during nonspeech pause times is as effective as masking during speech; there seems to be a residual effect on speech during the following periods of no-masking; and finally, low-frequency masking is more effective than high-frequency masking in reducing stuttering. It is clear that a simple explanation will not account for the effects of masking on the speech of stutterers.

EVALUATIONS

Evaluations of masking in research and clinical application have shown that its use results in a reduction in stuttering, usually in the form of a smaller number of stuttering spasms, and in the severity (duration) of the occurrences. In therapy, masking has been applied as a punishment or aversive stimulus, contingent on the occurrence of stuttering. It also has been applied in a facilitating form to coerce a slower rate with changes in prosodic elements of speech. In-clinic use was followed by out-clinic utilization of portable units, and several clinicians have reported beneficial, albeit mixed, results. Attitudes toward the use of masking are divided. Sheehan (1970, pp. 272-73) referred to it in very definite terms as being based on ". . . the not very illustrious genealogy of the quacks."

> Commercial exploiters of mechanical devices have attempted to clothe the discredited methods of a sorry past with the raiment of modern experimental psychology. They are quacks in Wundt's clothing. The hands are presented like the hands of Skinner or Wolpe, but the voice is the voice of Bogue.

Van Riper (1973) sharply criticized the use of masking as a basic fluency-inducing device. He pointed out the possible abusive uses of it as an accessory timing device to complement avoidance in stuttering and the possible amalgamation of masking into postponement systems of stuttering defense. He noted that synchrony in manual timing of masking, where the client triggers the noise too soon or too late, is a problem, except for the few who seem to have an innate sense of their speech rhythm. Also, he reported that some stutterers (using the manual control) actually developed finger twitches (of the switch-control finger) as an associated behavior. Van Riper stated that stutterers tended to resent using the machine, did not adapt to its use, found it progressively unpleasant, and showed few transfer effects when not using it: "As a permanent prosthesis, it simply was not tolerable" (p. 124). Wingate (1976) listed the annoyance factor of masking noise, the continued bother of turning the control on and off (on manual units), the reduction of hearing acuity while wearing the unit, and the false "stigma" of what appears to be a hearing aid so that people treat the stutterer as a deaf person.

The attitudes expressed toward masking are definite and valid. Those who support its use are correct that certain stutterers respond very favorably to it, and those who criticize it are correct that it is limited in its fluency support; does not help all stutterers; and is a visible prosthesis with inherent drawbacks in its operation, transfer, and effects on prosodic elements of speech. There is, as usual, a middle ground of use, where masking is applied diagnostically and as a step or part of a step in a total therapy program. To summarize, it appears that uses of masking include the following:

1. Diagnostic evaluation of
   a. Dependence on auditory monitoring, awareness of tactile and kinesthetic feedback, reaction to auditory stress, reaction to fluency, sensitivity to loudness, rate response to masking, and attitude toward masking.
   b. Performance in reading, automatic speech, monologue speech, and conversational speech during masking.
   c. Specific effects of masking on the frequency, duration, types, locus, and struggle of stuttering spasms.
2. Early demonstration to the client that stuttering is malleable and/or that fluency is attainable.
3. In-clinic use to provide periods of fluency or reduced nonfluency, where other techniques (for example, GILCU, rate control, and prolongation) can be practiced with greater ease.
4. In-clinic use during role-play reenactment of past speech experiences or rehearsal for anticipated situations. It may also be coupled with desensitization activities.
5. In-clinic or out-clinic use with specific techniques, such as pullouts or preparatory sets, where the masking can focus attention on movement sequences rather than on auditory signals.
6. Out-clinic use to provide solo practice in fluency and/or to facilitate practice on other control techniques mentioned previously.
7. Out-clinic use in an ongoing format, with clinicians helping to plan the frequency and duration of use.

CLINICAL APPLICATIONS

Clinical applications of masking will be based on those reports previously summarized. Masking has not been used extensively because other techniques generally seem to work better. However, the client dictates the therapy, and we have seen that some responded either so well to masking or so badly to everything else that good use was made of masking. The suggestions following are a mixture of personal experience and borrowings from the experience of other clinicians.

Diagnostic applications of masking have been referred to earlier. As part of the routine evaluation process the client can be tested for auditory acuity, including the SRT (speech reception threshold). In addition, establishing the MCL (most comfortable loudness level) and RCL (range of comfortable loudness) measures will be useful if masking is planned. Although testing speech discrimination in noise might be interesting and possibly useful, we lack a base in communication research to apply any results directly to stuttering therapy and say whether a score is good or bad with reference to the use of masking in therapy. It would be useful if we had a reliable correlation between comprehension in noise and speech performance under masking.

Standard measures for frequency, severity, adaptation, and consistency of stuttering in different speech modes should precede masking evaluation. They will provide a comparison for later effects, and using masking first possibly could contaminate (by residual effects) the baseline measures. Proceed to an evaluation of masking by explaining what it is, but do not suggest what its effects on speech might be. Instruct the clients to try to speak in their usual fashion during masking. After fitting earphones, positioning the microphone, and so on, proceed as follows:

1. If your unit produces variable frequency bands, set for the broad band or for band pass that does not filter out frequencies below 1,000 Hz.
2. Explain the process (see step 3) to the clients. Say that you will continue making loudness increments until a level of physical discomfort is reached, but urge them to differentiate between dislike and irritation and real discomfort. Use a tape recorder to store all speech output.
3. Set the masking unit's intensity level at about 15-dB SPL over the earlier SRT level of the better ear.[1] Have the clients count from one to ten, read several sentences from any source, and respond to several questions requiring answers in sentences. Increase the loudness of the masking by 10 dB, repeating the process with different automatic speech, sentences, and questions.

[1]You may not have equipment that can be set at SRT score levels or even in known decibel increments. In such cases, put the earphones on yourself, and have the client read aloud while you progressively increase the masking level until it seems equal to the loudness of the client's speech. Use this as a starting point with the client. If the unit does have known decibel increments, use what there is and make note of dial settings.

Continue 10-dB increments until the clients indicate that a level of discomfort has been reached.

4. Turn off the recorder and the masking unit and remove the earphones. Interview the clients about personal reactions to masking and perceptions of its effects on speech. Ask them about the different levels of masking and how they think it would feel to use masking for a prolonged period of time. Explain that you want to recheck a few of the settings, and arrange the masking unit and tape recorder again.

5. Have the clients read and speak spontaneously at your baseline masking level, at the high level, and about midway between. Sample 200 to 300 words of reading and about three minutes of free speech at each level. Instruct them to try to use a normal loudness level, ignore the masking, and not to try to hear their own speech through the masking.

When the testing is finished, you will want to play back the tapes, evaluate them in comparison to earlier baseline measurements of speech, and consider the following:

1. % SW, SW/M (where appropriate), average spasm duration, and any severity index used.
2. Comparisons of syllable duration and pause lengths in baseline and masked nonstuttered speech.
3. wpm or any other rate measurements used in baseline evaluations.
4. Loudness, pitch, inflection, and syllable stress changes.
5. Any apparent residual effects on speech when masking is turned off.
6. Personal reactions to, and comments about, masking.
7. Observations of changes in the postures, preformations, or exaggerations in the movements of articulators.
8. Any tendency for the stuttering spasms to change in their type or location or form other variations.

Early therapy applications of masking have been mentioned previously. Actually, the diagnostic use of masking can serve several of these purposes. Some stutterers, especially those who are pessimists and "victims," profit motivationally from a demonstration that it is possible to stutter less or not at all. This is true particularly with young stutterers (where temporary, complete fluency may result) or with older and very severe stutterers who have become wearily accustomed to a lifetime of uncontrollable stuttering. As a motivational device, masking can be used in similar situations. However, remember that stutterers react differentially to masking. Do not predict results for them, because failure or poor response could damage your credibility and reinforce their feelings of inadequacy. As a demonstration of fluency, masking should be linked to a variety of fluency modes so that the clients can understand that fluency can come in different forms, and the clinician can evaluate effectiveness and reactions to the different modes. Comparisons of masking, metronome, unison speech, DAF, and any other techniques are suggested. It may help to link the fluency experiments with therapy dialogue, where the clinician reinforces positive statements by the clients and is nonresponsive or negative to statements that are not positive; that is, don't encourage clients to feel that they can sit back and let a machine do the work for them.

In using masking or other techniques, direct the attention of the clients to recordings of their speech, with and without the use of masking. Useful practice in self-analysis can occur in this process. Direct the clients to listen and relisten (video tape is extremely helpful) to samples in order to analyze changes that occur in stuttering behavior. This technique, of course, involves a familiarity with the usual stuttering pattern (which may have to be learned) and then refines analysis skills to detect changes that occur under masking. You also are teaching the idea that it is possible to stutter in different ways. Desensitization will be a concomitant of this process as the client functions analytically with the stuttering. In addition to the evaluation and comparison of the stuttering patterns, masking can be used to direct analysis toward the nonstuttered speech characteristics. What happened to the client's rate, loudness, pitch, pause, syllable duration, and so on? These are changes the client should learn to watch for and analyze. In many cases, you might select several of those changes and have the client briefly use them (without masking) to see if they don't facilitate fluency. It is possible that you might develop patterns for future use in rate control, prolongation, pullouts, or preparatory sets.

In-clinic fluency practice with masking assumes you are planning a therapy program based on fluency facilitation, or you would not devote time to it. In order to give structure to use, you will want to establish goals for using masking and relate criteria to these goals.

Phase I: Establishment

1. Select a masking level that will be accepted by the client.
2. The client must learn to control manually the onset of the masking noise just prior to a speech attempt, turning the noise off when listening. If an automatic masker is used, the client will need to practice manually initiating noise for the first speech attempt or after a pause long enough to turn the noise off. You can have some clients initiate a vowel or "just phonation" to activate the masker, or even use the passive sigh-into-voicing method in order to get started with masking accompaniment. Until the client can manage the mechanical details and timing factors, wait for further development and practice.
3. Use continuous masking for five-minute practice periods on reading, monologue, and spontaneous conversation. Note which mode results in the least stuttering. Discuss the results with the client and determine, if you can, why any one of the modes is more fluent (if this is the case) than the others.
4. Concentrate on the speech mode from 3 that is most fluent. If they were relatively equal, use monologue. Practice until the client accumulates fifteen minutes under one of the following criteria:
   a. A 90 percent reduction in SW/M, compared to baseline measures.
   b. Five or fewer stutterings in the fifteen minutes.

Add the criterion that the stutterings are to be detected by the stutterer. You may want, for some clients, to modify this criterion (as well as any others) if they show a pattern of frequent, small stuttering spasms, as opposed to fewer spasms of greater severity.

5. Progress to Phase II in the speech mode you worked with in Phase I-4. Pick up the next speech mode and repeat I-4 with it while continuing into Phase II with the first speech mode. For variation, alternative five-minute units between the modes, keeping track of time and dysfluencies accumulated.

Phase II: Refinement

1. Basically repeat Phase I-4, but reduce the masking loudness level by approximately 10 dB.
2. Have the client pay attention to loudness, pitch, inflection, syllable duration, and so forth, trying to keep them as normal as possible.
3. Apply the same criteria as in Phase I.
4. When the criteria are met, progress to Phase III with the particular speech mode. When the second speech mode meets criteria in Phase I, move it into Phase II, and start the third speech mode in Phase I. This third mode may progress very rapidly. If the client displays no nonfluencies after five minutes, try moving to Phase II with the third speech mode.

Phase III: Stabilization

1. Experiment to find the lowest masking loudness level that will continue to provide fluency support; retain this as the preferred masking level.
2. Meet the fifteen-minute criterion, as before.
3. Continue emphasis on normalization of the speech pattern and on self-monitoring.
4. Bring other speech modes up to this phase as progress is made.
5. Note: Situational adaptation may contribute significantly to fluency and meeting criteria. This is acceptable now, but do not become falsely optimistic about progress.

Phase IV: Termination

1. With masking set at the preferred level established in Phase III, have the speech mode used until five minutes of stutter-free speech (or very small stutterings) accumulate.
2. Turn off the masking unit, but leave the earphones on. Instruct clients to try to keep the same speech pattern used during masking.
   a. On the occurrence of any stuttering spasm, the clients are to turn on the masking unit until they feel control has been reestablished and then turn it off.
   b. On the anticipation of stuttering, the clients may follow the instructions in 2a.
3. The criteria for success in this phase are several and variable.
   a. Clients turn on the masking unit after 90 percent or more of the stuttering spasms have occurred.

    b. Clients turn on the masking unit at the time of occurrence, or before, of 50 percent or more of the stuttering spasms. This criterion may be raised for some stutterers and lowered for others.

    c. The number of stutterings does not go over 10 percent of the baseline figure. With situational adaptation, this may be too easy a criterion to meet.

4. Typically, the client who responds well to masking will develop to the point at which the masking unit is used for the first five minutes of a therapy session and then, over time and in a steadily decreasing sequence, will be used less and less—depending on factors such as attitude, daily feelings and fatigue, and topics being discussed in therapy.

The client usually will report an improvement in out-clinic speech during these phases. Some therapy programs will use Phase IV to provide entry into other therapy techniques cited previously. It is also possible to phase out the masker and concentrate on strengthening and transferring the speech modifications, similar to the shaping program Leith and Chmiel (1980) report, which used DAF for shaping speech production.

OUT-CLINIC PROGRAMS

The clinician also may wish to continue use of masking into an out-clinic program.

Application of masking to out-clinic uses has been discussed previously. From past experience and information from other clinicians, we will recommend one of two approaches, depending on the type of masking unit used. For either type, manual or automatic, the client must be instructed in the operation and maintenance of the unit. Location of plugs and switches, battery life and replacement, care of wires and receivers, and operation of controls will have to be learned. For most models, the client will need to secure, or have made, skeletal earpiece inserts. The skeletal type of insert will allow better auditory acuity when the client is listening to other speakers. It is possible to use monaural receiver units, but best results are obtained binaurally. The physical arrangement of the masking unit will have to be determined and tried out. The laryngeal contact microphone, if it is an automatic unit, will be attached by an elastic or adjustable neckband or with special mounting tape sold by the unit's manufacturer or by tape-supply companies. Placement of the unit, pathways for the wires, and concealment will preoccupy the stutterer at first, and the clinician should provide assistance. (In our graduate stuttering course, each clinician is required to wear a portable masking unit for twenty-four to forty-eight hours in order to learn the use of and problems with the instrument.) Willingness of the client to wear the unit should be explored, along with identification of situations where activity or safety precautions would preclude wearing it. Out-clinic use of masking will be within the context of one of the following goals:

1. As a more or less permanent device to support fluent speech by the speaker.
2. As a temporary method to enhance the development of specific fluency facilitation patterns of speech.
3. As a temporary method to enhance the development of specific symptom control techniques to be used with stuttering spasms.
4. As a temporary method to encourage and require increased levels of tactile and kinesthetic monitoring of the speech mechanism.
5. As a temporary method in various aspects of therapy motivation, self-analysis, spasm variation, desensitization, or other areas of therapy.

All the foregoing have been discussed previously to some degree. Further development will be limited to the first goal, since the other four can reflect too many different emphases and organizations of therapy to cover here.

Continuous use of a portable auditory masking unit is a major decision by the clinician and by the client. It either reflects a decision to live "forever" with the speech support of an electronic unit, or it reflects a belief that the unit can be used on a decreasing scale as the stutterer gains confidence and ability in speech control. The client should understand the implications of the decision. If the client is willing to accept the probable outcome, therapy should progress through the following phases to accomplish the desired goal. As with other techniques in this book, these phases are not the only way to use masking. Many factors can alter the sequence, and the reader should not feel bound by them.

Phase I: Preparation

1. Discuss goals with the client and secure agreement on procedures. Plan the time frame of development, reporting, therapy phases, and so on. Preview the frustrations, problems, and embarrassments that could occur.
2. Practice the physical aspects of wearing the device, checking and maintenance procedures, and what to do in case of mechanical problems.
3. Make any decisions or plans about manual versus automatic triggering systems. If the automatic system is selected, practice application of the contact microphone, concealment, how to override the unit, and how to activate it on voiceless sounds.

Phase II: In-Clinic Practice

1. Determine the preferred setting and (if possible) the best frequency settings of the instrument.
2. Proceed through a simple sequence of increasing length and complexity of response. Decide ahead of time the criterion to meet before progressing to the next level, for example, no more than one SW/M at a severity level of

"mild" (less than one-second duration with no struggle or associated behaviors) for three minutes of performance at each step. Possible steps are
   a. Automatic speech in counting to 100, naming days and months, reciting memorized materials.
   b. Reading sentences.
   c. Reading material in paragraphs.
   d. Answering questions.
   e. Monologue topic speech.
   f. Asking questions.
   g. Making telephone calls.
   h. Talking with a third person in the room.
3. Practice general conversation while reviewing the result of 2a-h. Look for particular words or speech sounds that gave more trouble, and practice with them. Discuss whether telephone use requires removal of one earpiece. If necessary, consider use of easy onset and/or vowel prolongation to make getting started and continuation simpler.
4. Review and update the situational fear hierarchy so that the client can estimate masking needs according to situations. Use this discussion as further practice.
5. Spend at least one therapy session on outside assignments drawn from the hierarchy, with the clinician along. Evaluate and discuss success, problems, feelings, and auditors' reactions.
6. Use the input from 5 to develop a final plan for Phase III.

Phase III: Transition

As before, the following is only one way to proceed. There are many other possibilities that can be developed.

1. In the first week the client should wear the unit at all reasonable times, including relaxed times and days off.
2. The unit should be activated at the beginning of every speech situation. The client may deactivate it at any time and turn it back on at any time.
3. Adjustments in the settings of the unit can be made as the client wishes.
4. The report form such as Chart 11-1 is filled out daily or several times during the day if that is possible.

CHART 11-1 *Masking Use Report Form*

NAME: _____ DATE: _____

Situation Identification	Use of Unit		
	% of time on	No. of reactivations	Effectiveness
1.			
2.			
. . .			
20.			

5. The client returns to the clinic for a therapy session that week, bringing the reports. In addition to the issues raised by the client and the clinician, the following should be explored:
   a. Are there serious reservations about continued use of the unit? If so, can these be resolved?
   b. Are there any mechanical problems, wearing arrangements, or unit settings that need to be dealth with?
   c. Do any of the reported experiences indicate a need to revise the projected plan of use?

6. The second week of solo use is to be a replication of the first week, with any changes resulting from considerations under 5c. The client returns to the clinic, and evaluation is repeated. Ordinarily, clients will report that the unit is being turned off sooner and reactivation is occurring less often. Two weeks of use should allow identification of any particularly difficult situations, trouble words, or other special problems. These can be worked on in the therapy session.

7. At this point, the clinician will decide to continue the previous procedures, as amended, for a third week (or longer) or to proceed to the next step. Many individual factors can affect the decision, but suggested criteria are these:
   a. No major problems of attitude toward, and acceptance of, the method and the masking unit.
   b. No major problems with mechanical aspects or operator's use.
   c. Some reduction, at least 10 percent, in the time the unit is on. This will be an approximation since need, opportunity, situational difficulty, and other factors will vary.
   d. Stabilization or reduction in the dysfluencies produced by the stutterer, compared to the first week, with the same qualifiers as cited in 7c.

8. If the mutual decision is to proceed, the stutterer wears the unit full-time for the next two weeks but activates it only on perceived need. The previous report form can be adapted for use, and the client returns to the clinic each week.

9. At this point, the criteria from 7 are reapplied. If the answers are satisfactory, progress to Phase IV. If the criteria are not met, decide whether to solve the problems or terminate use of the unit. By this time the client may find the unit "too much trouble" to use, and you will have to do some serious work with attitude and motivation—which has been a major reason for the continuation of the weekly sessions.

Phase IV: Separation[2]

1. The client is instructed to decide when to wear the unit and when to activate it. Daily reports are discontinued.

2. After one week, the client calls the clinician on the telephone and makes a verbal report. After the second week, the client returns to the clinic for evaluation and planning.

3. If results have been satisfactory, shift the schedule to a four-week basis, where the client makes three weekly telephone reports and one clinic visit.

---

[2]Enrollment in a stuttering group for sharing, motivation, and problem solving can be done at any time in therapy but is particularly helpful in Phase IV or earlier in Phase III.

4. If results have been satisfactory, move to a monthly visit (no telephone reports, except at the client's need) for three months.

5. If results have been satisfactory, shift to a quarterly (three-month) visitation schedule, for six months.

6. If results have been satisfactory, terminate therapy with encouragement to return at any time or to call for consultation or assistance.

12

RHYTHM

Speech has its own intrinsic, individual pattern, which is not a paced rhythm. The limitations of neuron firing rate, impulse transmission speed, and the response and rest cycle of muscle fibers contribute to individual patterns, as do the facilitating and inhibiting interactions of brain stem and cerebellar centers. What we call rhythm in stuttering therapy is an artificial rhythm, usually with an atypical regularity and a pulse rate below that of normal speech. Although we will cite instances of irregular rhythm, most applications in therapy involve the timing of speech output to an external or an internal pattern that is absolutely regular. Technically, any device or behavior that produces a timing pattern is a rhythm method—singing, chanting, shadowing, unison speech, simultaneous talking and writing, metronome, and others. However, we will consider metronome and syllable-timed speech under rhythm and discuss certain other techniques in the final chapter.

The position of rhythm in speech therapy is, to say the least, anomalous. Boome and Richardson (1931) opposed it as quackery and as causing worse problems than before it was used. Barber (1940) regarded it simply as a distraction from stuttering. Bloodstein (1949) noted that any type of timing activity reduced stuttering, but he also suggested distraction as an explanation. Bluemel (1960) condemned rhythm because it distorted speech into an unusable pattern, and besides, it long had been associated with the quacks and their secret techniques. One of the more interesting comments was made by Van Riper (1973, p. 63):

> Any method which for at least a century and a half has failed so consistently to produce any real cure for stuttering and still manages to be used so widely must have something pretty vital in it. We think the vitality resides in the fact that it works. Yes, temporarily and unfortunately, it works.

As we will see, rhythm generally is reported as the most effective and rapid method for inducing fluency in stuttered speech. This has been known for over a century, yet the use of rhythm in current therapy dates back only twenty years or so—and many professionals still reject it.

The history of rhythm therapy for stuttering is vague until about two centuries ago. Historical reviews have traced it back to ancient Greece, but they tend to cite the years 1800 to 1830 as when it appeared in literature pertaining to stuttering (Klingbeil, 1939; Van Riper, 1973; Wingate, 1976). The best review probably is Wingate's. About 1830, Colombat de l'Isere published reports of a device called the *methonome* (Van Riper refers to it as the *mutonom*). This mechanism was shaped like an ancient lyre (a type of harp), where the strings or bars were stroked by a vertical arm of the wind-up pendulum. A sliding weight on the vertical arm controlled the rate of its movement and, hence, the beats per minute (bpm). A number of other professionals in France, England, and Germany used rhythmic patterns, but the method finally seemed to slide into relative obscurity. Robbins (1935) reported on significant differences between the rhythm of stuttered and fluent speech but recommended against the use of current (private school, mainly) rhythm techniques because the resulting speech was not normal. Johnson and Rosen (1937) found that rhythm was the most effective fluency inducer of twelve methods measured, but few professionals in the field responded (see later for further discussion). Barber (1940) varied the timing of syllable and word utterance and found that both significantly reduced stuttering, but nobody seemed to pay attention. Van Riper (1973) suggested that Van Dantzig (1940), in Holland, revived rhythm techniques. If so, the revival was quite muted and generally not noticed. This may have been due, in part, to professional prejudice or even to jealousy (Hutchinson, 1976).

RECENT HISTORY

After Van Dantzig, rhythm techniques more or less languished until a "new technique" was reported (Meyer and Mair, 1963) which involved the development of a miniaturized, behind-the-ears type of electronic metronome generator. Wingate (1976) noted that the development of rhythm at this time, and in the next twenty years, was marked by several unique factors:

1. It occurred mainly outside the United States.
2. Interest in this country generally was expressed outside the field of speech pathology.
3. Emphasis generally was on the therapeutic use of rhythm.
4. Rarely did any of the users build on previous use of rhythm.
5. The motivating force seemed to come from the development and availability of the electronic metronome.

Three years after the Meyer and Mair publication, Adler (1966) still referred to the ancient history of rhythm and not to recent developments. Wider use in Europe, particularly in England, developed rapidly (Beech, 1967), with a rejection of the noise-distraction explanation and historical credit given to Serre d'Alai and the isochrome, circa 1837. Rothman (1969), an osteopathic psychiatrist, published a report on the so-called Brady unit that could be worn as a behind-the-ear hearing aid (it was used to treat insomnia as well as stuttering). Brady (1971) reported on using the unit with twenty-three stutterers, citing favorable long-term (six months to three years) results for over 90 percent of the clients. Metronome use was recommended favorably in several European countries (Watts, 1973); but the Rothman and Brady reports had small impact on the American scene.

During the 1960s and 1970s, rhythm techniques were adopted by some of the behavioralists and transformed into programmed sequences (Ingham, 1975a; Ingham & Andrews, 1973b; Jones & Azrin, 1969), although it was noted that "In general, there was a paucity of data from therapists using rhythmic speech" (Ingham, 1975a, p. 385). Boberg (1976) described an intensive program that used rhythmic (syllable-timed) speech as one of its components. Dalton and Hardcastle (1977) reflected the waning (Cheasman, 1983) of rhythmic therapies in England when they admitted that rhythm quickly induced fluency but resulted in an abnormal speech pattern. Wingate (1976, p. 164) commented extensively on developments in rhythm therapy, noting that advances have been largely mechanical, and the basic principles of application have not changed:

> Rhythm therapy is now "behavior therapy," changes that occur are "conditioned," fluency is "shaped." At best the terms are innocuous in that they refer to nothing that was not known or done before. At the same time, their use reflects either ignorance of, or indifference to, what is known about rhythm and stuttering.

As we can see, rhythm moved on an uneasy course, and still does, between efficiency and relapse, respectability and quackery. Other opinions will be examined later. Nevertheless, it is a method or collection of methods that seems able to provide fluency improvement with great speed and with comparative ease. The fact that it has been associated now with behaviorists is of no more significance than its earlier association with quackery for decades; the application, rather than the technique, is important. Further review of this technique certainly is warranted.

RHYTHM RESEARCH

Research relative to rhythm has concerned both the basic patterns of stuttering and the artificially imposed pacing effects. A number of clinicians have hypothesized that stutterers have a disturbance in motor control or timing, speech monitoring, motor planning, or sensory feedback. Many, many studies have been devoted to these topics. It has been suggested that stutterers are less accurate than nonstutterers in timing speech programs, although there was considerable overlap between stuttering and nonstuttering groups. Also, stutterers dismissed from therapy were more accurate timers than were stutterers still in therapy (Cooper & Allen, 1977). On the production side, stutterers have been shown to have a slower neural response time (lip movement) to visual and auditory stimuli, greater frequency of eye fixations, regressive and progressive eye movements during silent reading, and slower phonatory response time to auditory stimuli than to visual stimuli (Brutten & Janssen, 1979; McFarlane & Prins, 1978; McFarlane & Shipley, 1981). An interesting, brief review of research relating to neurological function and coordination for speech can be found in the article by Andrews et al. (1983) and in Kent's (1983) comments on their propositions. The thrust of these reviews is to support, at least in part, the idea that some stutterers have a constitutional weakness in the planning, timing, and/or control of speech.

Although rhythm has been used with stutterers for centuries, very few clinicians were encouraged to investigate it, probably because of the quackery associated with it for so long. The dominance of applied rhythm was investigated by Azrin et al. (1968), who reported that either manual bar pressing or vocalizations in the presence of a regular stimulus beat tended to synchronize with the rhythm of that stimulus beat. F. H. Silverman (1971a) simply compared normal and metronome speech (at thirty-two bpm), reporting a significant reduction in all dysfluency types (except prolongations, which were low from the outset), for both stutterers and nonstutterers. In looking at different types of approaches, Johnson and Rosen (1937) compared variations in rate, loudness, pitch, and tempo (twelve conditions in all) in terms of their effects on stuttering, starting with a baseline average of 7.6 percent stuttering for eighteen subjects. The conditions of singing, metronome speech, talking in time to arm swinging, and talking in singsong (all strongly rhythm-based) resulted in stuttering percentages of zero (for singing) to 0.09 for singsong speech. Metronome speech yielded 0.06 percent stuttering.

Other comparative studies, more recently, have underscored the efficiency of rhythm procedures. Ost et al. (1976) compared metronome treatment to shadowing, finding that the former produced less stuttering after dismissal. A comparison among DAF, metronome, and masking noise indicated that all three significantly reduced stuttering while the subjects were reading, but only metronome significantly reduced stuttering during spontaneous speech (Hutchinson & Norris, 1977). Another study compared TO, noise, DAF, a contingent "wrong," and metronome during talking (Martin & Haroldson, 1979). Reported were an 80 percent reduction in stuttering frequency and a 46 percent reduction in spasm severity for metronome use. Only the TO condition was better, and both were two or three times more effective than the other methods. Hayden et al. (1982b) compared the effects of rhythm and masking on nonstutterers as well as stutterers in measuring speech initiation time. They reported that masking slowed SIT scores, whereas rhythm accelerated them. In a related study (Hayden et al., 1982a), it was reported that VIT scores were accelerated significantly by masking and also by rhythm, and that rhythm voice initiation time was significantly faster than during masking. In a study of comparison overkill, Andrews et al. (1982) evaluated three stutterers under fifteen conditions—including talking and writing, singing, choral reading, shadowing, arm swinging, syllable-timed speech, dialect, talking to an animal, two conditions of talking alone, relaxation, masking, slow rate, response contingent stimuli, and a combination of prolongation and DAF. They reported that all the conditions were responded to individually at times, but all generally reduced stuttering significantly. The conditions tended either to lengthen phonation duration (singing, choral reading, shadowing, prolongation and DAF) or to reduce rate (talking and writing, relaxation, slow rate, arm swinging, syllable-timed speech, prolongation and DAF). Unfortunately, the small subject population reduces the results to the level of interesting speculation.

Other studies have evaluated "arhythmic rhythm" against a regular metronome and normal conditions (Fransella & Beech, 1965). Although their experimental design limits acceptance of results, it was reported that arhythmic beats did not facilitate fluency. Haney (1976) reported that gradually increasing the rhythm pace, and then fading the intensity, did not result in a significant return of dysfluencies. Hutchinson and Navarre (1977) reported that metronome rhythm with stutterers and nonstutterers resulted in an increased airflow rate for nonstutterers and a decrease for stutterers, and both groups showed lower peak pressures and greater pressure durations during rhythmic speech production.

Research has suggested the possibility of a constitutional fault in at least some stutterers. Rhythmic pacing of speech apparently overcomes or compensates for most of the dysfluency factors, although we cannot assert exactly why this happens. In comparing rhythm techniques, especially metronome, to other fluency-inducing methods, we found many instances where rhythm seems to provide the most, or very high levels of, fluency for stutterers, and even for nonstutterers. Within the limits of normative research on age, sex, etiology, loudness, duration, frequency, and other factors, it appears that rhythmic pacing is one of the most effective fluency-development systems available to clinicians today. The questions relative to why it is effective and the acceptability of the created speech patterns remain to be explored.

REASONS FOR RHYTHM EFFECTS

Explanations for rhythm effect are hazy and spread in two directions. One area of interest concerns why it is effective, and the other, how it is effective in reducing dysfluency. Bloodstein (1972) suggested that distraction or simplification of motor planning (or both) could explain why rhythm is effective. Many earlier clinicians also cited distraction as the primary explanation. However, Beech and Fransella (1968) compared rhythm and distraction phenomena and concluded that the former does not function as a distraction. They also stated that its effects were not based on any tendency to reduce speech rate, but it may operate significantly *to make more predictable* the point at which any following vocalization will occur. In a subsequent study Beech & Fransella (1969) found that high predictability of following words was accompanied by significantly fewer production errors and by a shorter latency time before utterance, although subject variability was quite large. Dijk (1973) also rejected the distraction explanation, saying that the stutterer must concentrate on his or her speech in order to time it to the other source. Watts (1973) summarized current research and concurred that distraction is not a significant factor. In examining the bpm rate of metronome research, he found that there was a consistent pattern in that slower rates were more effective than normal or faster rates. Wingate (1969) hypothesized that rhythm organizes stress patterns, focusing on syllabic nuclei and emphasizing phonation. Finally, Watts also found support for the hypothesis that rhythm provides a pacing, or timing, vehicle to signal the initiation of a syllable, a word, or even a phrase (depending on the frequency and duration of the signal pulses). Kent (1983) also suggested that rhythm reduces temporal or timing uncertainty, allows more time to plan timing patterns, and generally simplifies the complex task of connected speech discourse. The problems that remain are to discover whether other parameters are involved and to explain why rhythmic effects are not approximately uniform across all stutterers.

VALUES OF RHYTHM THERAPY

Evaluation of rhythm divides into two categories—research studies concerning the stability and acceptability of rhythmic effects on speech and evaluative comments based on clinical experience, empirical research, or research by other professionals. F. H. Silverman (1971b) reported on a rationale for the use of the hearing-aid metronomes, that rationale being mainly to break into the fear-avoidance cycle of stuttering and to encourage the speaker to develop fluency experiences. Trotter and Silverman (1974) reported on four studies of metronome use with stutterers. Time periods for use varied from eighteen days to a year. For most time periods, effectiveness did not decrease, but Silverman's daily use resulted in some decrease after the first three months. Two years later, F. H. Silverman (1976) reported on personal use of a portable (spectacles) unit for three years. He reported securing a great reduction in severity and frequency of stuttering for about six months. However, over the next two years, the efficacy of the device gradually decreased. Poppen et al. (1977) reported on rhythm use with one stutterer, indicating that continued use of the unit resulted in a deterioration of fluency that changes in the bpm rate did not help. Apparently not all stutterers respond well to the use of rhythmic pacing. Meyer and Comley (1969) fitted forty-eight stutterers with portable metronome devices. Of the forty-eight clients, seventeen failed to respond to the method, and they were the more severe stutterers. The authors reported that unilateral use seemed to produce better speech results than did bilateral devices, and the clients did not like to use the bilateral devices in public. In general, clinicians could tell "almost immediately" if a client was going to respond to rhythm therapy.

The acceptability of rhythm-paced speech seems to place the method in a different status for many clinicians. Ingham and Andrews (1971) compared the results of DAF therapy to that of syllable-timed speech. Both showed similar improvements in stuttering frequency. Stutterers in the syllable-timed program, however, continued to show secondary characteristics, had a lower optimal rate of speech, and tended to break down in fluency when that optimal rate was surpassed. Reactions of listeners have been reported by several studies. In comparing unaided speech to metronome pacing, judges noted the reductions in stuttering in metronome speech but were negative toward some of the aspects of paced fluency (Silverman & Trotter, 1973). As stuttering increased in severity, so did listeners' acceptance of paced speech. Runyan and Adams (1979) sampled listeners' judgments of speech samples from six types of therapy programs, matching fluent samples from stutterers to similar speech samples from nonstutterers. In every instance, for each type of therapy (including metronome), the listeners could separate fluent speech of stutterers from normal speech of nonstutterers.

Mallard and Mayer (1979) found that when listeners observed videotapes of three stutterers, each talking as usual, talking at 100 wpm, and talking at 70 wpm, 78 percent to 96 percent of the judges preferred paced speech on two subjects, and 57 percent preferred stuttering in the third client. The authors noted that the third stutterer paced in a "staccato, machine-like manner." They advised clinicians to prevent the development of abrupt initiation and termination of syllables by clients and not to allow transfer of very slow rhythm rates to outside situations. Jones and Azrin (1969) may have made a contribution earlier to "naturalness." They kept the off beat period constant at one second but varied the duration of the on period of the stimulus tone. The stutterer was allowed to speak as long as the tone was on. They found an inverse relationship between stuttering and stimulus duration, up to a duration of about two seconds, and also an increase in naturalness and rapidity of speech.

Concerning professional attitudes, Pellman (1947) objected to the use of rhythm because he thought it intensified the feelings of inferiority and damaged one's self-concept. Van Riper (1971, p. 997), although admitting the initial efficacy of rhythm, was adamant about its values (or problems):

> Unfortunately, most of these distractions give small permanent relief because once their novelty is lost their interference with the stuttering stimuli becomes less effective. Indeed, through the reinforcement they achieve, distracting motor rituals can become incorporated into the abnormality.

Sheehan (1975), as we would expect, refers to Van Dantzig as having "exhumed the corpse" of rhythm, and he proceeds to criticize rhythm in scathing terms. Andrews et al. (1980) commented that as a treatment, rhythm is "unloved" because clients dislike its strict cadence, it does not deal with associated behaviors, and its effects tend to deteriorate over time. However, some researchers have suggested that our frequent rejection of rhythm may not be based completely on a foundation of research and professional objectivity. It is possible that at least part of the rejection relates to the fact that there is no obvious, satisfactory explanation for its effectiveness and its immediate results tend to diminish with time; moreover, there may be a degree of jealousy because rhythm requires no skilled clinician in its direct use (Beech & Fransella, 1969).

What we have is a technique that is one of the most effective, if not the most effective, in supporting fluency. It also acts with great speed and provides extensive opportunities for self-direction to the client. Applications can be made in group or individual formats, intensive or spaced schedules, and across a range of in-clinic and out-clinic activities. At the same time it is a technique that is not applicable to all stutterers and can be misused if pretherapy evaluations are slighted. The fluent speech produced initially is quite atypical of normal speech patterns, and transfer to normal speech can be quite difficult. Finally, with prolonged use the rhythm method may, to varying degrees, lose some of its effectiveness. The degree to which these pluses and minuses can be balanced, and what improvements are possible, will be addressed in the next two sections on applications in therapy.

USES OF RHYTHM

Applications of rhythm to therapy will concentrate on uses of rhythm in the last fifty years and will be followed by recommendations for current evaluation and clinical use. Barber (1940) compared various types of rhythmic devices, having stutterers read while

Walking, one syllable or word uttered per step.
Tapping one foot on the production of each word.
Arm swinging on each word or syllable.
Hand-wrist swinging on each word.
Using a singsong production, accenting alternate syllables.
Accenting every third word.
A light flashing for the production of each word.
A metronome sounding for each word, 92 and 184 bpm.
Tactile stimulation on each word.

Barber reported that accenting every third word was least effective, and walking and using the metronome reduced stuttering the most. All conditions significantly reduced stuttering. This wide range of effectiveness is supported by Wingate's (1976) statement that word rhythm can be as effective as syllable timing, even to the extent of keying short clauses and phrases to the rhythm. He also noted that absolute regularity of the rhythmic source is not necessary.

Van Dantzig's (1940) method of syllable tapping was an interesting combination of rhythm pacing, talking in concert with limb movement, suggestion, and development of mental imagery. After initial explanations and demonstration, the client rests one hand (palm down) in a relaxed curve (as if playing the piano) on a flat surface, such as a table top. On each syllable, utterance is timed by tapping one finger on the table top, starting with the little finger, progressing to the thumb, and starting back with the little finger again. If an utterance is interrupted by a repetitive stuttering spasm, the client is to

1. Suspend the tapping effort, but hold the finger in place.
2. Lower the hand and forearm toward the table top, while extending the fingers, but keeping the tapping finger in contact with the flat surface.
3. Keeping the tapping finger in contact, slowly raise the hand and forearm, timing this with a release of the stuttered syllable.

If the interrupting spasm is primarily tonic, the stutterer presses down with the tapping finger while stretching the hand and forearm, straining them with the tonic spasm, shortening the latter by timing it with the limb movement. These exercises are carried out to mastery level, progressively, in reading, reciting, answering questions, and spontaneous speech. As ability develops, the client is taught to hide the finger movements behind a book, behind the back, in a pocket, and so on. Those clients who do well can be taught to substitute mental visualization of the tapping process in place of the physical act.

Andrews et al. (1964) reported on using syllable-timed speech with thirty-five stutterers. Before initiation of therapy, baseline fluency levels were established and evaluations made for neurotic traits. Clients then were taught syllable-timed speech in which all stress and syllable contrasts were eliminated. Clients started by repeating sentences modeled by the clinician; they then progressed to reading and, finally, to spontaneous speech, using the syllable-timed utterance. This establishment phase usually took about two hours, children taking a little longer because of unfamiliarity of some of them with the concept of the syllable. Clients now were talking at about eighty spm (syllables per minute). Group therapy was used over the next two weeks to stabilize syllable-timed speech, explore attitudes and anxieties, and begin outside practice. Group sessions dropped to a weekly schedule for the next ten weeks as transfer of syllable-timed speech developed. Clients were advised to use normal speech, switching to syllable-timed utterances only when they stuttered. Following dismissal, the severity groups all showed a resurgence of stuttering and then stabilized over the following year. Two groups with baseline severities of 21 percent to 36 percent SW dropped to about 1 percent SW at dismissal and then rebounded to 7 percent to 10 percent SW in the next nine months. The five children (age eleven) started at 20 percent SW, dropped to 0 percent SW, and then went back up to about 1 percent SW in the ensuing months. The researchers also noted that syllable-timed therapy worked better when the "whole" person was considered in therapy, that refresher therapy during the sixth to ninth months in the postdismissal period might be valuable, that those clients who responded best had very few neurotic traits, that the amount of improvement toward normality (not just reduction in percent SW) was greater for the moderate than for the severe stutterers, and that the best progress was made by the children and by those over twenty-two years of age.

Brandon and Harris (1967) also stressed strongly the value of group activity in a program that ran 150 minutes per day for two weeks, followed by two sessions per week for three months, phasing down to weekly sessions, and finally dropping to quarterly sessions for group discussion and refresher practice on syllable-timed speech. They started with unison production of sentences and moved in carefully graded steps of difficulty in reading and speaking. Controlled outside assignments were conducted with the therapist, and later with another group member replacing the clinician. Eighteen clients were rated as successful (60 percent or greater improvement in fluency) and ten were rated as failures. The authors reported that intelligence and age (in disagreement with Andrews) had little relation to outcome of therapy. A low score on neurotic traits and a high level of extroversion appeared to relate to poor performance. Stutterers who showed least improvement appeared to have low anxiety and to have the following characteristics: relaxed, confident, cheerful, outgoing, friendly, sociable, and egocentric. Brandon and Harris felt that these traits reduced conditionability and learning drive.

Meyer and Comley (1969) reported on their use of rhythm with forty-eight stutterers, starting with word pacing and falling back to syllable timing for those who had trouble getting started. An optimal bpm rate was established for each client rather than a uniform rate. They divided the clients into three groups, which continued group therapy for purposes of problem solving, relaxation activity, and role-playing simulation. One group used a monaural portable metronome outside, the second group used a binaural unit, and the third group acted as unaided controls. Overall, 35 percent of the stutterers failed to master the rhythm technique, the majority of these being from the least fluent, "hard blocking" stutterers. These clients showed no significant improvement by the termination of therapy but improved significantly during the follow-up phase. The authors concluded that improvement under rhythm does not seem to be affected by the use or nonuse of portable units, that bilateral portable units generally are unacceptable to stutterers, and that stutterers will not all react similarly to rhythm—some failing to respond at all.

Wohl (1968) felt that the metronome reduced anxiety levels in general and inhibited awareness of speech and sensitivity to stress. Alford and Ingham (1969)—in combining syllable-timed speech with a token reinforcement system, negative practice, and parent training for home activity with children—felt that improved results could be expected with these additions to basic rhythm procedures. Plomley et al. (1971) structured a twenty-one day intensive program combining syllable-timed speech, contingent use of DAF, and situational practice for different groups, based on a token reinforcement pattern. They reported that clients who received both techniques (DAF and syllable-timed speech) could speak at normal and supranormal speech rates and maintain fluency, but syllable-timed-only clients could not maintain fluency at rapid rates of speech. On occasions where stuttering occurred, the first group generally produced sound and syllable repetitions only, whereas the syllable-timed-only group displayed secondary spasm patterns.

Ingham et al. (1972) combined syllable-timed speech, group psychotherapy, increased stuttering to heighten motivation, and a TRS (token reinforcement system), used mainly to reduce stuttering and improve rate.

Different combinations of these were used with fifty-eight adult stutterers divided into groups. The researchers reported that the token system and syllable-timed program resulted in the greatest changes in speech rate and in the percentage of stuttered syllables, whereas increased stuttering (negative practice) and psychotherapy sessions seemed unrelated to improvement—within the extremely limited definition they seemed to apply to "improvement."

J. P. Brady has extensively developed the rhythm therapy proposed by Meyer and Mair (1963), discussed earlier. His initial work (1968; 1971; 1972, with C. N. Brady) established a program in which the stutterer is counseled that rhythmic speech is a temporary method used to approach nonstuttered utterances, that it will adapt quickly to normal speech rhythm, and that it will be important to practice and learn in real situations outside the clinic to assure transfer and stabilization. Each client's optimal metronome rate is determined. Brady suggests that severe stutterers may have to go as low as forty bpm, whereas moderate stutterers may be able to double that. Also, severe stutterers may have to start with syllable timing, whereas less severe clients do well with a word-timed rate. Initially, the stutterer is led through progressive increases in the bpm rate. This fluctuates as the complexity of speech tasks increases (dropping back in bpm temporarily with each increase in speech complexity) and as the clinician works to develop normal aspects of stress, inflection, pausing, and so on. When feasible, the client can utter more than one syllable or word per beat, use beats to time pauses, and otherwise move away from cadenced speech. Therapy is weekly, with home practice sessions of thirty to forty-five minutes daily. When work involves more complex speech and emphasizes normalization of production, Brady sets a goal of 100 to 160 syllables (or short words) per minute without significant stuttering. Also, the home practice sessions should include an auditor in these advanced stages. Therapy then moves from the in-clinic metronome to a portable unit, temporarily dropping back to earlier demand and complexity levels as needed. A situational fear hierarchy is developed, and the client works through it, using therapy sessions for support, planning, and analysis. When the client is fearful of a particular situation (see later) or finds paced speech too artificial to accept, in-clinic simulation and normalization practice are used to attack both problems. The goal at this stage is fluent speech and general relaxation in all speech situations. Metronome use is faded out in the next stage, often with relapses, returns of fears, and other problems. Brady attempts to have the client develop an imaginary metronome, but if the client insists, prolonged use of the portable unit is allowed. Follow-up is necessary because of frequent regressions. Companion therapies can include DAF, desensitization, or any other comparable methods.

It has been suggested (Fiedler & Standop, 1983) that because of ". . . a great many training sessions required . . . stutterers often express an aversion to this procedure and perceive it at times to be as conspicuous as stuttering itself . . . the method should be reserved for the severest stuttering configurations" (p. 119). Previous comments about poor response of severe stutterers to pacing should be remembered. Brady (Brady & Brady, 1972) reiterated support for the use of the portable metronome but cited the need to develop a better relaxation association with the pacing effect. He later described (Brady, 1973) a procedure in which the client is taught relaxation on a progressive system (see Chapter 5), where major muscle groups are tensed and relaxed in a set sequence. Verbal suggestions and relaxing monologue from the clinician reinforce relaxation. All the instructions and subsequent monologue are accompanied by a soft-tone metronome at sixty bpm, speech and activity being coordinated to the pace of the beat. Brady suggests making a tape cassette of the first session, or one of the early successful ones, and having the client conduct his or her own in-clinic session by using the tape. The tape can be also used in home practice. Using a portable metronome, the client can transfer relaxation to situations where anxiety and tension have previously prevented control of stuttering or the normalization of speech. Brady estimated that five to ten MCR (metronome-conditioned relaxation) sessions are sufficient for the average client to achieve deep relaxation in just a few minutes. Using the tape cassette, the client may need only the first session with the clinician and can carry the rest of acquisition alone.

Wohl (1968), who does not hesitate to be right, or at least positive, cites rhythm therapy as the answer to a clinician's urgent need, since any technique seems to leave the stutterer with a gap between in-clinic success and out-clinic performance in real situations where fear breaks down the learned system. Wohl begins with twenty therapy sessions to teach relaxation. She then moves into a sequence to measure anxiety and sensitivity and to construct a fear hierarchy. This is followed by an extensive desensitization process. As part of it, the client fills out report forms on distressful situations, providing Wohl with ongoing evaluation material. This report form, according to Wohl, controls the client's efforts to seek sympathy from the clinician for all the suffering caused by stuttering. Wohl studies the speech and behavior patterns of the client and selects the desired therapy system. She feels that rhythm is a habit to be learned, and then unlearned, recommending the use of different signal forms to minimize habituation. Wohl states that at all times, best results are obtained from clients who have a family history of stuttering. She notes that some patients become so frustrated by the charting, the analysis, and by her refusal to listen to what she feels are inappropriate, paranoidlike verbalizations common to all adult stutterers that they may reject treatment, display temper, and even show catastrophic behavior. Wohl also feels that the metronome relieves anxiety in the clinician and in the client's relatives.

In an expansion of therapy procedures, Wohl (1970) begins by stating that it is correct to divide stutterers into four fairly equal groups of festinating, phonatory blocking, oral blocking, and ataxic-like stuttering, with about 4 percent falling into psychiatric categories. Evaluation procedures should avoid any show of investigation but be used mainly to measure baseline dysfluency characteristics. A minimum personal history is needed, and self-disclosure by the client should be discouraged, since the speech clinician generally cannot handle it. In treatment, clients are told that they will be offered ten therapy sessions. If performance is satisfactory, another ten visits will be offered. Sessions should be as close together as possible, preferably daily. For one time, and not again, the clinician summarizes the aversive spectra of stuttering in general and any particulars specific to the client. A pamphlet of printed instructions for out-client practice is provided, and no deviation or error by the client is encouraged. The client must provide the metronome. The client is told that no specific speech rate is required, and syllabic speech or any similar "mutilation" will not be learned. Wohl, believing that less than 1 percent of the stutterers actually need formal training to learn stress-time speech, allows the client to set the speech rate and bpm pace. The treatment steps are too microscopically chronicled to repeat here.

Initial training[1] starts with mental counting, using the metronome as a pacing cue and then turning it off. This progresses to oral counting, variations in counting, series counting, and then serial production of other automatic speech sequences. Thirty-two steps are invoved. The next seventeen steps relate to walking and moving parts of the body in time to metronome rhythm, followed by fifteen steps concerned with graphic movements. The latter start with parallel pencil strokes in rhythm, then other lines, and finally to glyphic-type marks. The client moves to alphabet letters, and ends with words and familiar writing. Stuttering is approached directly by covering the first twenty-eight steps. The client starts by listening to the metronome, uttering beat-synchronized nonsense syllables, varying rate, naming in increasing numbers, developing word strings and, finally, using sentences. Extensive practice is required for getting restarted after normal pause breaks. With the use of the portable metronome and development of a situational fear hierarchy, transfer is facilitated. Wohl requires the client to turn the device off when not speaking, so behind-the-ear units are not recommended. The client is told to obey rules or treatment will be discontinued, and the clinician must show a "positive and unrelenting" attitude or progress will be reduced. About twenty hours of Jacobson-type relaxation, performed earlier, is coupled with classic desen-

---

[1]This set is intended for festinating speech, walking, and writing. Whether all parts or only certain sections are used depends on presented needs at the time of therapy.

sitization procedures to provide for situation transfer. Ultimately, the client either will outgrow any need for the portable unit or (in a few cases) will develop a pattern that incorporates the metronome on a permanent basis.

Coppola and Yairi (1982) reported on using rhythm with three stuttering preschool children (ages three to five). Two were rated as moderate stutterers, and one as severe. They were seen for three forty-five minute therapy sessions each week for five weeks. The basic therapy sequence started with metronome demonstration and familiarization. While varying bpm rates from 80 to 120, the clients practiced saying compound words (in preference to two one-syllable words or other two-syllable words). Picture cards were used as stimuli. Therapy then progressed as follows:

1. Six sessions were used to practice two-syllable words, using picture cards and starting each session with the familiar compound word practice. In the sixth session, each child selected his or her preferred bpm rate. This varied from 104 to 112 bpm and was used subsequently in the following steps.
2. At the individual bpm rates, children practiced phrases of three single-syllable words, moving next to three-syllable phrases.
3. Using various stimuli, the children worked on four-to-six-syllable sentences, the clinician modeling if the child had difficulty in pacing.
4. When children were able, generally, to go without modeling, practice shifted to controlled spontaneous speech.
5. In the last three sessions, use of the metronome was phased out progressively.

The authors reported a good fluency development and spontaneous generalization. The children varied in their basic abilities to follow a paced rhythm, and all the children periodically grew bored and had to have breaks in the routine.

The studies cited summarized, in some detail, a variety of approaches to metronome rhythm in therapy. The capacity to speak in an cadenced rhythm requires minimal practice, and most clients adapt to it quickly. Some do not. Most of the programs involve considerable attention to other aspects of speech therapy, as well as to dealing with attitude, anxiety, and tension. It is possible to use rhythm as a preliminary step in therapy, as a bridging technique between in-clinic and out-clinic procedures, and as a continuing method to be taught for consistent use on a self-directed basis following dismissal. The next section will suggest some constructs for evaluation.

CLINICAL APPLICATIONS

Preliminary Steps

Recommended applications of metronome therapy start with the suggestion that certain questions should be answered before initiation. Subsequent events can change an early answer, but one should hesitate to apply a therapy technique "just to see what happens." On that basis, ask the following:

1. Is the metronome technique to be used as a primary procedure or as an adjunct?
2. What outcome is expected if the technique is successful?
3. What are the fallback options if the approach does not work?
4. What other therapy activities should precede, coincide with, and follow metronome work?
5. What information about the client suggests that metronome therapy is the preferred, or at least a recommended, approach?

The final question implies evaluation for selecting candidates. Would that our knowledge was so precise! However, to normal evaluation activities, one might include the following areas of inquiry or testing if rhythm techniques are possible in therapy:

1. Standard test(s) of auditory acuity to assure that the client hears auditory stimuli within a normal range.
2. Inquiry about prior training and experience in singing, acting, public speaking, and other areas emphasizing control of speech production and monitoring of output.
3. Inquiring about musical experience in playing instruments of various kinds or experience and training in singing. This could emphasize tonal awareness, timing, and monitoring.
4. Observation of gait and motor coordination. Formal motor testing is not suggested, but try to classify the client broadly in terms of his or her general motor coordination. Markedly poor coordination may be contraindicative for rhythm therapy or perhaps suggest (for example, Wohl) that special rhythm training might help the client.
5. Related to 4, observation of the writing behavior of the client and the accuracy of the product. Again, no specific relationship is implied, but such observations might contribute to the overall picture of the client as a motor performer.
6. Observation of response to changes in auditory monitoring, designed to evaluate tactile and kinesthetic awareness, adaptation, and compensations adopted by the client. Use of masking noise and DAF are two possible stimuli.

These points are exploratory and not based on clearly established criteria. It has been reported that some stutterers will not have the coordination needed to pace the production of words or syllables (Hutchinson, 1976), and related information may be helpful in selection and planning.

7. Observation of performance on tests of rhythm perception and production, such as the Seashore tests series or other tests of the ability to identify, separate, or reproduce rhythmic patterns.
8. Observation of direct response to rhythmic intervention. Use a metronome or tape recording of metronome beats at 40, 80, and 120 bpm rates. Tell the stutterer to listen initially to the beat sound for four or five beats and then to

utter one word per beat. Once started, the client continues uttering one word per beat until the task is completed. At 40, 80, and 120 bpm, check the following productions:

a. Twenty monosyllabic words.
b. Twenty two-syllable words.
c. Ten short sentences.
d. About one minute of paragraph reading.
e. About one minute of monologue on any topic.

If the client has extensive timing problems after 8a, try dropping from one word to one syllable per beat. Separate instances of stuttering from any difficulty in maintaining the set pace. It also is appropriate to try to problem solve for any difficulties that arise. If the client seems to do well with rhythm, repeat several of the test areas in 8, turn off the beat signal, and have the client continue at the same pace as if the signal were still present.

9. Evaluation of personality characteristics (Brandon & Harris, 1967) by routine methods. At the least, rate the client on the following descriptive adjectives on a 1 to 10 scale, where 10 is "most like this" and 1 is "least like this":

outgoing	sociable	independent
relaxed	confident	cheerful
cooperative	nonfrustrated	dominant

You can also ask the client for a self-rating and have ratings done by family members or close friends. Supposedly, and this is conjectural, the higher the score, the lower the probability of a favorable response to this style of therapy. If reliable, this formula may not have anything to do with rhythm, per se, but may reflect low motivation and/or dislike of rigid types of therapy.

10. Consideration of the client's age (Andrews et al., 1964). It is possible that younger stutterers respond faster and with better long-term results. Unfortunately, we do not have longitudinal measures to establish cutoff points.

11. Consideration of the severity of stuttering. Moderate to mild stutterers may have the best chance of achieving fluent and normal-sounding speech, but severe stutterers may be more accepting of the program's structures and the nonnormal sound of cadenced speech.

12. Consideration of the type of stuttering spasm (Hutchinson, 1976; Meyer & Comley, 1969). It has been suggested that stutterers with laryngospasm predominance and those who tend toward strongly tonic spasms may respond less well to the initiation of rhythm therapy.

13. Consideration of personal reactions. Don't respond to most first responses. Initial objection to or intolerance for rhythm may fade when the client considers alternatives; and early acceptance can give way to frustrated irritation for a variety of reasons.

Because of the uncertainty of most of the foregoing items it is not possible to add up a score and identify a cutoff point for low-risk application of rhythm therapy. Certainly, research in these areas could be very helpful to the clinician. On a personal basis, it would appear that a severe stutterer with predominantly oral, tonic stuttering spasms; with apparently good motor coordination and average or better sense of rhythm; and tending to the average or low side of previously mentioned personality traits might respond best to rhythm therapy. However, one could also argue that a client possessing the opposites of the foregoing might most need a therapy that would improve and reinforce rhythmic capacities.

In previous sections I have specified a number of metronome approaches in considerable detail. To minimize redundancy, further applications will be stated briefly. First, metronome selection should be considered. I recommend against mechanical (wind-up) types because the bpm rate changes as they run down, and the beat can fluctuate at lower rates. Electronic units are preferred, especially those that produce both an audible click or tone and a light flash, which can be used separately or in combination. If funds are available, the table-top standard model should be supplemented by a portable unit called a *micronome*, or *pacemaster* (Fiedler & Standop, 1983). It also is possible to use a haptometronome, which is worn in contact with the body (for example, the wrist) and delivers an inaudible tactile pulse. For flexible use and transportation, it may be helpful to record on an audio tape cassette ten minutes each of 40, 50, 60, 70, 80, 90, 100, 110, and 120 bpm rates (you will want a 90-to-120-minute cassette). On the cassette, mark the footage meter reading for each rate. One clinician told me she recorded a different cassette for each rate and then let the client borrow the appropriate one for home practice. With these preparations you can move through the following phases.

Phase I: Planning

1. Complete an evaluation to determine the person's rhythmic capacities and to consider factors that might affect clinical decisions.
2. Determine the intended use(s) of the program:

   a. Simple demonstration of fluency possibilities or speech variation, with some other remedial approach to follow.
   b. Use of rhythm as a major technique to obtain fluency and transfer it to out-clinic use. Decide whether to use a planned phase-out or whether the client will decide. Other procedures (for example, relaxation or desensitization) may precede or accompany the rhythm method.
   c. Use rhythm, at the appropriate time, to support fluency techniques such as breathstream management, relaxation, and rate control.
   d. Use rhythm to help implement or transfer symptom-control techniques such as pullouts, preparatory sets, and speech monitoring.
   e. Use particular methods, techniques, or situations in special ways.

Phase II: Familiarization

The metronome is introduced and demonstrated, the clinician modeling different rates. Examples of syllable and word timing are given (for children, you may need a tangential activity to clarify the syllable concept).

1. Instruct the client to listen each time to the metronome for five to six beats and then to perform whichever task is requested from the following list, in time to the beat.

   a. Tap finger.   c. Nod head.
   b. Tap foot.   d. Move jaw.

   After the client has performed one item for eight to ten beats without problems, shift to the next task. If necessary, model during the preliminary five to six beats each time.

2. Repeat 1 at a faster rate. Starting at 40 bpm and then using 80 and 120 bpm should be adequate, but smaller increments can be used if the client has trouble shifting.

3. Repeat 1, but inform the client that you will change bpm rates during the performance. Don't try to trip up the client by changing too frequently; you just want preliminary monitoring and practice in shifting to different bpm rates.

4. Repeat 1, but inform the client that you will turn off the unit several times. When that occurs, the client is to continue the rhythmic performance until stopped. Try various rates. After five to ten solo beats, turn the unit back on and observe the client's timing response. Note: With children, metronome use can be built into games. Marching and other forms of physical enthusiasm also can be used.

5. Evaluate overall responses and reactions, and decide whether or not to

   a. Terminate and switch to another technique.
   b. Continue to the next phase.
   c. Plan a tangential program to develop better rhythm, awareness, and coordination before continuing.

Phase III: Establishment

The purpose of this phase is to establish the production of speech in time to metronome pacing. Fluency is desired, but pacing on fluent speech is the goal. The following steps can be edited and amended, depending on the client's response.

1. At progressive metronome rates, have the client produce nonsense syllables ranging across articulation locations (/bʌ/, /dʌ/, /lʌ/, /kʌ/). Ignore any dysfluencies, although you can remind the client to concentrate on moving to the beat. When this task is performed well, move on.

2. Repeat 1, but after the first five productions of any syllable, turn the unit off and have the client continue at the same pace for five more productions.

3. Repeat the rate progression and on/off practice from the first two steps, with the client using a list of monosyllabic words that you have provided. If the stutterer has shown strong phonemic emphases in stuttering, you might try to

minimize these presentations in the early part of practice. Try for CVC combinations rather than words that have accessory consonants (such as *brute* and *rust*). Treat dysfluencies as in 1.

4. Provide a list of two-syllable compound words (for example, *sunset, whitewash, airport*):

   a. Have the client produce one syllable per beat, with one or two beats between each word.

   b. Have the client produce one word per beat, with one or two beats between each word. Each syllable is stressed equally.

   Repeat this process until the client can time productions without error. Dysfluencies should show a reduction of at least 50 percent from baseline measures. If they do not, consider a tangential relaxation program. Some clients will have trouble with word pacing and will find it necessary to stay with syllable timing in this and subsequent steps until they (usually) are able to move on.

5. Repeat step 4, but arrange words in groups of five. First, turn the metronome off (prewarn the client) after the fourth word, so the last word is uttered without timing support but at the same pace. After several successes (continuation of timing and equal stress), turn the unit off after the third word and evaluate, and then turn it off after the second word.

6. Repeat step 4, but use two-syllable units (one or two words) that may function in communication, such as

Hello!	Are you?	Get up!	I will.
Who, me?	I am.	Try it.	What for?

   Apply the same fluency criterion as in step 4.

7. Use the word units from 6, but make utterances (in cadence) for the client to respond to, for example:

CLINICIAN	CLIENT
Are you going to the picnic?	Who, me?
I'd like to have a car.	What for?
Are you going to town?	I am.

   After demonstrated success, advise the client that you will turn off the metronome after your utterance; have the client maintain the same cadence and stress in the response. If problems occur, return to full pacing.

8. In this step, use strings of three to five syllables. Avoid words that are hard to pronounce or those proven to be stutter-provoking. Try for phrases, such as

I can go.	Good morning, Mary.	That will be all.
How much is it?	What time is it?	

   If the client employs standard phrases, names, or terms in business, family, or social life, try to use them. At first, pace everything, and check whether syllable-timed or word-timed speech is adequate (because of real speech approximation). When the client is stable in production, use the metronome for the first two or three productions and then turn it off. Be sure that your own speech is in cadence. Repeat the stimulus-response pattern from step 7.

9. With or without the metronome, go back over the previous phrases and

practice variations in inflection, stress, and pausing. If it is "better" to have two syllables on one beat and pause, encourage experimentation. If dysfluencies occur, switch the metronome on and have the client briefly return to a steady pace and stress pattern.

10. At this point, work with the client on an ELU (extended length of utterance) approach, where reading of progressively longer sentences, and then paragraphs, is used. Follow with, or mix along the way, spontaneous speech that lags behind the ELU level of reading. In practice, turn off the metronome as much as possible, and practice variations in timing, stress, and inflection. At this point, work until the dysfluency rate is down at least 70 percent from baseline measures. Experiment with the client to establish the bpm rate he or she is most comfortable with (this can be done earlier). At the same time, identify a slower "recovery rate" that can be used if trouble develops.

Phase IV: Stabilization

The purpose of this phase is to extend and stabilize the pacing ability of the client, secure further dysfluency reduction, and prepare for major transfer work.

1. The client starts each session with two to three minutes of reading with 100 percent metronome use. The first minute should be at "recovery rate," and the rest of the time at the preferred rate. If relaxation has been taught previously, this is a good time for reintroduction and practice during the metronome activity; if not taught previously, Brady's suggestions (Brady & Brady, 1971) about making an audio tape cassette of relaxation and pacing for home practice might be useful.

2. Provide reading material in which the first five words of each sentence have been underlined. The client reads aloud, producing underlined words in cadence and completing the rest of the sentence in his or her usual speech pattern. Accumulate fifteen minutes of successful practice; the return-to-normal completions can have a fair amount of metronome effect in them.

3. The client reads aloud without the metronome but with timed speech. The clinician records and guides the client's self-analysis on the playback of tapes. Any dysfluencies are analyzed against timing patterns, and the client is taught that dysfluencies are to become signals to slow down, relax, and pace speech production. Continue practice until the client can accumulate ten minutes' reading time with no more than five mild stutterings.

4. Provide topic cards, or ask questions, for the client to respond to in monologue. Ask the questions in a cadenced rate, or activate the metronome while the client reads the topic card. The client uses paced speech in the monologue until five minutes of speaking time accumulates. Strict timing can be eliminated then, except for the following occasions:
    a. The first three or four words of the initial utterance and after significant pauses in speech.
    b. When speaking rate becomes too fast; this criterion will have to be developed with each client. In such an event (fast rate), the client paces the next three to four words to reset the rate.
    c. For five to ten words following any dysfluency. At first, the clinician evaluates and signals along with the client but phases out as the client takes over the task. Appropriate evaluations of prosodic elements are

made to improve normalization of speech. After the point at which the client takes over major evaluation and consequent responsibility, success for this step is an accumulation of fifteen minutes of monologue with no more than five mild dysfluencies and no more than five omissions in evaluation. Except for pacing initial words, for pause breaks, and after dysfluencies, the client is encouraged to drop pacing; however, timing can be used to the extent that the client feels a need for it.

5. In this phase, converse spontaneously with the client. Beyond several minutes of practice at the beginning of each session, no cadenced speech is used except for timing utterances on three to five words following any dysfluency. Beyond that, the extent of pacing is up to the client. Continue practice until the client accumulates thirty minutes of speech with no more than ten mild dysfluencies and no more than ten evaluation errors. For evaluation errors, add five minutes to the accumulation requirement.

Phase V: Transfer

Transfer activities do not wait until the end of Phase III. If therapy is conventionally scheduled one to three times weekly, transfer work should start at about the level of step 5 of Phase II, with home practice assignments (preferably two fifteen-minute periods daily) of activities previously performed adequately during in-clinic sessions. The client usually will need to purchase a metronome or use a cassette tape of recorded beats.

1. If necessary, review and practice relaxation procedures.
2. Structure (or restructure) the client's situational fear hierarchy, and select several of the easy ones.
3. Discuss the selected situations with the client, and help with planning. Rehearse for out-clinic use by engaging in simulation activities, where the client can practice cadence control, evaluation, and relaxation. If necessary, work for desensitization by reciprocal inhibition or implosion.
4. Decide on the number of times situations are to be tried and what the evaluation criteria should be.
5. Plan a temporary, daily system of written reports that can be brought back to the clinic.
6. When the client has completed four or five replications of each of the initial situations successfully, arrange a continuing meeting schedule. If the therapy program uses a miniature portable metronome, Phase III would introduce it by step 3. The client should be trained to use it as an initiating mechanism, after pauses, and at or after dysfluency occurrences. In Phase IV, activities would be the same but would involve use of the portable unit.

Phase VI: Maintenance

The prior phase ordinarily will last for three to six months. Maintenance typically should continue for another eighteen months. Its purposes are to provide clinical support and guidance while the client takes responsibility for controlling speech. If available, and if not already in operation, membership in a stutterers group can be of significant assistance.

1. The client has weekly group meetings and individual sessions with the clinician. Formal reports are dropped, and the client works on progressing through the situational hierarchy list from Phase IV. Simulation rehearsal, desensitization, relaxation, growth in self-evaluation, and normalization of speech are common targets. This period typically lasts for six months, although it can be shortened.

2. During the second six-month period, the client maintains weekly group meetings, but individual clinician sessions drop to a monthly basis, unless otherwise agreed upon. Telephone contact is made by the client during "off" weeks if there is no stutterers support group; agree on a reporting day and time, and contact the client if she or he fails to do so (do this only twice). Activity centers around the hierarchy list, problem solving, and (particularly important) maintaining levels of motivation. If the client is responsive, a behavioral contract can be developed.

3. During the final six months, the client agrees either to monthly review sessions (no required telephone calls) or to two quarterly sessions with monthly telephone calls (clinician will not initiate). Continued group participation, if any, is up to the client. Try to schedule the client to talk to several new clients, a new stuttering group, and/or interest groups or classes. The client is counseled about relapse dangers, deliberate practice of pacing to keep skills sharp, and periodic evaluation of changes in the hierarchy list. Availability of the clinic for refresher work or problem solving is noted, but not stressed to the point where the client feels that the clinician is predicting a relapse.

This summary has been written as if metronome rhythm was to be the only remedial procedure used, except for excursions into relaxation and desensitization. However, the reader is reminded that rhythm pacing can be used in a variety of therapy contexts and for differing periods of time. Finally, it is emphasized again that the foregoing steps are not prescriptive. They were put together for a stutterer who is fairly severe and adapts rather slowly to rhythm pacing. Many factors could change the rate of progress, the completeness with which each step is followed, and the stringency of criteria.

13

Other Therapies

A penalty involved in writing a book that delineates specific techniques of therapy in extended detail is that one runs out of space before running out of techniques. In the preceding chapters, not all the reasonable variations and applications of the various methods were discussed, yet the coverage allocated to them resulted in there being a number of methods for which adequate space is not available for more than basic coverage. In fact, some techniques cannot be discussed at all.

In this chapter, as the final one, I will attempt to fit a number of therapy methods under the rubric of "other techniques." In order to make them fit, research reviews have beeen truncated, and assignments for clinicians and clients have been eliminated. To the extent possible, therapy applications have been described in detail. However, a number of the methods are sufficiently lacking in current popularity and/or in specification of methodological details that only general information about them can be provided. To the extent that available resources are known, the reader is supplied with references to books or articles where more detailed information can be obtained. In many instances, clinical experience of the reader will add dimensions for which space is lacking here.

The selection of these techniques is related to several possible factors. Some of them are ones with which I have had minimal experience and could secure limited information about. In a few instances, the space allocated reflects my opinions concerning value. Regardless of reasons, an effort was made to present a reasonable sampling of available information and to present the positive and negative attitudes concerning various techniques.

CHORAL SPEAKING

The background of choral speaking, or unison speech, derives from ancient times, when theatrical performance was supplemented, explained, or commented on by unison speaking of secondary performers. For generations (and in some areas today) it was used in education for learning, practicing responses, developing pronunciation, and so on. At one time, so-called diction specialists used it extensively. In choral speaking there occurs a uniformity of speech production that seems to submerge many individual differences. Falck (1969) suggested that it was effective with stutterers because it overcomes ". . . inhibiting doubt in the ability to produce normal speech" (p. 85). Eisenson (Eisenson & Wells, 1942) proposed that reduction in responsibility for communication might explain stutterers' improvement. Barber (1939) stated that the distraction aspect could overcome any fear and anticipation related to speech. Pattie and Knight (1944) suggested that unison reading, although it does not have the even rhythm of a metronome, may impose a rhythmic pattern on the subject, acting as a pacer. Perhaps the most tenable explanation is that choral speaking makes it possible for the stutterer to improve speech timing and coordination and management of the communication triad—respiration, phonation, and articulation. This leaves us without a definitive explanation, but we have done much therapy with less explanation many times before.

Research in choral speech has been limited. Johnson and Rosen (1937) reported on the effects of choral reading with eighteen stutterers. Seventeen subjects did not stutter at all, and the one hold-out reduced dysfluencies. Barber (1939) also evaluated eighteen stutterers in fourteen choral reading situations. Her ingenuity was remarkable, as she had two stutterers and one nonstutterer read together, one stutterer and one nonstutterer read together, two stutterers read together, and so on. Subjects also read while the other sound source (stutterer, nonstutterer, phonograph) produced nonsense syllables or a repetitive vowel. Sorting through all variations, it appeared that choral reading was most effective when the speakers read the same material, although almost any accompanying production (even mechanical noise) reduced stuttering. Eisenson and Wells (1942) compared readings when stutterers believed that their second effort of choral reading was being broadcast to a next-door audience. Choral reading, overall, reduced stuttering. On the second reading, with an invisible audience, eight subjects increased errors by an average of 6.4 (compared to the no-audience reading), seven subjects reduced errors further by an average of 3.7 compared to the no-audience reading, and four subjects exhibited no change. In other words, as we have seen before, situational anxiety is a variable factor in stuttering.

Pattie and Knight (1944) had stutterers read before a small audience under six conditions: alone, in unison with another present, and with other person on the telephone, reading the same material; a repeat of the preceding two conditions, but with each reader having different material. For the unison readings the average adaptation effect was 22 percent (from initial to final solo reading). The two readings of dissimilar material showed stuttering reductions of 39 percent by telephone link and 52 percent when together. When both read the same material, dysfluency reductions were 84 and 90 percent. Ingham and Carroll (1977) matched stutterers' fluent utterances from solo and choral readings, asking judges to differentiate between them. The listeners were able to separate choral from solo reading performances with only four of nine stutterers (that is, the speech productions sounded approximately the same). In a follow-up study with only three stutterers (Ingham & Packman, 1978), judges could differentiate the solo from the choral speech of the two subjects. They also reported that choral reading seemed to show a marked increase in wpm rate, an increase due apparently to sharp reduction in dysfluency rate rather than to any real increase in the rate of utterance. Finally, Adams & Ramig (1980) evaluated stutterers and nonstutterers during choral reading, in terms of vowel duration, vocal SPL, sustained phonation across word boundaries, and dysfluency frequency. Results indicated no general change in SPL; but if a subject's SPL began below that of the companion reader, the SPL of the former tended to rise (the reverse was not true). Overall, subjects tended to shift vowel duration toward that of the companion reader, but only stutterers showed a significant reduction in vowel duration during choral reading (compared to solo reading). This might be considered contradictory to Ingham and Packman's (1978) finding, just cited. However, the authors caution against comparing different modes of choral reading. Phonation continuation across word boundaries showed no consistent influence from choral reading.

Applications of unison speech to therapy are varied. In 1953, I used it with a college-age stutterer through an auditory training unit with duplicate microphones, headsets, and volume controls. Sitting apart, we started with my attenuator set so that my speech overrode his own. By degrees, my signal was faded until he could remain fluent without my support. Cherry and Sayers (1956) reported that choral reading was effective whether identical, dissimilar, or gibberish companion material was read. With reference to gibberish, they noted that phonetic sequence, timing, and other common language factors tended to persist. Van Riper(1959, 1971, 1973) noted the fluency effect of unison speech and advised the clinician to be prepared to ignore any stuttering occurrences and to maintain a normal reading pattern. Falck (1969) advised the following sequence in using choral speech:

1. The clinician leads off by repeating a selected phrase, each time with clear pronunciation and easy production.
2. When he or she is ready, the client joins in and they repeat together. If dysfluencies occur, the clinician continues without alteration until the client can tie in.
3. Once the client is stable in fluency, the clinician fades her or his production away (quickly or slowly) until the client is speaking alone.
4. Any work on rate, inflection, and so on can be modeled by the clinician.

Gregory (1968) provides a useful description of choral reading for the advanced, young stutterer. Using a tape recorder for playback of progress to fluency, the clinician and child work from word lists to paragraph material. After basic fluency is achieved, choral reading is mixed with spasm analysis, negative practice, voluntary stuttering (for example, bounce), and revised motor speech patterns. Other techniques, such as relaxation, can be integrated with the choral speaking activities.

Decisions to use choral speech in therapy revolve around the same goals and criteria cited for metronome rhythm therapy. It seems that some of its best uses are with children, and I have observed that many adolescents and adults seem to feel that it is "childish." Nevertheless, a suggested sequence for use with older stutterers follows.

Phase 1: Evaluation

1. Repeat evaluation procedures cited previously for other sections, omitting parts that involve other specific techniques.
2. Instruct the client to speak in unison with you as you count to twenty. Count slowly, evenly, and with slight prolongations. Do this two or three times, recording for analysis (record the client, not yourself).
3. Have the client read a paragraph of at least five hundred words aloud for about three minutes, recording and noting dysfluencies. Tell the client that you now will read it aloud and he or she is to join you. Make your voice dominant at first, and then fade to match the client. If the client's production is fluent, or mostly so, slowly fade your production further (warn client of this prior to reading) until the client finishes the final thirty seconds alone.

Evaluate the client's ability to blend into choral reading, and time utterances to coincide with yours. Even at this point, dysfluencies should be reduced noticeably. During the paragraph reading, try small variations in rate, inflection, and other variables to see how quickly the client picks up and accompanies you accurately.

Phase II: Establishment

Different physical arrangements can be used. The clinician and client can use dual microphone and earphone sets. The clinician can start "live" in front of the client and then shift to the side of or behind the client. The clinician can tape-record the stimulus material in advance and function as an observer and guide. Work can be individual or group or both. Various electronic units have the capacity to play repeatedly the same stimulus material. If you need to amplify your own production, many adaptations of milk cartons, paper tubes, stethoscopes, portable audiometers, and other resources can be used. Clients' variables, and your own resources will suggest possibilities. For these reasons, the following examples below are quite tentative and intended to illustrate a progression rather than to recommend a particular sequence.

1. Use a word list and read 50 to 100 words at a steady pace, without marked pauses between words. The client reads along. Count the dysfluencies that occur.
2. Read a list of ten to twenty sentences with the client, recording the client. Play back and analyze dysfluencies in terms of frequency, severity, location, phoneme, or other factors. As a model, do not stop when the client stutters, but go ahead and finish the sentence.
3. Utter phrases for the client to repeat with you. The client listens the first time and accompanies you as you slightly overproduce the second time, speak normally on a third production, and fade to quiet voice the fourth time. Record and analyze as before.
4. Read a paragraph that will last approximately two minutes. During the first thirty seconds, overproduce your speech. During the next half-minute, drop to normal voicing and speak quietly for the last minute. Record and analyze.

Use these procedures for several sessions to establish a basal fluency level. Usually, on paragraph reading, the client should reduce dysfluencies by 90 percent or more. If reduction is less than 50 percent, it is necessary either to solve the problems or to consider switching to another technique.

Phase III: Development.

The client has demonstrated that she or he can be relatively fluent in connected reading. In this phase, you want to increase the fluency and the self-confidence, incorporate other aspects of therapy, and bring in transfer elements (see later). Inclusion of other therapy aspects will be guided by your initial plan and personal preferences.

1. Begin each session with five to ten minutes of activities repeated from Phase II. This step will help start each meeting from a familiar fluency base.

2. Repeat step 2 from Phase II, but vary by dropping out after the first three or four sentences.

3. Repeat step 3 from Phase I, but drop out on the fourth production.

4. Use a paragraph of about 600 to 800 words in length. Practice choral reading while you supply the following models of speech:
   a. Normal speech.
   b. Quiet voice.
   c. Whisper.
   d. Syllable-timed.
   e. Word-timed.
   f. Easy onset.
   g. Prolongation.
   h. Continuous phonation.
   Take time as needed to explain and demonstrate these (or other) methods. After the client has adjusted to each one, have him or her complete the last fifteen to thirty seconds of the paragraph alone, using that particular technique. Record and play back for discussion. The intent of this step is to test and develop flexibility in the client for listening and production variation. However, you also can use it to test the efficacy of different fluency techniques.

5. Repeat step 3 in Phase I, using the different speech modes just listed; have the client finally repeat alone. Analyze and discuss as before.

6. Use paragraph reading in the normal speech mode. As you read, fake mild to moderate stuttering spasms without high tension levels, associated behaviors, or struggle. Vary repetitions, prolongations, and stoppages, occasionally combining types. Make them slow and long enough (temporally) so that the client has time to pick up and coincide with you. This step helps the client increase awareness and monitoring and models a relaxed form of stuttering. Be sure to follow typical patterns concerning when and where you stutter. Play back and discuss. You can precede this step (or replace it) with insertion of unusual, not bizarre, changes in inflection, rate, and so on, or by adding various other production modes.

7. Repeat step 6, but on each faked stuttering spasm, shift it into one of the production modes listed in step 4. Move slowly so that the client can coincide with you.

8. Repeat step 7, but have the client read alone. If any spasms become real, she or he continues them until they return to voluntary control and can be completed as planned. The clinician can step in during escaped fakes, coincide with the spasm, increase his or her own volume, and "lead" the client out of the spasm—but the goal is the client's self-control.

At this point the client typically is fluent, or nearly so, during reading and has developed an ability to vary speech in different ways. Awareness and monitoring skills usually have improved markedly. Pseudostuttering practice has helped in desensitization, modeling of simpler stuttering patterns, and practice in using different production modes to anticipate or retrieve fluency failures.

Phase IV: Application

This phase will not be spelled out since individual preferences will dictate application. Most approaches will follow one of three orientations:

1. Continuation and expansion, with special emphasis on Phase V transfer activities, of fluency practice from choral reading exercises. The client becomes more and more aware of what fluent speech is and how it is produced. The clinician may engage in specific shaping activities.
2. Use of choral modeling and practice to develop a particular fluency technique or combination of techniques. The clinician might want to combine slow rate, easy onset, and prolongation, starting each session with unison practice and returning to it whenever necessary.
3. Use of choral reading and practice to develop skills in symptom modification and control. The clinician can model and guide, fading out by degrees. The client can develop control progressively, and ultimately, become a model for the clinician to coincide with.

Phase V: Transfer

This phase can start with the first therapy sessions, but typically it would begin in Phase II. In programs where option 1 of Phase IV is selected, transfer activities will be the primary source for spreading fluency, and these will be particularly applicable to children.

1. Supply the client with a cassette tape that has preprinted materials (provide copies to client) recorded on it and also has repeated phrases and sentences for the client to practice. Recommend two or three ten-minute practice periods per day, with reports due on performance and problems.
2. Provide printed sentence lists and paragraphs for home practice with other persons (if possible, have that person, or persons, visit the clinic for brief instruction; if not possible, you can record the instructions and demonstrations on audio tape). Other persons also can read to the tape recorder, and the client can use the tape and script for repeated practice at his or her convenience. The client practices reading with different persons. Introduction of other readers into in-clinic sessions also can be used.
3. Have the client record brief advertisements from radio or television and practice unison speech with the playback.
4. As you progress through the phases, shift outside the activities, printed matter, and prerecorded material so that home assignments reflect previous clinical activity.
5. Use the situational hierarchy list as described in the metronome section.
6. Utilize group support and a maintenance phase-out program as suggested in the metronome section.

In using choral speaking, I have not found it to be particularly effective as a total or major therapy component, except with some children, where certain environmental manipulations could support transfer of fluency or control activities. With older stutterers it has been more effective as a stage of therapy or as an adjunct to other techniques.

SHADOWING

The definition and history of shadowing is, at best, vague. Beech and Fransella (1968) define it as monitoring aloud what some other person is saying. Others have called it "tracking." Recently, some clinicians have referred to it as "O'Riley Therapy," after the corporal on "M.A.S.H." Basically, shadowing involves a first speaker who reads or speaks spontaneously from or about material not available to the second speaker. The second speaker attempts to repeat what the first person says, usually one to two syllables (words) behind. Presumably, context predictability for phonemic sequence, grammatical order, and following-word predictability (along with pauses for catching up) allow shadowing to occur. Subject familiarity also may be a factor. Cherry (1953) is accorded credit by many for having been the first to identify and investigate shadowing, although Freund (1966) referred to reports of its use in Germany before 1900. Apparently Marland (1957) created the label *shadowing*, to refer to the process. Certainly, Cherry has earned primary credit in this area. Cherry (Cherry, 1957; Cherry et al., 1955; Cherry & Sayers, 1956) reported on using shadowing with stutterers, hypothesizing that the client's sensory perceptions were shifted largely from self-production to the patterns of the first speaker. Cherry reported that having a listener repeat audio tape material, concurrently, in ". . . a subdued or whispered voice . . ." is very easy to do. The resulting speech, according to Cherry (1957, p. 279),

> . . . tends to be in irregular detached phrases . . . [usually] in a singularly emotionless voice as though intoning. . . . He mouths the words like an automaton and extracts little semantic content, if any.

Emotional content is lost, and retention of information or directions heard is unusually poor.

Explanations of shadowing have not been particularly helpful to our understanding of it. Wingate (1969) considered the possibility that the first speaker somehow serves as a model, but he could not explain how this would function. He felt that the semimelodic, intoning characteristic of the second speaker's voice emphasizes phonation and continuity of phonation above other characteristics. Along with prosodic elements, Wingate suggested that the second speaker is exercising the foundation of oral communication—vocalization, intonation, prosody—with less information on the suprastructure of meaning and feeling. Subsequently (Wingate, 1976) he pointed to a significant reduction in rate as a possible factor. In general, he felt that the factors operating in choral speech and singing also apply to fluency in shadowing speech.

Fransella (1971) evaluated the effect of stutterers' knowing when an utterance would occur and found large individual differences in the resulting frequency of stuttering. Yovetich et al. (1977) reported that in dichotic listening, where the secondary message was dysfluent, stutterers made significantly more shadowing errors than did nonstutterers. Also, the listening ability of second speakers may be involved, since it has been reported that listening accuracy of (nonstuttering) subjects was related to their scores on rhythm perception (Sergeant, 1961). These studies emphasize the point that we lack essential research to describe thoroughly variables involved in shadowing, and we are not even close to explaining how it works.

Applications of shadowing have been limited, particularly as compared to techniques such as choral speaking or rhythm. Cherry et al. (1955) reported on the use of shadowing with five severe stutterers, moving them through an imitation of modeled intonation and rhythm patterns and through progressively faster rates. He reported a "striking improvement" in all five cases after two to four weeks of therapy. Marland (1957) used shadowing with preschool children who were combined clutterers and stutterers. She felt its primary value lay in training new listening habits and altering patterns of speech production. The predictability, and great importance of, home practice with shadowing was emphasized.

Limited use of shadowing (Walton & Mather, 1963) with one stutterer was reported. After forty-eight sessions, in-clinic speech was very fluent, but transfer did not occur. An additional forty-seven sessions centering on systematic desensitization seemed to provide the means for the stutterer to cope adequately with out-clinic fluency needs. A more positive report resulted from work with thirty-eight stutterers who received a mixture of shadowing and anxiety reduction (Kelham & McHale, 1966). The writers achieved an overall success with approximately 74 percent of the clients, noting that lower age and number of sessions seemed to be correlated positively with fluency. Kondas (1967) reported on shadowing use with twenty subjects, ranging in age from eight to twenty years. In the first two sessions, therapy centered on correct breathing habits. Shadowing was introduced in the third session, followed as soon as feasible by daily practice assignments at home. Four clients, after ten to fifteen shadowing sessions, were switched to desensitization procedures. Follow-up evaluations indicated that 70 percent of the clients were "cured" or "much improved," and Kondas recommended the treatment for further use. However, there also have been reports (Kondas, 1968) of extreme variations in stutterers' responses when shadowing was shifted among repeated readings of the same text, massed reading of the same text, shadowing with the new texts, and shadowing with the same texts.

Peins et al. (1970) described a tape-recorded self-therapy program for stutterers, including shadowing along with masking. Subsequently (Peins et al., 1972) a tape-recorded program was compared to a "standard therapy" group and a nontherapy control group. The tape program included shadowing along with various other practice techniques. The standard therapy (weekly meetings) worked on avoidance behavior, attitude change, and speech alteration. After six months, the tape therapy group showed more (eleven of twelve clients) improvement than did the standard therapy (eight of twelve clients) group. The control group had one improve, one worsen, and seven show no change.

Sergeant (1961) sounded a discouraging note in reporting that at 60-dB loudness and 102-spm rate (normal speech rate usually is $200+$ spm), the intelligibility scores for second (shadowing) speakers only averaged 68 percent. With extensive practice (sixteen sessions) some subjects could reach 80 percent intelligibility. This study, aimed at a very demanding telecommunication situation, tended to minimize context values, tended to omit clinicians' shaping activity, and was limited to its practice sessions.

A negative note was sounded by Ingham and Andrews (1973b), who reported that shadowing seems to require combination with other techniques in order to be effective, although they criticized the methodological inadequacies of the studies they reviewed. Bloodstein (1969) grouped shadowing (along with syllable-timed speech and similar techniques) under the "distraction" tag, distraction that will lose its value over time. Van Riper (1973) was willing to consider shadowing as a reinforcement of normal speech for very young stutterers who have no avoidances. However, he questioned its value with adult stutterers because of the lack of transfer. Fiedler and Standop (1983, p. 111) perhaps summarized the attitudes of many clinicians in placing shadowing with other speech aids,

> . . . which while in use may lead to conditional failure reduction, are generally only a step, although an important one . . . they may restore to the stutterer once again the feeling that his or her speech disorder is not entirely hopeless. This, above all, is an essential precondition for continuing often wearisome work in therapy.

Use of shadowing will not be developed here beyond the level of recommendations. I have used it only a few times and hesitate to make extensive suggestions. Criteria for using shadowing are unknown to me, in any formal sense. Research suggests that youth, simpler stuttering syndromes, and a capacity for perception of rhythm patterns may relate to better results. It is possible that opportunities for home practice, a client's tendency to introversion, and involvement of other techniques also should be considered. In using shadowing, certain general procedures can be suggested:

1. Observe the client, especially at first, for signs of undue tension and stress. Some people 'relax and shadow,' whereas others make it hard work.
2. With reference to 1, schedule breaks in shadowing activity to allow for relaxation. Time the breaks according to the overt needs of the client.
3. Change material often enough so that the client does not slip into unison

speech through familiarity; some clients will show a positive talent for this, using context and predictability as clues.

4. Plan carefully how you will use shadow fluency; what techniques are to precede, accompany, and/or follow shadowing; and what your course of action will be if shadowing does not produce satisfactory results after the first four to eight hours of in-clinic effort.

When the decision has been made to use shadowing, explain what you want the client to do, and demonstrate shadowing by using no prerecorded material or having a colleague come in briefly (see rate levels). After the client understands what is to be done, start with very simple levels.

1. Have a prerecorded tape of your reading at a very slow rate of fifty to sixty wpm. Reading material should be simple, with familiar words, and somewhat paced in timing (that is, minimize subgroup rushes of syllables). Instruct the client to
   a. Listen to the voice, not to oneself, talking.
   b. Repeat what is said, lagging behind by one to two words (two to three syllables).
   c. Keep one's own (client's) voice at a quiet level or even, at first, at a whisper. The tape can be used several times, as long as the client does not slip into unison speech.

2. Repeat step 1 with different taped samples until the client can shadow effectively. Interrupting dysfluencies should be observed and evaluated but separated from the overall shadowing criteria. When the client can shadow effectively, move to the next step.

3. Read aloud, "live," at the slow rate. Instruct the client to copy your production—rate, rhythm, inflection, duration, stress, and so on. Be sure that you maintain the slow rate, and keep production variables to a minimum. It may help if you use a microphone circuit and both of you wear earphones, to accentuate your speech to the client and for you to avoid being influenced by the other person's speech. Continue until shadowing is performed consistently.

4. Repeat step 4, but introduce the following variations as the client's performance warrants:
   a. At a slow rate, introduce normal variations and slight exaggerations of loudness, inflection and so on.
   b. At the slow rate, use more complex material from magazines and newspapers.
   c. With simple material, increase the rate to 60 to 80 wpm and then to 80 to 100 wpm. Then reintroduce the variations suggested in 4a and 4b.

5. Have a colleague, client's friend, or someone from the client's family read aloud for recording. Family or friends of the client are preferred, since they now will be "trained" for transfer practice. Use materials of varied complexity, and have them read at several wpm rates cited earlier.

6. Introduce other persons into the therapy session and have them read aloud. Start with simple material and the slow rate, changing as the client improves.

Up to this point, some clients could move through all the steps in just a few therapy sessions. Most will require about four to ten sessions, and a few will take twelve to twenty sessions. By completion of step 6, the client should be able to shadow a variety of materials at slow and moderate rates. In addition, there will have been some reduction in the intoning quality of speech, with more normalization of production. In the next steps you want to increase flexibility and make some use of the fluency the client has developed.

7. At a rate of about 100 wpm, concentrate on further development of prosody and normalization of speech. Use live-voice first readers, and record the client (keep the first reader away from the microphone). Play back and shape the client's productions toward normalcy.

8. Increase wpm rates until the client has trouble shadowing. Then discuss rates, securing agreement from the client on a rate that is acceptable and also provides for accurate shadowing.

9. Repeat previous steps, introducing other models and variations in complexity.

Transfer of shadowing is difficult in the broad sense of the word but simple in terms of out-clinic practice assignments. Taped exercises can be prepared with little difficulty and should be initiated by the time that step 2 is in process. If family members or friends can come in for brief training sessions, their speech variety is quite useful. Also, this frequently has the effect of improving speech models at home (particularly useful for children). With some trial runs in the clinic, clients can use opportunities such as television newspersons (not sportscasters) and particular roles in movies or broadcast plays for practice.

When the client reaches a combined level of effective shadowing and fluent speech, the clinician usually should have subsequent methodologies in process or prepared. It is unlikely that spontaneous generalization will occur above elementary school ages. Modeled speech patterns can be used for shaping, or specific fluency techniques (for example, easy onset or prolongation) or symptom controls (pullouts or preparatory sets) can be taught and practiced through shadowing. Also, the derived in-clinic fluency can be used to allow easy movement to the next level of therapy. It seems doubtful, and just as well, that shadowing bears the seeds of a future revolution in therapy for stuttering.

ROLE PLAY

Role play, sometimes called *behavior rehearsal*, is used both with children and with adults. It has strong ties to the psychodrama therapies for emotional disorders and to simulation activities for legal, corporate, interview, and other strategies. Role play can be used as a fairly simple rehearsal vehicle for the client to practice particular techniques before out-clinic use. The clinician can use role play to explore, and alter, attitudes or emotions toward oneself, others, and particular situations. Desensitization and implosion therapies frequently use role play. Emotional release, development of insight, self-instruction, self-consequation, and other skills can utilize role play. It can be used with adolescent stutterers on group or individual bases (Bryngelson et al., 1944; Chapman, 1959). Preschool children, although not more fluent, produce more speech when conversing with a puppet instead of an adult (Martin et al., 1972b). Pollaczek and Homefield (1954) reported effective use of masks with elementary school children, using the masks to facilitate willingness to speak and for freedom of expression. Honig (1947) recommended role play as a part of warm-up activities to focus on problems particular stutterers perceived in speech situations and to apply to prospective stressful situations group members faced. Other clinicians also have suggested role play for a range of purposes (Goldsmith, 1973; Lemert & Van Riper, 1958; Murphy & Fitzsimmons, 1960; Van Riper, 1973; Rustin, 1978).

In role play, the participants tend to identify with their role and treat it as pseudoreal, even though they know it is not real (Higgins et al., 1983). This can be an asset or a liability. Trojan (1965) exemplifies the potential liabilities (for speech pathologists) in his "kinetic discharge" therapy. This role play (or psychodrama) approach is designed for psychopathic, psychoneurotic stutterers and requires formal psychotherapy training for the clinician. Role play opens the opportunity for emotional release and/or the elicitation of psychological problems above the level of the average clinician's training and experience. This possibility leads some to oppose role play therapy, but this point of view is overly conservative and biased. Therapy for stuttering (or any communicative disorder) *is* psychotherapy. Some behavioral therapists who insist that attitude adjustment is either irrelevant or inappropriate in stuttering therapy are guilty of hypocrisy. You cannot work with behavior in a categorized fashion, selecting and ignoring what you will work with. Each of us has a level of competence, and it grows as we grow. Part of that growth is a recognition of our limitations as compared to the needs of the client. In therapy, we do not focus on marital relationships, parental problems, neurotic practices, and so on, and if they become significant, we help the client decide whether or not special help is needed to deal with them while we concentrate on our priorities. To the extent that communication is involved, we are involved.

Role play is used best when it is a component of an overall therapy program. Maxwell (1982) has provided a model for combining cognitive therapy (relaxation and airflow) with group use of role play. Any type or form of therapy can encompass role play if time and physical arrangements are made for it. As with other techniques in this book, discussion of role play will concern its use with adolescents and adults. With many exceptions possible, the following suggestions are offered:

1. Clients usually show an initial reluctance or even resistance to role playing, whether situations are based on reality or on complete imagination. In most instances, initial embarrassment or resistance disappears after a short period of adjustment.

2. In most situations, role play should wait until a client and clinician relationship, or group identities, have started to develop. When the client is not sure about the reality situation and the other person(s) in it, role playing can be uncomfortable or even threatening.

3. The clinician, if part of a situation, should be careful to "live the role" and not try to be a clinician and a role player at the same time. In group situations, except for modeling, it usually is best if the clinician remains in the primary therapy role, also functioning as director and stage manager.

Fiedler and Standop (1983) provide an extensive model that can be applied in many therapy settings.

1. First, develop and rank a situational hierarchy. Selecting an item from the hierarchy, proceed to develop a scenario of the persons involved, the setting, the trend of speech exchanges, and typical outcome(s).

2. Work to specify exactly the problems the client perceives in the selected situation (or cluster of similar situations). Separate talking, social aspects, content, and so on.

3. Specify solutions to the identified problems. Practice the solutions in fragments, for example, use of preparatory sets or easy speech onset on certain productions, inhibition of particular struggle or avoidance devices, and what to do if a severe stuttering spasm occurs.

4. Place chairs, tables, and so on to simulate the layout of the real situation. Minor properties (newspaper, clipboard, cup) can be supplied. Decide the role the clinician (or other person) is to play, and provide an unwritten "script."

5. Emphasize to the client that first efforts are for practice and that mistakes are to be expected. Errors in performance, or in therapy techniques are expected and can be dealt with. Performance sessions beyond one or two minutes are not preferred because of fatigue, of technique application, and role consistency. Also, short sessions can be repeated more easily several times in succession.

6. Immediately following each performance, have the client(s) discuss several points:
   a. Feelings and experiences.
   b. Success in speech and technique.

7. In most instances, repeat the situation after planning based on evaluations in 6. Revisions can cover generalities, performance of the other person(s), and very specific applications toward speech goals.

8. Plan transfer to real situations, being very specific in areas stressed and action required.

As you can see, role play here is used as a rehearsal vehicle for transferring fluency or control skills to an out-clinic status. A similar format can be used for other purposes as well. Role play may move slowly at first, especially if the stutterer has strong feelings of inadequacy in speech situations. Gentle coaching, approval, and modeling may be needed for awhile. Audio and video recording is of great assistance in helping clients learn from role play, both for general and specific behaviors. Group therapy often is enhanced by role play, at times as a routine part of a weekly session. Finally, in periodic maintenance visits to the clinic by dismissed clients, role play can be useful in exploring particular problems and rehearsing solutions.

WHISPER SPEECH

Whisper speech has been reclaimed from the quackery dump site and used by a number of clinicians. Schwartz (1967) reported that compared to oral speech, whispering significantly increased the average duration of syllables—a condition targeted in many timing or rate control therapies. In a comparison of rehearsal effects on stuttering adaptation, Brenner et al. (1972) found that pantomimed speech showed the least effect, with whispering a close second, and oral rehearsal had the traditional adaptation effect. Moss (1976) also compared stuttering production effects of rehearsal, followed by reading aloud. Silent, pantomime, and whispered rehearsal had little effect on vocalized readings, whereas vocal rehearsal was followed by a significant reduction in dysfluencies. Bruce and Adams (1978) found that adaptation *during* repeated whisper readings was greater initially than adaptation on oral readings aloud, but a final oral reading (following the whispered rehearsals) rebounded to almost double the dysfluency level of the last oral readings following four consecutive oral readings. In other words, the first whisper and pantomime were not "recognized" as being sufficiently similar to normal, oral speech for a significant adaptation effect to occur. A similar comparison (Perkins et al., 1976), focusing on occurrence of dysfluencies, found that pantomime, and then whispering, greatly reduced stuttering, suggesting that simplification of phonation and respiration has a fluency-inducing effect. The introduction of artificial stress created no increase in stuttering during whispered and pantomimed speech or vocal speech, and the latter again had significantly more stuttering than the first two methods.

The effect of whispered speech may be distraction and novelty, as many have suggested, it may relate to an increase in consonant and vowel duration and decrease in rate (Starkweather, 1982), or it may relate to

motor simplification. It may relate to all of the foregoing. The vocal configuration for whispering is quite different from that for normal phonation.
Instead of the medial arytenoid surfaces being parallel or in contact, they
often are seen to be abducted posteriorly, creating an opening in the inter-
cartilaginous vocal fold area. This may be due to the relaxation of the
posterior cricoarytenoid and arytenoideus (interarytenoids) muscles, at
least in part, while the lateral cricoarytenoid probably does contract. Vocal
fold movements and closure seem to vary from some amount to none at all.
Whispering sharply reduces the length of speaking time on one breath and
essentially has no frequency or harmonic characteristics. Slight variations
in the aperiodic pseudoquality and the loudness of the whisper are possible. It is also possible that a whisper is not vocal fold abusive, contrary to
many opinions (Zemlin, 1980). The foregoing description reinforces comments about motor simplification, and also suggests the elimination of most
of the habitual respiratory and phonatory coordination patterns, and
therefore, probably supports an assumption of altered articulatory patterns.

The usefulness of whispered speech in stuttering therapy generally is
limited in the same way as that of singing, discussed subsequently. Shine
(1980) suggests modeling whispering for children in fluency therapy, progressing to a softly vocalized "easy speaking voice." He suggests that children who cannot whisper fluently should try an easy, prolonged, DAF-type
voice at first. Such applications are the general rule in therapy: Use whispered speech briefly as a way to move to another technique or as a low-cue
or minimal trigger practice mode for symptom control systems.

SINGING

Singing as an approach to stuttering therapy is totally unknown to many
clinicians. Wingate (1969) noted that singing had a very positive effect on
stuttering, and he later (1976) stated, "Undoubtedly singing is the most
widely known of the conditions having a salutary influence on stuttering"
(p.191). His grounds for use of the "most widely known" are not known,
unless he was selecting from the many conditions under which stuttering is
reduced or absent. He noted that compared to traditional speaking, singing is predominantly phonation, that rate is slowed down (mainly because
of increased phonation, particularly of sonorants), and that production is
usually louder. Miller (1982) also suggested increased duration of voicing
as an explanation of singing's effectiveness. Perhaps the latter is why so few
popular singers stutter. Wingate went on to relate increased duration to
vowel production and to suggest that ". . . the principal difference between
speaking and singing involves what happens with vowel production" (p.
194). Ramig and Adams (1980) reported that children and adults (stuttering and nonstuttering) both increased vowel and pause durations when

reading at artificially increased and decreased pitch levels. Wingate argued that singing was simpler than speaking, in that syllables were less complex; there were fewer variations in pitch, loudness, and timing; and there were fewer contrasts in stress. Also, there were richer harmonics, more open resonators, greater concentration of sound, and a need for better breath support and control. I am not sure how Wingate adds this all up and comes out with "simpler." Having survived years of formal vocal training, I would note that singing involves much more precise targets with a narrower acceptability range (again, many currently popular singers are excepted) than does oral speech. The difference lies perhaps in the answer to the question, "What is singing?" As we will see, singing therapy can cover genuine, melodic production of tunes and also intoning, semichanting productions of speech.

Starkweather (1982), in commenting on Wingate's contentions, noted that Wingate essentially is incorrect in minimizing a rhythm effect in singing because the song's beat often does not correspond to syllables of the lyrics. He states, very correctly, that syllables may not be *on* the beat, but they usually are timed closely in reference *to* the beat. They even may be set carefully to the off-beat. Van Riper (1982) also emphasized the importance of ". . . the correspondence of the timing of syllables with the musical notes" (p. 245). Exceptions among the many styles and popular modes of singing can be found, but singing generally will follow a beat, or pace the syllables of lyrics, with reference to a rhythmic pattern, especially on the stressed syllables. Starkweather also expanded Wingate's emphasis on vowel prolongation, in that all steady-state areas (nasals, silent periods, semivowels), as well as vowels, show the most lengthening. He felt that consonant lengthening was proportionately as great, or more so, than the lengthening of vowels. Finally, Starkweather pointed out that Wingate's vocalization hypothesis ignores the fact that whispering (non-voice) can reduce stuttering significantly. Johnson and Rosen (1937) noted the fluency effect of singing but ascribed it to distractions. It also was suggested, in addition to changed vocal patterns, that familiarity with a song's words and tune was involved in reducing stuttering. Wingate (1976) in reviewing research, rejected this latter statement, saying ". . . familiarity with either the words or the tune is relatively immaterial in regard to the effect of singing on stuttering" (p. 196).

Colcord and Adams (1979) compared stutterers to nonstutterers on reading and singing, reporting that stutterers, while significantly reducing dysfluencies, also increased voicing duration without particularly altering either the average or peak vocal SPL measures, whereas fluent speakers showed significant changes in both. Singing also may increase the fundamental frequency range of stutterers, which research has shown is significantly less than that of nonstutters (Healey,1982). Another consideration may be in the fundamental pitch itself, since research suggests that speaking in either an artificially high or low pitch significantly reduces stutterers' dysfluencies, with a lowered pitch being more effective than an elevated pitch (Ramig & Adams, 1981). Overall, we have no definite answers to the questions about singing effectiveness in reducing stuttering. The changes in voicing may be a direct factor or an agent leading to other effects (for example, rate) that are as, or more, significant.

An extensive review of singing applications can be found in Van Riper's text (1973) and also in an article by Galloway (1974). Van Riper suggests that there is greater popularity of singing-type techniques in Europe. Despite his basic scepticism, he reports positively on several procedures he viewed. Galloway vigorously attacks singing therapy for its lack of transfer, for being motorically different from speech, for being incompatible with other techniques, and for being subject to the same habituation process (and resurgence of stuttering) that other novel utterance methods suffer from. He states that neither the past history of therapy results nor the present research base can justify the use of singing therapy for stuttering. Nevertheless, it is used.

As indicated earlier, I received formal vocal and instrumental training and feel (hope) that my musical sense is pretty well developed. Beyond several specific applications that follow, I have not found singing therapy superior to, and usually not as effective as, other methods that are available. Uses with which I am familiar are these:

1. With children, as an initial fluency-inducing and relaxing step, when the client clearly enjoyed it and performed well.
2. With children, as part of a program to develop a better sense of timing, rhythm, and body coordination.
3. Briefly, with mature stutterers, as part of an overall program to develop awareness and control of phrasing, breathing, pause timing, and inflection and stress variations.
4. With mature stutterers, as an initial step, leading to unison speech or other rhythmic types of procedures.

Beyond childhood, it seems that many stutterers find singing embarrassing or just very difficult to do. Before using it, I would suggest evaluating the range of the clients and their abilities to perceive differences in pitch, quality, rhythm, and loudness. If these abilities are below average, singing probably should be limited to an intoning or chanting style of production.

MONOTONE

Monotone speech has been an occasional therapy technique for many years. Its dysfluency- reduction effect has been reported (Bloodstein, 1950) as one of the novel speech modes that can be used. Speculation has revolved around the reasons for its effect. Wingate's (1970) first hypothesis of rate reduction was considered, but he modified it (Wingate, 1981) to provide for fluency effectors where rate reduction was not a significant factor. An excellent study by Adams et al. (1982) compared ten stutterers to controls in normal and in monotone reading. Subjects did not practice the use of monotone. All stutterers and eight of the nonstutterers reduced fundamental frequency, all reduced vocal SPL, and none significantly altered (reduced) reading rate during monotone speech. There was a significant reduction in stuttering, on a group basis, during monotone reading. The two stutterers who did not reduce their fundamental frequency also did not reduce their dysfluencies, and probably they actually were not reading in monotone. It was felt that monotone simply was an aspect of the concept that motor simplification tends to reduce stuttering and did not relate to any rate hypothesis.

Without practice first, people will tend to fall into a stereotyped, rather than a monotone, pattern in which pitch and loudness levels and variabilities are redundant, whether or not reduced. Early stages of slow rate, prolongation, continuous phonation, and other techniques tend to show a similar pattern of stereotyped production. Clients tend to find monotone speech boring, and its use is arguable when considering other techniques that are available.

When monotone is used, it often helps to start with an oscillator (or audiometer) set near the F_o of the individual and have the person match the steady tone heard through a pair of earphones. As skill develops, the earphone signal can be attenuated progressively, being increased at need. The clinician should learn to produce truly monotone (not stereotyped) speech, in order to model. Later, as the client continues monotoning, the clinician can move back to normal prosody. There usually will be no strong rationale to maintain use of monotone speech for any great length of time in the schedule of a therapy program.

BOUNCE

The bounce technique was known widely in stuttering therapy from 1940 to 1960 and still is in use to some extent. It goes back many decades. The method is associated particularly with Johnson's stuttering therapy (1946) and has been called the "Iowa bounce" (Van Riper, 1958). Johnson described the bounce as a ". . . streamlined pattern of nonfluency . . ." (p. 463) to be substituted for stuttering. After in-clinic practice, the client introduces it into daily speech, starting with easy situations, using it liberally on neutral words (that is, pseudostuttering) as well as on those words where stuttering is anticipated. Over time, the neutral word bounces can be reduced as the client gains tolerance for public nonfluency. This technique supposedly changes the client from a stutterer to a "nonfluent individual" who will have less and less inclination to stutter. Gregory (1968) reports use of the bounce technique, among other methods, and stresses that use of the schwa vowel in bouncing the first syllable is inappropriate and counterproductive (for example, saying *guh-guh-guh-get* instead of *ge-ge-ge-get*).

The bounce simultaneously is a mode of voluntary pseudostuttering and a control technique for real stuttering. As the latter, it combines relaxation, syllable timing, motor rehearsal, and other elements of therapy. It can be used on any phoneme but is particularly applicable to plosive sounds where easy onset, prolongation and so forth are more difficult to initiate. One possible production sequence for using the bounce can be summarized as follows:

1. Consciously relax the speech areas and inhale normally to provide adequate breath support. If the bounce will occur during ongoing speech, slow down production of the previous two or three words to allow for preparation.
2. Release the airstream, following with an easy vocal attack so that the first production is slightly prolonged and breathy.
3. Produce the first syllable of the target word. Be sure that the vowel uttered is the one that will be used in the final utterance of the word (no schwa vowel unless appropriate). Exceptions can occur; for instance, bounce on the word *street* can require particular productions.
4. Syllables or phonemes are produced with an easy, effortless repetition in which sound and intersound intervals are constant and the same. Stress or other speech elements are minimized.
5. Bouncing continues until the speaker feels that relaxation and control are sufficient for completion of the word. This may be two bounces, or twenty.
6. The word is spoken as a paced continuation of the bounce, without any perceptible difference between any one repetition and the final one. The rest of the word can be uttered with whatever degree of normality is appropriate as long as the shift from bounce to word is not disturbed at the last second.

Errors in bounce production usually revolve around failure to start with an easy and relaxed production, irregularity in the timing pattern of the ongoing bounce, and "jerking" or hurrying out of the bounce into the word. During in-clinic practice, a metronome can be used for initial time-rate support. Unless out-clinic use of the bounce for voluntary stuttering is planned in order to increase tolerance and acceptance, the in-clinic practice usually concentrates on progressive reduction of the number of bounces needed before fluent completion is possible—although practice in out-clinic extended bouncing may help reestablish a control that is slipping. Some clinicians take the bounce reduction to the point where the client slows down and/or pauses and then *mentally* bounces before uttering the word. If situations turn out to be particularly difficult or a fluency crisis occurs suddenly, the client can employ the number of bounces needed to assure or regain control over the dysfluencies. The bounce often works quite well for many stutterers, but some clients do not like its obvious and automatonlike quality. It is, of course, subject to careless abuse, automatization, and incorporation into a habituated stuttering pattern—as are all symptom and fluency techniques. I have used it many times and find it best as an ancillary technique when the client is having symptom or fluency-control problems with particular phonemes or phoneme combinations.

EASY ONSET

Easy onset travels under a variety of names and is used in a number of different ways. It probably owes its use, as do many techniques, to the real or anticipated difficulty the stutterer has in getting started on an utterance (Van Riper, 1973, p. 341):

> It is on sounds, syllables, and words that the stutterer feels he has had his past troubles thousands and thousands of times. Somehow we must find some ways to keep those cue perceptions from generating the specific abnormal preparatory sets. . . .

Easy onset also can be restructured from reciprocal inhibition orientations, with a link to relaxation and breathing patterns. To varying degrees, easy onset attempts to produce an utterance without haste, tension, or pressure so that stuttering does not occur. It may be as simple as light consonant contact or airway dilation or a complex of relaxing and coordinating the triad of respiration, phonation, and articulation. In its various forms, it can include aspects of prolongation, continuous phonation, whisper, legato, rate reduction, breath control, and light contacts.

As a simple form, light consonant contact requires that the stutterer slight the constriction and contact degrees of consonant production. It also has been taught as a type of ventriloquism (Froeschels, 1950, 1952a), and some have taught it with the aid of a bone prop (a short prop of bone or plastic, slotted at each end to fit over the upper and lower central incisors, separating the dental arches according to the length of the prop). The resulting speech, at its extreme, is of the "hot potato" variety at first, and can even sound like no more than a production of exaggerated vowel strings. As the stutterer shapes toward a more normal contact, speech intelligibility and normal qualities improve. In the stutterers I have seen use light contacts, syllable rate tended to reduce noticeably, and vowel prolongation tended to increase as they searched for the best degree of consonant contact. It has been used as "the only way of speaking" (particularly by quacks), and often then ultimately becomes incorporated into a returned stuttering pattern. I have used it in cancellations, pullouts, preparatory sets, spasm alteration, relaxation, and rate-control therapies—focused only on the probable or actual stuttering spasm.

In its possible combinations, any of the following levels of involvement can be used:

1. Production of consonants with lightened contacts of lips, tongue, and palate against articular surfaces.
2. Emphasis on simultaneous or breathy vocal attacks, as opposed to hard glottal attacks. This may be accompanied by vowel prolongations, continuous phonation, equalization of vocal stress, or insertion of starter sounds to get the articulators moving.
3. Timing of respiration in coordination with phonation and/or deliberate release of air prior to vocalization. Relaxation and stabilization of the respiratory process also can be involved.

Irwin (1972) described an easy stammer therapy in which she instructs the client to slow down, decrease tension, and prolong sounds. It is used on all words at first and then shifted toward consistent use on particular words. Use development follows an ELU (see later) pattern. Irwin recommended it for any type of stutterer, at any age, and reported that follow-up indicates good maintenance results. Lockhart and Robertson (1977) reported on a therapy program emphasizing hypnotherapy (the mild stutterers received hypnotherapy only) and involving an easy onset type of speech control. Therapy begins with monosyllable words initiated by bilabial plosives and produced in a semibounce where the initial phoneme is repeated twice in an easy, relaxed manner and the word is uttered on the third repetition. Tensing and relaxing the articulators, followed by production, is used on the same words, and the words then are put into phrases. This sequence is repeated, taking sounds in their various homophenous groupings until the client has progressed through the various speech sounds. Relaxation and easy vocal attack are emphasized when necessary. Paragraph reading, backward text reading, and monologue practice are followed by special attention to trouble words and work on rate and prosody. It was reported that fluency usually was stabilized in thirty to forty weekly sessions. Hypnosis was used weekly for the first eight sessions and approximately on a monthly basis after that.

Weiner (1978) reported on "Vocal Control" therapy in which thirty-four clients received Jacobson-style relaxation and, as needed, desensitization and reinforcement techniques. Basic breathing exercises for breath support and glottal relaxation were provided. Weiner stated that any voice problems (vocal fry, constricted resonance, and so on) were corrected, noting that "every stutterer" typically needs work with vocal quality. Easy onset was taught by eliminating strong glottal strokes and developing gradual onset of vocal vibration. About 65 percent of the stutterers reduced articular hypertonicity through the respiration and phonation techniques. For the remainder, easy onset was extended to include a type of light consonant contact, biofeedback awareness and control, desensitization, and/or covert positive reinforcement to reduce anxiety. Therapy extent ranged from 21 to 118 sessions, and thirteen clients still were in therapy when the report was published. Pretherapy fluency percentages for twelve dismissed clients ranged from 97.5 percent to 75 percent. Follow-up fluency measures ranged from 100 percent to 80 percent.

A consistent user of easy onset in his shaping program has been Webster (1974, 1977, 1979), who uses computer-monitored shaping targets. Saint Louis (1979) reported that the semiautomatic approach makes it simple for the stutterer to self-teach appropriate levels of vocal onset and reduce initial tension levels on utterances. The availability of equipment, software, maintenance, and clinician training reduces the applicability of this approach. Perkins (1973b; 1983; Perkins et al. 1979) has utilized easy onset techniques in his rate control therapy, stressing flexibility to meet the spasm characteristics and particular needs of various clients. Many other clinicians apply easy onset to various degrees, in various formats, and at different points in therapy. I favor it primarily in symptom therapy as a voluntary nonfluency (not, as some name it, a "fluency" technique), in control techniques, and in rate control therapy as a method of actuating the timing elements of speech production.

Easy onset is not the same thing as light contact, relaxed speech, or other labels that have been used. Easy onset is the coordination of an adequate breathstream through relaxed vocal folds so that the air and/or phonation slightly precede articulator movement, which is made with reduced tension and in a continuous manner to link sounds within and across the syllable(s) of a word. It is discussed in the chapter on breathstream therapy; the chapter on relaxation and desensitization; the several chapters on cancellations, pullouts, and preparatory sets; and the section of this chapter on monitoring and prolongation. It actually is not one technique as much as it is a possible emphasis resulting from a combination of techniques. It should not be used as an only-therapy procedure since the dangers of relapse and incorporation into a revived stuttering pattern are too great to risk.

PROLONGATION

Prolongation of sounds to control spasms or to induce fluency is involved in a number of therapy techniques. Methods such as rate control through DAF, continuous phonation, singing, and others promote or require prolongation of speech sounds. It is an old technique. Fiedler and Standop (1983, p. 102) summarize Gutzmann's approach to therapy in Germany (circa 1920), where the client is instructed to "Prolong the first vowel of an utterance and connect all words of a sentence with one another as though all of it was one word."

Van Riper (1973, p. 81) refers to rate control and the prolonging of vowel sounds as "Another hoary old method . . . exhumed from the grave where it belongs." He traces the technique back to France and Germany, in the nineteenth century, and then updates to the popular use of rate control and prolongation by a number of respected clinicians from 1910 to 1940. Whitten (1938) describes self-use of prolongation as part of a symptom control program that includes attitude and personality readjustment procedures; and Gifford (1940) makes extensive use of prolongation in her therapy programs. There have been contemporary practitioners since then. Webster (1972) makes extensive use of prolongation in his shaping program, and Mowrer's rate control program (Mowrer & Case, 1982) results in prolongation effects. The Schwartz (1976) airflow program also involves prolongation to a significant degree. The review by Andrews et al. (1983) discusses the value of prolongation in facilitating fluency, but Wingate (1983) finds no particular factual base or deduced superiority over other techniques to recommend prolongation.

Prolongation may be applied to increase the duration of vowels (and consonants) within word boundaries or to function as a continuous phonation, where word boundaries are reduced or eliminated. The techniques can be limited to the initial sounds of words or to all vowels in a word or include all consonants as well (by carrying over voicing from the preceding sound). Elsewhere in this text, research has been reviewed suggesting that the vocal initiation time (VIT) measures for stutterers is slower than that for nonstutterers (Metz et al., 1979) and that having to shift from nonvoicing to voicing in sound formation is positively related to stuttering (Adams & Reis, 1971). Stuttering also seems to occur more frequently after a pause (when voicing must be reinitiated) and when the sound initiating a word is followed by a voiced sound (Wall et al., 1981). Prolongation tends to stabilize these variables to a greater degree, perhaps simplifying motor planning and switching. It also creates a reduction in speech rates, tends to reduce prosodic variations, and allows for better timing of sequential production efforts. Whether expanded vocalization is a major producer of fluency or whether it is a product of other changes is not clear. Helps and Dalton (1979) illustrate the combination use of prolongation in an intensive therapy program in which the stutterers prolonged syllables and continuant consonants, used a light consonant contact to elongate plosives, and worked on continuous voicing.

Variations in definition and application tend to confuse a description of prolongation. As noted in the previous paragraph, it means different things to different clinicians. Also, it varies from being a byproduct or effect of a particular technique to being a targeted behavior that is practiced for learning. Jones (1977) describes "legato speech" in a way that combines prolongation, continuous phonation, and easy vocal onset. Helps and Dalton (1979), as described, combine other elements. In my own discussion of prolongation the following eclectic definition will be applied:

> Prolongation technique involves increasing the production duration of speech sounds, with appropriate adjustments in the rate of speech, in articulator movements and contacts, in the timing of syllable and pause durations, and in characteristics of prosody. Phonation across voicing boundaries, within or between words, also may occur.

Peins et al. (1972) utilized legato-style procedures in their tape-recorded therapy program for home self-therapy. Watts (1971) used DAF to initiate a vowel prolongation program, finding effective reductions in stuttering but noting that the method made burdensome demands on self-control. Andrews (Andrews 1973; Ingham & Andrews, 1973b; Andrews, 1974a; Andrews et al., 1980) reported on a number of prolongation applications, usually as part of an intensive program and on an in-hospital basis. Reinforcement systems, group work, and carefully planned transfer activity also were involved. The writers reported use of DAF for modeling and initial practice to achieve prolongation, and (see later) they carried the client through carefully graded rate increments as prolongation was decreased. It was felt that this prolongation system was superior to the use of rhythm techniques. Curlee and Perkins (1969) described a rate control therapy in which DAF was used to force rate reduction through prolonging syllables. Irwin (1980) reported on an "easy stutter" program which placed heavy emphasis on prolongation.

Sample programs can include the Irwin sequence just cited. The "easy stuttering" is a faking, where the first syllable of the word is prolonged. If a plosive is involved, the client uses a light consonant contact on the phoneme and slides into a prolongation on the following vowel. On occasions where a plosive is followed by another consonant, the second consonant is treated as part of the first unit, with prolongation occurring on the following vowel.

The program initially has the client read for thirty minutes daily, faking a prolongation and easy stutter on the first word of every line. This is duplicated the next week, with a familiar person present. After that, with the same person, the client works on real stuttering spasms, stopping and then prolonging initial syllables. When daily practice is effective, transfer starts to outside situations, using a ranked fear hierarchy. As the heirarchy progress continues, the client maintains but reduces the daily practice. On a discriminative basis, the client reduces the duration of prolongation (minimal length should be about 150 msec).

Irwin used client-applied measures of improvement, without reference to clear baseline data, in reporting on twenty-six of eighty-seven clients. Those clients reported results that averaged around "very good improvement."

Franck (1980) reported on a therapy program involving group instruction in prolongation with airflow and light consonant contact. The clients start at a 60-spm rate and progress in 30-spm increments. During three two-hour sessions, they are expected to reach 150 spm in conversational speech, also receiving practice in speech analysis and relaxation. Clients then move into groups of about thirty and meet one and one-half hours per week. They are allowed to continue for up to six months. The group sessions practice the five spm rates (60, 90, 120, 150, 180), work on relaxation, and perform varied speech activities. Those who are ready then move, in groups of fours, into a sixty-hour, five-day, intensive program with three clinicians per group to help. Starting at a low spm rate, clients move through a rigorously demanding series of rate increases, where no nonfluencies are allowed and self-monitoring is stressed. Criteria are specific and applied strictly. The program, according to the authors, is very fatiguing to clinicians and requires staff availability, large therapy space, and special equipment. However, only 2 percent of the clients fail to complete the program.

The results of prolongation therapy, or therapy utilizing prolongation, have been variable. Frayne et al. (1977) used naive listeners to judge ten stutterers who had completed an Ingham and Andrews type of program some six to eighteen months earlier. On the parameters used (rate, smoothness, hesitations, intonation), the listeners generally perceived stutterers as normal speakers. Franck (1980) reported that at the end of the intensive phase of therapy (before maintenance), 96 percent of the clients were completely fluent. However, 73 percent felt that they did not sound like other fluent speakers, 74 percent still had to consciously and deliberately use control techniques, 27 percent felt that they sounded artificial, and 21 percent were embarrassed when they were using the controls. A covert measure (telephone call by a stranger to "interview" about opinions on available therapy) indicated that 67 percent of those contacted (forty-five) had measured fluency levels below 80 percent during the conversation, and 34 percent had measured fluency levels below 50 percent. Overall, 55 percent of the clients indicated that they were maintaining a significant level of improvement.

In comparison studies, Andrews (1974a) reported that two years after dismissal, stutterers who received fluency reinforcement and prolongation training were maintaining better fluency than were clients who received fluency reinforcement only. Another report (Helps & Dalton, 1979) compared syllable-timed speech to prolongation, measuring about six to twelve months after the completion of intensive therapy in syllable-timed or in prolongation methods. The syllable-timed group showed a 20 percent improvement, compared to an average improvement of 61 percent for the prolongation group. Members of the prolongation group who entered follow-up therapy raised their fluency average to 86 percent.

Van Riper (1973, p. 84) expressed strong doubts about the permanence of claimed improvements.

> Moreover, there may be real dangers in training a stutterer to prolong his vowels. . . . Some of the severest stutterers we have ever known were those whose major abnormality consisted of interminably long vowel sounds.

He continued to emphasize the dangers of teaching children to prolong, noting that mature stutterers can always return to their old way of stuttering when "retarded speech" fails them. He stated that prolongation failed many years ago when we lacked the "magic of the machine" and taught prolongation directly, and there is no reason now to think the results will be any better. He ended his commentary with, ". . . if this were the route to fluency, the age old problems would long ago have been solved" (p. 85).

Despite Van Riper's criticisms and some of the statistical data from follow-up studies, prolongation seems to function as well as most techniques and better than some. Several fairly specific sequences have been referred to previously, so I will limit further discussion to general suggestions. The reader is reminded of other sections on easy onset, airflow, relaxation, and so forth, as they would relate to prolongation.

1. Confirm or establish a good respiratory pattern to provide support for the greater usage of air often involved in prolongation.
2. Confirm or teach (either initially or concurrently) an adequate relaxation so that initiation and continued smooth sound transitions are facilitated.
3. Teach an easy onset to sound production, stressing release of the breathstream and use of light consonant contacts.
4. Practice prolongation on vowel-initiated words at first, and then use words starting with consonants.
5. On consonant initiation, begin with voiced continuants such as /n/, /z/, /r/, and so on, before trying voiceless ones.
6. Practice separately on plosives, stressing, a light contact that drags or stretches slightly so that the contact acquires a movementlike characteristic.
7. Move to prolongation on entire words, introducing continuous phonation if it is needed.
   a. Start with all-voiced, all-continuant words, such as

renown	morning	zone	northern
revere	mover	zinger	ringing
reason	merry	navy	

   b. Add words that have unvoiced, nonplosive sounds.
   c. Add plosives.
8. Provide practice phrases and sentences, initially loading them with voiced phonemes, and move toward conversational speech.

9. Use samples, models, DAF, metronome, or other methods to teach the clients levels of spm rate production until they can equate length of prolongation to (at least) slow, moderate, and normal speech rates. Insist that clients are able to monitor themselves and change prolongation and rate patterns. Ingham (1984) was worried that clinicians today overfavor rate control therapies to the exclusion of other possibilities, but rate control is integral in many approaches.

10. When basic skills have been acquired, always devote time to prosodic elements and "normal"-sounding speech.

11. Provide practice, guidance, and modeling in decreasing the frequency and duration of prolongations, targeting early sentences, initial words, feared words, and words following significant pauses.

12. Use a situational fear hierarchy list in transfer-planning activities.

13. Use group activity if available, particularly for sharing problems, problem solving, and monitoring.

14. Before dismissal, schedule an "advanced skills" booster session to occur three to six months after termination. Describe it as being routine for skills refinement and problem solving rather than for protection against relapse.

As with other techniques, evaluate performance on a continuing basis for abuses, patterns of error, and whether or not prolongation is the best technique for a particular client.

MISCELLANEOUS PROCEDURES

Extended Length of Utterance (ELU)

Extended length of utterance (ELU) was the keystone of nearly all sensible therapy many, many years before it was "discovered," placed in a behavioral frame, dressed up in learning terminology, and hung up for self-admiring applause. It is a program sequence based on the old maxim that we learn best in small steps. Articulation therapy has practiced ELU for centuries, starting with isolated sounds and progressing through syllables, word position, phrases, sentences, and so on. Stuttering therapy, regardless of symptom or fluency orientation, follows the same pattern in most techniques—move from the simple to the complex, from easier to harder. However, the practitioners of ELU have structured stages to a degree ignored by most clinicians in the past. On a similar plane, gradual increase in length and complexity of utterance (or GILCU) is a systematization of the linguistic and situational variables that move speech from simple to complex and easy to difficult levels. Ryan's GILCU program (1971, 1974) is an excellent example of the method. The most complete example of ELU planning probably is Costello's (1980) program, in which she describes twenty-three steps to reach a six-word string and then converts to fluency time for nonstuttered speech (starting with five seconds and ending with five minutes of continuously fluent speech). Each step must be performed ten consecutive times without error (stuttering) before progressing to the next step. Step failure (and design of a branch step) occurs after five consecutive failures in any one step or failure to meet the passing criteria for any single step over a period of three therapy sessions. Branch steps, in difficulty level, fall between the last step passed and the current step just failed.

As noted earlier, ELU is hardly a revolutionary development. However, its importance lies in actually planning carefully for a stutterer in graded levels of difficulty, with predetermined criteria for what constitutes success. There are two limitations to GILCU and ELU. One is the danger that some clinicians will apply example programs literally to a variety of clients, without adjusting timing, criteria, or stimuli. The second limitation is the possibility that some clinicians will assume that length of utterance (or situational complexity) meet the needs of the client. Some clients will need substeps. Specific word fears may be important for some clients and not for others. Perceptions of situational complexity vary from client to client. The lure of one-program-fits-all is not intended by the developers and should be guarded against.

Any ELU or GILCU program can be integrated with any fluency or symptom approach and with any specific therapy technique. The concept itself can be applied to any habit reduction or skill acquisition. Usually, specific programs of reinforcement and/or punishment accompany the step procedures since, in and of themselves, the steps lack significant effects on stuttering. These approaches simultaneously are reminders that very few things are new under the sun—and that any procedure can be revised, improved, be given structure, and then applied in ways that facilitate measurement of progress.

Time Out (TO)

Time out (or TO) also has been in the therapy room for many years. I am sure that some Neanderthal child was exiled to silence in a deserted corner of the family cave as a behavior modification device. Costello (1975) provided an excellent review of TO research up to that time, establishing it as an aversive stimulus. When its use becomes contingent on the occurrence of stuttering, it will decrease the frequency of dysfluencies. Haroldson et al. (1968) simply activated a red signal light upon the occurrence of any stuttering. While the light was on (ten seconds) the client was not allowed to continue speaking. Stuttering frequency was decreased markedly, although relapses tended to occur during postexperimental periods. Adams and Popelka (1971) compared standard (five readings) stuttering adaptation to readings with ten-second TO contingencies after each stuttering. As expected, adaptation on repeated readings occcurred but not nearly to the extent it occurred on the TO readings. Martin et al. (1972a) used TO puppetry with stuttering children, where the puppet withdrew for ten seconds following each stuttering. Fluency results were reported to be excellent (two subjects), although the possible confounding effect of puppet use could not be evaluated.

Martin and Haroldson (1979) compared TO to contingent use of "wrong" after each stuttering and to continuous use of separate masking noise, of DAF, and of metronome rhythm. Each experimental condition lasted for thirty minutes. When %SW and stuttering duration were considered, TO effected the greatest reduction; more than a third of the subjects increased %SW during "wrong," and over 50 percent increased spasm duration under masking. Interestingly, those showing the greatest reductions under TO also showed large reductions under DAF and metronome. The authors reminded us that unlike the noncontingent conditions, TO does not seem to change materially the pitch, loudness, or prosodic elements of the stutterer's speech.

Costello (1980) provided an excellent example of combining TO with a sequential therapy program (see section on ELU). She described how, when stuttering occurred, the clinician was to say "stop" and to turn away for ten seconds. When the penalty time was up, the clinician turned back to the stutterer and acted as a good, reinforcing listener. The client did not have to restart from the stopping point. Costello also noted, very wisely, that for the last ten minutes of each session, TO was dropped and the clinician just became a good listener. At first, stuttering tended to increase during the final period, but fluency began to stabilize by the sixth session. Instruction in monitoring, fluency development, and so on was inserted. With each session, the TO segment was reduced and the non-TO final period expanded. Time-out procedures can be applied by the client (James, 1983) but are less effective than when administered by the clinician. Clients are not as reliable in assessing TO penalties and, given the option, elected fairly brief TO penalty periods. Whether this reflects clients' weakness, or clinician perfectionism is undetermined.

In applying TO, be sure you have a preliminary baseline measure (preferably for each session) against which effects can be measured. Be sure that the TO length is adequate for penalty but does not waste time; for example, the Curlee and Perkins (1969) TO of thirty seconds seems inappropriately long (especially sitting in the dark). Signals and any accompaniment (light, "stop," "wrong," turning out lights) should be adequate for the purpose but should not embarrass, amuse, or irritate the client too much. Consistency is very important, and you should define criteria very clearly for the client—and apply them every time. Finally, an increasing non-TO period can be a reward as well as aiding in transfer. Time out can fit into most therapy programs and be very useful in facilitating rapid learning or change. Whether it is truly penalizing, breaks performance into small strings of motor planning, allows relaxation, or simply breaks into the self-reinforcement of dysfluency is not as important as the fact that it seems to be very effective, crosses age barriers, and seems to affect all stuttering subgroups.

Speech Monitoring

Speech monitoring has been applied in more than one way. At times it is used to instruct the stutterers to listen to the speech of nonstutterers in order to become aware of the frequency with which they are not fluent, as well as to become aware of stuttering spasms (Ryan, 1971; Shames & Florance, 1980; Van Riper, 1973). It also can be applied more intensely (Van Riper, 1973) to organize an in-depth monitoring on type, severity, and location of spasms, along with associated behaviors and personal feelings. Monitoring can be taught as a technique to check on the use of acquired fluency methods (Boberg, 1980a; Curlee & Perkins, 1969) as a progressive sequence in making the client responsible for his or her own speech pattern.

People, fluent or stuttering, differ in their level of self-awareness. Fictional characters, and current comedians, can mix up words with apparent unawareness. Most of us have friends who will for example, say, *tread* for *thread* and vice versa, unaware they have committed any error. I am sure that stutterers show the same spread of awareness levels. Add to that the possible emotional levels blocking speech awareness and the "gray out" phenomenon, and it should be considered that most stutterers probably need work on monitoring.

Van Riper (1958, 1973) described a method of "high stimulus speech monitoring" in advanced cases of stuttering to monitor fluency and to detect developing stuttering tensions. It seems to be associated particularly with preparatory sets. The method can be described as a gentle form of speech chewing or as a combination of prolongation and continuous phonation where consonants (even plosives) are made with a sliding, dragging contact. One client described it as spreading peanut butter on the articulators and, without using his hands, trying to remove the sticky substance as he talked. Van Riper (1958) reported that clients fatigued rapidly in using this technique, and some found it irksome. My experience has been similar. However, in short intervals, I have found it to be a useful checking device, and especially useful when a client is having trouble or fears that trouble may occur. There may be a residual effect, but this is completely speculative; when I would work with a number of stutterers in the same day with high-stimulus speech monitoring, my wife could detect it in my speech (even though I wasn't "doing" it) when I arrived home that evening. As stated, this is speculative and could be limited to certain types of individuals. Steps involved in using the monitoring can be as follows:

1. Practice on phrases of two to four words, without any plosives. Slow the rate, establish an airstream, prolong vowels, and on consonants "stretch" them by

moving the articulators through the production. Muscle pressure will increase, but the movement should be continuous so that tremors or stoppages do not develop.

2. Add plosive words to the practice, moving through their production rather than uttering them as stops. This will produce a slightly sloppy, elongated plosive, but it will not be particularly noticeable to the listener.

3. Practice on sentences.

4. Move to monologue. In this stage, concentrate on
   a. Restoring any losses in prosodic elements and normalizing rate.
   b. Encouraging the client not to monitor every word but only "important" words. This usually happens spontaneously as rate and prosody develop.

5. Practice conversational exchange.

6. Use assignments. Mix short ones (for example, telephone call to a store) with longer situations. Brief situations should be monitored 100 percent, whereas longer ones should be experiments in what level of use is best for the particular individual.

7. In planning maintenance programs, propose consistent and decreasing use of high-stimulus speech monitoring, perhaps in the following sequence:
   a. For the first month, use monitoring in three situations every day and evaluate speech.
   b. In the second month, apply monitoring to one extended situation each day, evaluating as before.
   c. In the third month, use the monitoring once each week in an extended situation and carefuly evaluate the status of fluency.
   d. For the next three months, use monitoring one day each month, in at least half the speech situations that day. Take the opportunity to assess status.
   e. Return to the clinic for a report, overall review, and discussion of any needs after this six-month period.

Speech monitoring also is applied to check on fluency. Curlee and Perkins (1969) trained the client to judge performance in rate control, as well as feelings of self-confidence, and to self-consequate the results of the evaluations. Shames and Florance (1980) proposed a specific program of monitored and unmonitored speech.

1. After the client has acquired ability in continuous phonation and several rates of speech, the clinician practices using an overt signal to vary the rate of the client's speech. Results are recorded, played back, and analyzed until the client recognizes the differences between fast and slow rates and good and poor performances.

2. The client becomes responsible for self-signaling, moving to the use of a covert signal.

3. The client practices moving toward a normal rate.

4. The clinician will signal periodically after a good job of target production, and the client can stop monitoring for the next four to five words (off-time increases as performance improves).

5. The. client takes over the monitoring of speech, rewarding him- or herself with increasing periods of unmonitored speech. The client now is responsible for all aspects of monitoring and self-consequating the evaluations from monitoring.

Shames and Florance commented that after awhile, periods of unmonitored speech start to take on the characteristics of the controlled, monitored speech. Boberg (1980a) reported on a program (intensive) in which analysis, prolongation, attitude change, and cancellation were used. Self-assessment monitoring, using audio and video equipment, was taught throughout therapy. The client purchased a wrist digital counter and was responsible for tallying cancellations, rate (200 ±40 spm), and prosody errors and for producing speech at or below 1 percent SW. The clinician kept a covert tally. The client had to succeed, without monitoring error, for three consecutive sessions. A failure at any time required three new successful sessions. If there was a second failure, the client dropped back to the previous phase and met criteria there before trying self-monitoring again. The next phase involved working on varying the rate (especially in feared situations). Signal practice was used to shift easily from slow rate to normal rate and so on. Two successful clinician-directed sessions had to be followed by two successful client-directed sessions. Transfer of control and monitoring involved twelve outside situations devised by the clinic, plus ten situations that were particular to the client. All situations were recorded (at least five minutes, cumulative). The tape was evaluated and more work planned, or the client was scheduled for dismissal and maintenance.

Starkweather (1980) questions the possible overuse of monitoring, saying ". . . the use of elaborate programs of rate control or monitoring is not necessary, at least not with adults" (p. 375). He argues that if therapy has been effective in removing avoidances, the therapy instructional program, clinician modeling, and practice are all that are needed. Starkweather is correct if we assume extremely effective generalization and avoidance elimination that will remain in effect once the client is separated from the support of a clinician. It is hard to become enthusiastic about digital counters and calculating percentages against word estimate, but basic monitoring capacity is desirable. Until we can predict who will use it, dump it, forget, and backslide; and use it, regress, and panic; or other possibilities, it is better to possibly "waste" some time and teach a thorough monitoring procedure.

COMMENTARY

There is no space for detailed consideration of hypnotism, drug therapy, CO_2 therapy, gesture speech, IPC therapy, nondirective therapy, personal construct analysis, and many more. Of the techniques presented, it is impossible to discuss all the different ways a technique could be varied or contexts in which it could be used. My opinions, therefore, have intruded to a considerable degree. I have tried to separate my personal biases from results of published research and the opinions of others, but I accept the onus of my opinions. The goal of this book is to provide explanations and

procedural steps for as many techniques as possible. Because of my foregoing comments about omissions and restrictions, I would be glad to hear
from any readers who know of another way to use some of the techniques
that have been discussed or would like to communicate about methods that
were not covered. My one orientation is based on the idea that therapy for
communication disorders is essentially an alteration in the interpersonal
behavior of others toward others. When we change speech, we change the
persona, no matter how slightly. If there were no other reason, this would
make skill in technique an important variable. As we learn to do the things
we ask our clients to do, and communicate with other professionals about
it, we can aspire to do well the things that we do.

References

ADAMCZYK, B. (1959). Use of instruments for the production of artificial feedback in the treatment of stuttering. *Folia Phoniatrica*, 11:216-18.

ADAMCZYK, B., KUNISZYK, W., & SMOTKA, E. (1979). Influence of echo and reverberation on the speech process. *Folia Phoniatrica*, 31:70-81.

ADAMCZYK, B., SADOWSKA, E., & KUNISZK-JOZKOWIAK, W. (1975). Influence of reverberation on stuttering. *Folia Phoniatrica*, 27:1-6.

ADAMS, M. R. (1976). Some common problems in the design and conduct of experiments in stuttering. *Journal of Speech and Hearing Disorders*. 41:3-9.

ADAMS, M. R. (1977). A clinical strategy for differentiating the normally nonfluent child from the incipient stutterer. *Journal of Fluency Disorders*, 2:141-48.

ADAMS, M. R. (1978). Further analysis of stuttering as a phonetic transition defect. *Journal of Fluency Disorders*, 3:265-71.

ADAMS, M. R. (1982a). A case report on the use of flooding in stuttering therapy. *Journal of Fluency Disorders*, 7:343-54.

ADAMS, M. R. (1982b) Fluency, non-fluency, and stuttering in children. *Journal of Fluency Disorders*, 7:171-85.

ADAMS, M. R. (1983). Learning from negative outcomes in stuttering therapy: I. Getting off on the wrong foot. *Journal of Fluency Disorders*, 8:147-53.

ADAMS, M. R. & HAYDEN, P. (1976). The ability of stutterers and nonstutterers to initiate and terminate phonation during production of an isolated vowel. *Journal of Speech and Hearing Research*, 19:290-96.

ADAMS, M. R., & MOORE, W. H. (1972). The effects of auditory masking on the anxiety level, frequency of disfluency, and selected vocal characteristics of stutterers. *Journal of Speech and Hearing Disorders*, 15:572-78.

ADAMS, M. R., & POPELKA, G. (1971). The influence of "time out" on stutterers and their disfluency. *Behavior Therapy*, 2:734-39.

ADAMS, M. R., & RAMIG, P. (1980). Vocal characteristics of normal speakers and stutterers during choral reading. *Journal of Speech and Hearing Research*, 23:457-69.

ADAMS, M. R., & REIS, R. (1971). The influence of the onset of phonation on the frequency of stuttering. *Journal of Speech and Hearing Research*, 14:639-44.

ADAMS, M. R., RIEMENSCHNEIDER, S., METZ, D., & CONTURE, E. (1974). Voice onset and articulatory constriction requirements in a speech segment and their relation to the amount of stuttering adaptation. *Journal of Fluency Disorders*, 1:23-29.

351

ADAMS, M. R., RUNYAN, C., & MALLARD, A. R. (1975). Airflow characteristics of the speech of stutterers and nonstutterers. *Journal of Fluency Disorders*, 1:4-12.

ADAMS, M. R., SEARS, R. L., & RAMIG, P. R. (1982). Changes in stutterers and nonstutterers during monotoned speech. *Journal of Fluency Disorders*, 7:21-35.

ADLER, S. (1966). *A Clinician's Guide to Stuttering*. Springfield, Ill.: Charles C Thomas.

ALFORD, J., & INGHAM, R. J. (1969). The application of a token reinforcement system to the treatment of stuttering in children. *Journal of the Australian College of Speech Therapists*, 19:53-57.

AMMONS, R., & JOHNSON, W. (1944). Studies in the psychology of stuttering: 18, The construction and application of a test of attitudes toward stuttering. *Journal of Speech Disorders*, 9:39-49.

ANDREWS, G. (1973). Stuttering therapy: How simple can an effective treatment program become. *Australian Journal of Human Disorders of Communication*, 2:44-46.

ANDREWS, G. (1974a). The etiology of stuttering. *Australian Journal of Human Communication Disorders*, 2:8-12.

ANDREWS, G. (1974b). The measurement of stuttering, *Australian Journal of Human Communication Disorders*, 2:6-7.

ANDREWS, G., & CRAIG, A. (1982). Stuttering: Overt and covert measurement of the speech of treated subjects. *Journal of Speech and Hearing Disorders*, 47:96-98.

ANDREWS, G., CRAIG, A., FEYER, A., HODDINOTT, S., HOWIE, P., & NEILSON, M. (1983). Stuttering: A review of research findings and theories circa 1982. *Journal of Speech and Hearing Disorders*, 48:226-46.

ANDREWS, G., & CUTLER, J. (1974). Stuttering therapy: The relation between changes in symptom level and attitude. *Journal of Speech and Hearing Disorders*, 39:309-11.

ANDREWS, G. B., GUITAR, B., & HOWIE, P. (1980). Meta-analysis of the effects of stuttering treatment. *Journal of Speech and Hearing Disorders*, 45:287-307.

ANDREWS, G., HARRIS, M., GARSIDE, R., & KAY, D. (1964). The inhibition of stuttering by syllable-timed speech. G. Andrews & M. Harris (eds.). *The Syndrome of Stuttering*. The Spastics Society Medical and Educational Unit. London: Heinemann.

ANDREWS, G., & HARVEY, R. (1981). Regression to the mean in pretreatment measures of stuttering. *Journal of Speech and Hearing Disorders*, 46:204-7.

ANDREWS, G., HOWIE, P. M., DOSZA, M., & GUITAR, B. E. (1982). Stuttering: Speech pattern characteristics under fluency inducing conditions. *Journal of Speech and Hearing Research*, 25:208-15.

ANDREWS, G., & INGHAM, R. J. (1971). Stuttering: Considerations in the evaluation of treatment. *British Journal of Disorders of Communication*, 6:129-38.

ANDREWS, G., & TANNER, S. (1982). Stuttering: The results of five days treatment with an airflow technique. *Journal of Speech and Hearing Disorders*, 42:427-29.

AVARI, D. N., & BLOODSTEIN, O. (1974). Adjacency and prediction in school-age stutterers. *Journal of Speech and Hearing Research*, 17:33-40.

AZRIN, N., JONES, R., & FLYE, B. (1968). A synchronization effect and its application to stuttering by a portable apparatus. *Journal of Applied Behavioral Analysis*, 1:283-95.

AZRIN, N. H., & NUNN, R. G. (1974). A rapid method of eliminating stuttering by a regulated breathing approach. *Behavior Research and Therapy*, 12:279-86.

AZRIN, N. H., NUNN, R. G., & FRANTZ, S. (1979). Comparison of regulated breathing versus abbreviated desensitization on reported stuttering episodes. *Journal of Speech and Hearing Disorders*, 44:331-39.

BACHRACH, D. L. (1964). Sex differences in reactions to delayed auditory feedback. *Perceptual and Motor Skills*, 19:81-82.

BAKEN, J. R., McMANUS, D. A. & CAVALLO, S. A. (1983). Prephonatory chest wall posturing in stutterers. *Journal of Speech and Hearing Research*, 26:444-50.

BAR, A., SINGER, J., & FELDMAN, R. G. (1969). Subvocal muscle activity during stuttering and fluent speech. *Journal of the South African Logopedic Society*, 16:9-14.

BAR, H. (1940). A quantitative study of the specific phenomena observed in stuttering. *Journal of Speech Disorders*, 5:277-80.

BARBARA, D. A. (1965). *Questions and Answers on Stuttering*. Springfield, Ill.: Charles C Thomas.

BARBER, V. (1939). Studies in the psychology of stuttering: XV. Chorus reading as a distraction in stuttering. *Journal of Speech Disorders*, 4:371-83.

BARBER, V. (1940). Studies in the psychology of stuttering: XVI. Rhythm as a distraction in stuttering. *Journal of Speech Disorders*, 5:29-42.

BAYLY, R. B. (1965). Comments from a stutterer. *Today's Speech*, 13:2-3.

BEAUMONT, J., & FOSS, B. (1957). Individual differences in reacting to delayed auditory feedback. *British Journal of Psychology*, 48:85-89.

BEECH, H. R. (1967). Stuttering and stammering. *Psychology Today*, 1:48-51, 61.

BEECH, H. R., & FRANSELLA, F. (1968). *Research and Experiment in Stuttering*. London: Pergamon Press, 1968.

BEECH, H. R., & FRANSELLA, F. (1969). Explanation of the rhythm effect in stuttering. B. Gray & G. England (eds.). *Stuttering and the Conditioning Therapies*. Monterey, Calif.: The Monterey Institute of Speech and Hearing.

BELMORE, N. F., KEWLEY-PORT, D., MOBLEY, R., & GOODMAN, V. (1973). The development of auditory feedback monitoring: Delayed auditory feedback studies on the vocalizations of children aged six months to 19 months. *Journal of Speech and Hearing Research*, 16:709-20.

BENDER, J. F. (1939). *The Personality Structure of Stuttering*. New York: Pitman Publishing Co.

BERECZ, J. M. (1973). The treatment of stuttering through precision punishment and cognitive arousal. *Journal of Speech and Hearing Disorders*, 38:256-67.

BERLIN, S., & BERLIN, L. (1964). Acceptability of stuttering control patterns. *Journal of Speech and Hearing Disorders*, 29:436-41.

BERNSEN, D. A., & BOCKOUEC, T. D. (1972). *Progressive Relaxation Training: A Manual for the Helping Professions*. Champaign, Ill.: Research Press.

BERRY, M. F., & EISENSON, J. (1945). *The Defective in Speech*. New York: F. S. Crofts & Co.

BERRY, R. C., & SILVERMAN, F. H. (1972). Equality of intervals on the Lewis-Sherman Scale of Stuttering Severity. *Journal of Speech and Hearing Research*, 15:185-88.

BLACK, J. (1951). The effect of sidetone delay on vocal rate and intensity. *Journal of Speech and Hearing Disorders*, 16:50-56.

BLACK, J. (1955). The persistence of the effects of delayed sidetone. *Journal of Speech and Hearing Disorders*, 20:65-68.

BLOOD, G. W., & SEIDER, R. (1981). The concomitant problems of young stutterers. *Journal of Speech and Hearing Disorders*, 46:31-33.

BLOODSTEIN, O. (1949). Conditions under which stuttering is reduced or absent: A review of literature. *Journal of Speech and Hearing Disorders*, 14:295-302.

BLOODSTEIN, O. (1950). A rating scale of conditions under which stuttering is reduced or absent. *Journal of Speech and Hearing Disorders*, 15:29-36.

BLOODSTEIN, O. (1960). The development of stuttering, I: Changes in nine basic features. *Journal of Speech and Hearing Disorders*, 25:219-37.

BLOODSTEIN, O. (1969). *A Handbook on Stuttering*. Chicago: National Easter Seal Society for Crippled Children and Adults.

BLOODSTEIN, O. (1972). The anticipatory struggle hypothesis: Implications of research on the variability of stuttering. *Journal of Speech and Hearing Research*, 15:487-89.

BLOODSTEIN, O. (1975a). *A Handbook on Stuttering*. Chicago: National Easter Seal Society for Crippled Children and Adults.

BLOODSTEIN, O. (1975b). Stuttering as tension and fragmentation. J. Eisenson (ed.). *Stuttering, a Second Symposium*. New York: Harper & Row.

BLOODSTEIN, O. (1979). *Speech Pathology: An Introduction*. Boston: Houghton Mifflin.

BLOODSTEIN, O., & SHOGAN, R. L. (1972). Some clinical notes on forced stuttering. *Journal of Speech and Hearing Disorders*, 37:177-86.

BLUEMEL, C. S. (1957). *The Riddle of Stuttering*. Danville, Ill.: The Interstate Publishing Co.

BLUEMEL, C. S. (1960). Concepts of stammering: A century in review. *Journal of Speech and Hearing Disorders*, 25:24-32.

BOBERG, E. (1976). Intensive group therapy program for stutterers. *Human Communication*, 1:29-42.

BOBERG, E. (1980a). Intensive adult therapy program. W. H. Perkins (ed.). *Strategies in Stuttering Therapy*. J. L. Northern (ed.). *Seminars in Speech, Language and Hearing*. New York: Thieme-Stratton.

BOBERG, E. (1980b). (ed.). *Maintenance of Fluency: Proceedings of the Banff Conference*. New York: Elsevier.

BOLAND, J. L. (1953). A comparison of stutterers and non-stutterers on several measures of anxiety. *Speech Monographs*, 20:144.

BOOME, E. J., BAINES, H. M. S., & HARRIS, D. G. (1939). *Abnormal Speech*. London: Methuen.

BOOME, E. J., & RICHARDSON, M. A. (1931). *The Nature and Treatment of Stammering*. London: Methuen.

BOUDREAU, L. A., & JEFFREY, C. J. (1973). Stuttering treated by desensitization. *Journal of Behavior Therapy and Experimental Psychiatry*, 4:209-12.

BRADY, J. P. (1968). A behavioral approach to the treatment of stammering. *American Journal of Psychiatry*, 125:843-48.

BRADY, J. P. (1971). Metronome-conditioned speech retraining for stuttering. *Behavior Therapy*, 2:129-50.

BRADY, J. P. (1973). Metronome-conditioned relaxation: A new behavioral procedure. *British Journal of Psychiatry*, 122:729-30.

BRADY, J. P., & BRADY, C. N. (1972). Behavior therapy of stuttering. *Folia Phoniatrica*, 24:355-59.

BRANDON, S., & HARRIS, M. (1966). Stammering, an experimental treatment programme using syllable-timed speech. *Speech Pathology Diagnosis: Therapy and Practices*. Report of the National Conference of Speech Therapists. Edinburgh: E. & S. Livingston.

BRANDON, S., & HARRIS, M. (1967). Stammering, an experimental treatment programme using syllable-timed speech. *British Journal of Disorders of Communication*, 2:64-68.

BRANKEL, V. O. (1961). Pneumotachographic studies of stuttering. *Folia Phoniatrica*, 13:136-43.

BRENNER, N. C., PERKINS, W. H., & SODERBERG, G. A. (1972). The effect of rehearsal on frequency of stuttering. *Journal of Speech and Hearing Research*, 15:483-86.

BRESTOVICI, B. (1978). Stuttering and stoppages in speech. *Defaktol*, 12:11-21. In *dsh Abstracts*, 508, 18:97.

BROWN, S. (1937). The influence of grammatical function on the incidence of stuttering. *Journal of Speech Disorders*, 2:207-15.

BROWN, S. (1938). Stuttering with relation to word accent and word position. *Journal of Abnormal and Social Psychology*, 33:112-20.

BRUCE, M. C., & ADAMS, M. P. (1978). Effects of two types of motor practice on stuttering adaptation. *Journal of Speech and Hearing Research*, 21:421-28.

BRUTTEN, E. J. (1963). Palmar sweat investigation of disfluency and expectancy adaptation. *Journal of Speech and Hearing Research*, 6:40-48.

BRUTTEN, E. J., & GRAY, B. B. (1961). Effect of a word cue removal on adaptation and adjacency: A clinical paradigm. *Journal of Speech and Hearing Disorders*, 26:385-89.

BRUTTEN, E. J., & SHOEMAKER, D. J. (1967). *The Modification of Stuttering*. Englewood Cliffs, N.J.: Prentice-Hall.

BRUTTEN, G. J. (1973). Behavior assessment and the strategy of therapy. Y. Lebrun & R. Hoops (eds.). *Neurolinguistic Approaches to Stuttering*. The Hague: Mouton.

BRUTTEN, G. J., & JANSSEN, P. (1979). An eye-marking investigation of anticipated and observed stuttering. *Journal of Speech and Hearing Research*, 22:20-28.

BRYNGELSON, B. (1935). Sidedness as an etiological factor in stuttering. *Journal of Genetic Psychology*, 47:205-17.

BRYNGELSON, B., CHAPMAN, M., & HANSEN, O. (1944). *Know Yourself—A Guide for Those Who Stutter*. Minneapolis, Minn.: Burgess Publishing Co.

BRYNGELSON, B., & RUTHERFORD, B. (1937). A comparative study of laterality of stutterer and nonstutterer. *Journal of Speech Disorders*, 2:15-16.

BURGRAFF, R. I. (1974). The efficacy of systematic desensitization via imagery as a therapeutic technique with stutterers. *British Journal of Disorders of Communication*, 9:134-39.

BURKE, B. (1975). Variables affecting stutterers' initial reactions to delayed auditory feedback. *Journal of Communication Disorders*, 8:141-55.

CANTER, G. J. (1971). Observations on neurogenic stuttering: A contribution to differential diagnosis. *British Journal of Disorders of Communication*, 6:139-43.

CHAPMAN, M. (1959). *Self Inventory (Group Therapy for Those Who Stutter)*. Minneapolis, Minn.: Burgess Publishing Co.

CHASE, R., SUTTON, S., FIRST, D., & ZUBIN, J. (1961). A developmental study of changes in behavior under delayed auditory feedback. *Journal of Genetic Psychology*, 99:101-12.

CHEASMAN, C. (1983). Therapy for adults: An evaluation of current techniques for establishing fluency. P. Dalton (ed.). *Approaches to the Treatment of Stuttering*. London: Crom Helm.

CHERRY E. C. (1953). Some experiments on the recognition of speech with one and two ears. *Journal of the Acoustical Society of America*, 25:975-79.

CHERRY, E. C. (1957). *On Human Communication*. Cambridge: Massachusetts Institute of Technology Press.

CHERRY, E. C., & SAYERS, B. McA. (1956). Experiments on the total inhibition of stammering by external control, and some clinical results. *Journal of Psychosomatic Research*, 1:233-46.

CHERRY, E. C., SAYERS, B. M., & MARLAND, P. (1955). Experiments on the complete suppression of stammering. *Nature*, 176:874-75.

CIAMBRONE, S. W., MARTIN, R. A., & BERKOWITZ, M. (1983). A correlational study of stutterers' adaptation and voice initiation times. *Journal of Fluency Disorders*, 8:29-38.

CODE, C. (1979). Genuine and artificial stammering: An EMG comparison. *British Journal of Disorders of Communication*, 14:5-16.

COLCORD, R. D., & ADAMS, M. R. (1979). Voicing duration and vocal SPL changes associated with stuttering reduction during singing. *Journal of Speech and Hearing Research*, 22:468-79.

CONTURE, E. G. (1973). Comments on "Effects on stuttering of changes in audition." *Journal of Speech and Hearing Research*, 16:753-54.

CONTURE, E. G. (1982). *Stuttering*. Englewood Cliffs, N.J.: Prentice-Hall.

CONTURE, E. G., McCALL, G., & BREWER, D. W. (1977). Laryngeal behavior during stuttering. *Journal of Speech and Hearing Research*, 20:661-68.

COOPER, C. S., & COOPER, E. B. (1969). Variations in adult stutterer attitudes towards clinicians during therapy. *Journal of Communication Disorders*, 2:141-53.

COOPER, E. B. (1971). Integrating behavior therapy and traditional insight treatment procedures with stutterers. *Journal of Communication Disorders*, 4:40-43.

COOPER, E. B. (1972). Recovery from stuttering in a junior and senior high school population. *Journal of Speech and Hearing Research*, 15:632-38.

COOPER, E. B. (1977). Controversies about stuttering therapy. *Journal of Fluency Disorders*, 2:75-86.

COOPER, E. B. (1982). A disfluency descriptor digest for clinical use. *Journal of Fluency Disorders*, 2:355-58.

COOPER, E. B., & THOMPSON, M. P. (1971). Accuracy of stutterer perceptions following self-observation through video recordings. *Journal of Communication Disorders*, 4:119-25.

COOPER, M. H., & ALLEN, G. D. (1977). Timing control accuracy in normal speakers and stutterers. *Journal of Speech and Hearing Research*, 20:55-71.

COPPOLA, V. A., & YAIRI, E. (1982). Rhythmic speech training with preschool stuttering children: An experimental study. *Journal of Fluency Disorders*, 7:447-57.

COSTELLO, J. (1975). The establishment of fluency with time-out procedures: Three case studies. *Journal of Speech and Hearing Disorders*, 40:216-31.

COSTELLO, J. (1980). Operant conditioning and the treatment of stuttering. W. H. Perkins (ed.). *Strategies in Stuttering Therapy*. J. L. Northern (ed.). *Seminars in Speech, Language and Hearing*. New York: Thieme-Stratton.

CRANE, S. L., & COOPER, E. B. (1983). Speech-language clinician personality variables and clinical effectiveness. *Journal of Speech and Hearing Disorders*, 48:140-44.

CROSS, D. E. (1977). Effects of false increasing, decreasing and true EMG biofeedback on the frequency of stuttering. *Journal of Fluency Disorders*, 2:109-16.

CROSS, D. E., & LUPER, H. L. (1979). Voice reaction time of stuttering and non-stuttering children and adults. *Journal of Fluency Disorders*, 4:59-77.

CROSS, D. E., & LUPER, H. L. (1983). Relation between finger reaction time and voice reaction time in stuttering and nonstuttering children and adults. *Journal of Speech and Hearing Research*, 26:356-61.

CROWE, T. A., & COOPER, E. B. (1977). Parental attitudes toward and knowledge of stuttering. *Journal of Communication Disorders*, 10:343-57.

CRYSTAL, D. (1980). *Introduction to Language Pathology*. Baltimore: University Park Press.

CULLINAN, W. L. (1963). Stability of consistency measures in stuttering. *Journal of Speech and Hearing Research*, 6:134-38.

CULLINAN, W. L., & PRATHER, E. M. (1968). Reliability of "live" ratings of the speech of stutterers. *Perceptual Motor Skills*, 27:403-9.

CULLINAN, W. L., & SPRINGER, M. T. (1980). Voice initiation and termination times in stuttering and non-stuttering children. *Journal of Speech and Hearing Research*, 23:344-60.

CURLEE, R. F. (1980). A case selection strategy for young disfluent children. W. H. Perkins (ed.). *Strategies in Stuttering Therapy*. J. L. Northern (ed.). *Seminars in Speech, Language and Hearing*. New York: Thieme-Stratton.

CURLEE, R. F. (1981). Observer agreements on disfluency and stuttering. *Journal of Speech and Hearing Research*, 24:595-80.

CURLEE, R. F., & PERKINS, W. H. (1969). Conversational rate-control therapy for stuttering. *Journal of Speech and Hearing Disorders*, 34:245-50.

CURLEE, R., & PERKINS, W. (1973). Effectiveness of a DAF conditioning program for adolescent and adult stutterers. *Behavioral Research and Therapy*, 1:395-401.

CZUCHNA, P. E. (No. 9). Guidelines. M. Fraser (Dir.). *To the Stutterer*. Memphis, Tenn.: Speech Foundation of America.

DALTON, P., & HARDCASTLE, W. J. (1977). *Disorders of Fluency and Their Effects on Communication*. London: Edward Arnold.

DANILOFF, R., SCHUCKERS, G., & FETH, L. (1980). *The Physiology of Speech and Hearing*. Englewood Cliffs, N.J.: Prentice-Hall.

DANZGER, M., & HALPERN, H. (1973). Relation of stuttering to word abstraction, part of speech, word length, and word frequency. *Perceptual Motor Skills*, 37:959-62.

DARLEY, F. L. (1964). *Diagnosis and Appraisal of Communication Disorders*. Englewood Cliffs, N.J.: Prentice-Hall.

DEWAR, A., DEWAR, A. D., & ANTHONY, J. F. K. (1976a). The effects of auditory feedback masking on concomitant moments of stuttering. *British Journal of Disorders of Communication*, 11:95-102.

DEWAR, A., DEWAR, A. D., AUSTION, W. T. S. & BRASH, H. M. (1979). The long term use of an automatically triggered auditory feedback masking device in the treatment of stammering. *British Journal of Disorders of Communication*, 14:219-30.

DEWAR, A., DEWAR, A. D., & BARNES, H. E. (1976b). Automatic triggering of auditory feedback masking in stammering and stuttering. *British Journal of Communication Disorders*, 11:19-26.

DICKSON, D. R., & MAUE-DICKSON, W. (1982). *Anatomical and Physiological Bases of Speech*. Boston: Little, Brown.

DIJK, M. B-V. (1973). "Distraction" in the treatment of stuttering. Y. Lebrun & R. Hoops (eds.). *Neurolinguistic Approaches to Stuttering*. The Hague: Mouton.

DONOVAN, G. E. (1971). A new device for the treatment of stammering. *British Journal of Disorders of Communication*, 6:86-88.

DOWNIE, A., LOW, J., & LINDSAY, D. (1981). Speech disorder in Parkinsonism—usefulness of delayed auditory feedback. *British Journal of Disorders of Communication*, 16:135-40.

DUNCAN, M. H. (1949). Home adjustment of stutterers vs. nonstutterers. *Journal of Speech and Hearing Disorders*, 14:255-59.

DUNLAP, K. (1942). The technique of negative practice. *American Journal of Psychology*, 55:270-76.

EDELMAN, G. M. (1981). Group selection as the basis for higher brain function. F. O. Schnett, et al. (eds.). *The Organization of the Cerebral Cortex*. Proceedings of a Neurosciences Research Program Colloquiem, Cambridge, Mass.: The MIT Press.

EGOLF, D. B., SHAMES, G. H., JOHNSON, P. R., & KASPRISN-BURRILLI, A. (1972). The use of parent-child interaction patterns in therapy for young stutterers. *Journal of Speech and Hearing Disorders*, 37:222-32.

EISENSON, J. (1958). *Stuttering, a Symposium*. New York: Harper & Row.

EISENSON, J. (1975). Stuttering as perseverative behavior. J. Eisenson (ed.). *Stuttering, a Second Symposium.* New York: Harper & Row.

EISENSON. J., & WELLS, C. (1942). A study of the influence of communicative responsibility in a choral speech situation for stutterers. *Journal of Speech Disorders,* 7:259-63.

ELDRIDGE, M., & RANK, B. K. (1968). *A History of the Treatment of Speech Disorders.* Edinburgh: E. S. Livingstone.

EMERICK, L. (1963). A clinical observation of the "final" stuttering. *Journal of Speech and Hearing Disorders,* 28:194-95.

EMERICK, L. (No. 9). Express yourself or go by freight. E. M. Fraser (Dir.). *To the Stutterer.* Memphis, Tenn.: Speech Foundation of America.

ERICKSON, R. L. (1969). Assessing communicative attitudes among stutterers. *Journal of Speech and Hearing Research,* 12:711-24.

ESPIR, M. L. E., & ROSE, F. C. (1970). *The Basic Neurology of Speech.* Oxford: Blackwell Scientific Publications.

FAIRBANKS, G., & GUTTMAN, N. (1958). Effects of delayed auditory feedback upon articulation. *Journal of Speech and Hearing Research,* 1:12-22.

FALCK, F. J. (1969). *Stuttering: Learned and Unlearned.* Springfield, Ill.: Charles C Thomas.

FALKOWSKI, G. L., GUILFORD, A. M., & SANDLER, J. (1982). Effectiveness of a modified version of airflow therapy: Case studies. *Journal of Speech and Hearing Disorders,* 47:160-64.

FEW, L. R., & LINGWALL, J. B. (1972). A further analysis of fluency within stuttered speech. *Journal of Speech and Hearing Research,* 15:356-63.

FIEDLER, P. A., & STANDOP, R. (1978). *Stuttering, Integrating Theory and Practice.* Trans. by S. R. Silverman from *Stottern, Wege zu einer Intergarvien Theorie und Behandlung.* Urban & Schwarzenberk. Rockville, Md.: Aspen Systems Corp., 1983.

FISHMAN, H. C. (1937). A study of the efficacy of negative practice as a correction for stammering. *Journal of Speech Disorders,* 2:67-72.

FLANAGAN, B., GOLDIAMOND, I., & AZRIN, N. (1958). Operant stuttering: The control of stuttering behavior through response-contingent consequences. *Journal of Experimental Analysis of Behavior,* 1:173-77.

FORTE, M., & SCHLESINGER, I. M. (1972). Stuttering as a function of time of expectation. *Journal of Communication Disorders,* 5:347-58.

FRANCK, R. (1980). Integration of an intensive program for stutterers within the normal activities of a major acute hospital. *Australian Journal of Human Communication Disorders,* 8:4-15.

FRANSELLA, F. (1968). Self-concepts and the stutterers. *British Journal of Psychiatry,* 144:1,531-35.

FRANSELLA, F. (1970). Stuttering: Not a symptom but a way of life. *British Journal of Disorders of Communication,* 5:22-29.

FRANSELLA, F. (1971). The "rhythm effect" in stuttering as a function of predictability of utterance. *Behavioral Research and Therapy,* 9:265-71.

FRANSELLA, F. (1972). *Personal Change and Reconstruction: Research on a Treatment of Stuttering.* New York: Academic Press.

FRANSELLA, F. (1974a). George Kelly's personal construct theory. *Australian Journal of Human Communication Disorders,* 2:62-70.

FRANSELLA, F. (1974b). Personal construct theory applied to stuttering and measurement of change. *Australian Journal of Human Communication Disorders,* 2:70-75.

FRANSELLA, F. (1974c). The therapeutic or reconstruction process. *Australian Journal of Human Communication Disorders,* 2:76-85.

FRANSELLA, F. (1975). Personal construct theory applied to stuttering and measurement of change. *Australian Journal of Human Communication Disorders,* 3:6-18.

FRANSELLA, F., & BEECH, H. R. (1965). An experimental analysis of the effect of rhythm on the speech of stutterers. *Behavioral Research Therapy,* 3:195-201.

FRAYNE, H., COATES, S., & MARRINER, N. (1977). Evaluation of post-treatment fluency by naive subjects. *Australian Journal of Human Communication Disorders,* 5:48-54.

FREEMAN, F. J. (1979). Phonation in stuttering: A review of current research. *Journal of Fluency Disorders,* 4:79-89.

FREEMAN, F. J. (1982). Stuttering. N. J. Lass, L. V. McReynolds, J. L. Northern, & D. E. Yoder (eds.). *Speech, Language, and Hearing,* Vol. II. Philadelphia: W. B. Saunders.

FREEMAN, F. J., & ROSENFIELD, D. B. (1982). "Source" in disfluency. *Journal of Fluency Disorders,* 7:245-96.

FREEMAN, F. J., & USHIJIMA, T. (1975). Laryngeal activity accompanying the moment of stuttering: A preliminary report of EMG investigations. *Journal of Fluency Disorders,* 1:36-45.

FREEMAN, F. J., & USHIJIMA, T. (1978). Laryngeal muscle activity during stuttering. *Journal of Speech and Hearing Research,* 21:538-62.

FREUND, H. (1966). *Psychotherapy and the Problem of Stuttering.* Springfield, Ill.: Charles C Thomas.

FRITZELL, B. (1976). The prognosis of stuttering in schoolchildren. A 10-year longitudinal study. E. Loebell (ed.). *Proceedings XVI International Congress of Logopedics and Phoniatrics, Interlaken 1974.* Basel: Skarger.

FROESCHELS, E. (1950). A technique for stutterers—"ventriloquism." *Journal of Speech and Hearing Disorders,* 15:336-37.

FROESCHELS, E. (1952a). Chewing method as therapy. *Archives of Otolaryngology,* 56:427-34.

FROESCHELS, E. (1952b). *Dysarthric Speech.* Magnolia, Mass.: Expression Co.

FROESCHELS, E., & JELLINEK, A. (1941). *The Practice of Voice and Speech Therapy*. Boston: Expression Publishing Co.

GALLOWAY, H. F. (1974). Stuttering and the myth of therapeutic singing. *Journal of Music Therapy*, 1:202-207.

GAUTHERON, B., LIORZOU, A., EVEN, C., & VALLANCIEN, B. (1972). The role of the larynx in stuttering. Y. Lebrun & R. Hoops (eds.). *Neurolinguistic Approaches to Stuttering. Proceedings of the International Symposium on Stuttering*. The Hague: Mouton.

GENDELMAN, E. G. (1977). Confrontation in the treatment of stuttering. *Journal of Speech and Hearing Disorders*, 42:85-89.

GERSTMAN, H. L. (1983). The concatenation of stuttering to negative behavioral events: A clinical insight. *Journal of Fluency Disorders*, 8:168-74.

GIBNEY, N. (1973). Delayed auditory feedback: Changes in the volume, intensity and the delay intervals as variables affecting the fluency of stutterers' speech. *British Journal of Psychology*, 64:55-63.

GIFFORD, M. (1940). *Correcting Nervous Speech Disorders*. Englewood Cliffs, N.J.: Prentice-Hall.

GILLESPIE, S. K. & COOPER, E. E. (1973). Prevalence of speech problems in junior and senior high schools. *Journal of Speech and Hearing Research*, 16:739-43.

GOLDIAMOND, I. (1960). Effects of delayed feedback upon the temporal development of fluent and blocked speech communication. TR-2, AFCRC Contract AF 19(604)6127, Southern Illinois University.

GOLDIAMOND, I. (1965). Stuttering and fluency as manipulable operant response classes. L. Krasner & L. Ullman (eds.). *Research in Behavior Modification*. New York: Holt, Rinehart & Winston.

GOLDIAMOND, I. (1967). Supplementary statement to operant analysis and control of fluent and non-fluent verbal behavior. No. M.H. 08876-03, U.S. Department of Health, Education and Welfare, Public Health Service.

GOLDSMITH, L. (1973). Dramatic play in group stuttering therapy. Y. Lebrun & R. Hoops (eds.). *Neurolinguistic Approaches to Stuttering*. The Hague: Mouton.

GORDON, E., GORDON, L., SHAPIRO, M., MENTIS, M., & SUCHET, M. (1983). Biofeedback and stuttering. *South African Journal of Communication Disorders*. In *dsh Abstracts*, 466, 23:74.

GÖTTINGER, W. (1981). A differentiating description of "stuttering." *Sprache-Stimme-Gehor*, 4:67-73. 1980 In *dsh Abstracts*, 1668, 21:354.

GOTTLOBER, A. B. (1953). *Understanding Stuttering*. New York: Grune & Stratton.

GOVEN, P., & VETTE, G. (1966). *A Manual for Stuttering Therapy*. Pittsburgh: Stanwix House.

GRAY, B. B., & BRUTTEN, E. J. (1965). The relationship between anxiety, fatigue, and spontaneous recovery. *Behavioral Research in Therapy*, 2:251-59.

GRAY, B. B., & ENGLAND, G. (1972). Some effects of anxiety deconditioning upon stuttering. *Journal of Speech and Hearing Research*, 15:114-22.

GREENE, M. C. L. (1972). *The Voice and Its Disorders*. Philadelphia: J. B. Lippincott Co.

GREGORY, H. H. (1968). *Learning Theory and Stuttering Therapy*. Evanston, Ill.: Northwestern University Press.

GREGORY, H. H. (ed.). (1978). *Controversies About Stuttering Therapy*. Baltimore: University Park Press.

GRONHOVD, K. D. (1977). BRAT: Management of breathing, rate, airflow, and tension. *Journal of the American Speech and Hearing Association*, 19:654.

GRONHOVD, K. D., & ZENNER, A. A. (1982). Anxiety in stutterers: Rationale and procedures for management. N. J. Lass (ed.). *Speech and Language Advances in Basic Research and Practice*. New York: Academic Press.

GRUBER, L. (1971). The use of the portable voice masker in stuttering therapy. *Journal of Speech and Hearing Disorders*, 36:287-89.

GUITAR, B. (1975). Reduction of stuttering frequency using analog electromyographic feedback. *Journal of Speech and Hearing Research*, 18:672-85.

GUITAR, B. (1976). Pretreatment factors associated with the outcome of stuttering therapy. *Journal of Speech and Hearing Research*, 19:590-600.

GUITAR, B. (1979). A response to Ingham's critique. *Journal of Speech and Hearing Disorders*, 44:393-405.

GUITAR, B., & BASS, C. (1978). Stuttering therapy: The relation between attitude change and long-term outcome. *Journal of Speech and Hearing Disorders*, 43:393-400.

HAHN, E. F. (1943). *Significant Theories and Therapies*. Stanford, Calif.: Stanford University Press.

HAM, R., CANTRELL, J., & WALLACE, L. (1983). *A comparison of two delayed auditory feedback units and speaking rates of children and adults*. Unpublished research, Ohio University.

HAM, R., FUCCI, D., CANTRELL, J., & HARRIS, D. (1984). Residual effect of delayed auditory feedback on normal speaking rate and fluency. *Perceptual and Motor Skills*, 59:61-62.

HAM, R., & STEER, M. (1967). Certain effects of alterations in auditory feedback. *Folia Phoniatrica*, 19:53-62.

HAMRE, C. E., & WINGATE, M. E. (1973). Stuttering consistency in varied contexts. *Journal of Speech and Hearing Research*, 16:238-47.

HANEY, R. R. (1976). Modification of oral reading disfluency by a paced reading procedure: II. An experimental evaluation. *American Corrective Therapy Journal*, 30:75-79.

HANNA, R., WILFING, F., & McNEIL, B. (1975). A biofeedback treatment for stuttering. *Journal of Speech and Hearing Disorders*, 40:270-73.

HANSON, W., & METTER, E. (1980). DAF as instrumental treatment for dysarthria in progressive supranuclear palsy. *Journal of Speech and Hearing Disorders*, 45:268-76.

HAROLDSON, S. K., MARTIN, R. R., & STARR, C. D. (1968). Time-out as a punishment for stuttering. *Journal of Speech and Hearing Research*, 11:560-66.

HAYDEN, P., SCOTT, D., & ADDICOTT, J. (1977). The effects of delayed auditory feedback on the overt behaviors of stutterers. *Journal of Fluency Disorders*, 3:235-46.

HAYDEN, P. A., ADAMS, M. R., & JORDAHL, N. (1982a). The effects of pacing and masking on stutterers' and nonstutterers' speech initiation times. *Journal of Fluency Disorders*, 7:9-19.

HAYDEN, P. A., JORDAHL, N., & ADAMS, M. R. (1982b). Stutterers' voice initiation times during conditions of novel stimulation. *Journal of Fluency Disorders*, 7:1-7.

HAYNES, W. O., & ORATIO, A. R. (1978). A study of clients' perceptions of therapeutic effectiveness. *Journal of Speech and Hearing Disorders*, 43:21-32.

HEALEY, E. C. (1982). Speaking fundamental characteristics of stutterers and nonstutterers. *Journal of Communication Disorders*, 15:21-29.

HEALEY, E. C., MALLARD, A. R., & ADAMS, M. R. (1976). Factors contributing to the reduction of stuttering during singing. *Journal of Speech and Hearing Research*, 19:475-80.

HEINIGER, N. L., & RANDOLPH, S. L. (1981). *Neurophysiological Concepts in Human Behavior.* St. Louis, Mo.: C. V. Mosby.

HELPS, R., & DALTON, P. (1979). The effectiveness of an intensive group speech therapy programme for adult stammerers. *British Journal of Disorders of Communication*, 14:17-30.

HELTMAN, H. (1943). *First Aids for Stuttering.* Boston: Expression Co.

HENDEL, D., & BLOODSTEIN, O. (1973). Consistency in relation to inter-subject congruity in the loci of stuttering. *Journal of Communication Disorders*, 6:37-43.

HIGGINS, R. L., FRISCH, M. B., & SMITH, D. (1983). A comparison of role-played and neutral responses to identical circumstances. *Behavior Therapy*, 14:158-69.

HILLMAN, R. E., & GILBERT, H. R. (1977). Voice onset time for voiceless stop consonants in the fluent reading of stutterers and nonstutterers. *Journal of the American Speech and Hearing Association*, 16:610-11.

HIXON, T. J. (1973). Respiratory function in speech. F. J. Minifie, T. J. Hixon, and F. Williams (eds.). *Normal Aspects of Speech, Hearing and Language.* Englewood Cliffs, N.J.: Prentice-Hall.

HIXON, T., MEAD, J., & GOLDMAN, M. (1976). Dynamics of the chest wall during speech production: Function of the thorax, rib cage, diaphragm, and abdomen. *Journal of Speech and Hearing Research*, 19:297-356.

HIXON, T. J., SHRIBERG, L. D., & SAXMAN, J. H. (1980). *Introduction to Communication Disorders.* Englewood Cliffs, N.J.: Prentice-Hall.

HOLLINGSWORTH, H. L. (1939). Chewing as a technique of relaxation. *Science*, 90:385-87.

HONIG, P. (1947). The stutterer acts it out. *Journal of Speech and Hearing Disorders*, 12:105-9.

HOOD, S. B. (1973). Integration of directive and non-directive therapies for adults who stutter. *Ohio Journal of Speech and Hearing*, 8:28-35.

HOOD, S. B. (1974a). Clinical assessment of the moment of stuttering. *Journal of Fluency Disorders*, 1:22-34.

HOOD, S. B. (1974b). Effect of communicative stress on the frequency and form-types of disfluent-behavior in adult stutterers. *Journal of Fluency Disorders*, 1:36-47.

HOOPS, R., & WILKINSON, P. (1973). Group ratings of stuttering severity. Y. Lebrun & R. Hoops (eds.). *Neurolinguistic Approaches to Stuttering.* The Hague: Mouton.

HOWIE, P. M., WOODS, C. L., & ANDREWS, G. (1982). Relationship between covert and overt speech measures immediately before and immediately after stuttering treatment. *Journal of Speech and Hearing Disorders*, 47:419-21.

HULIT, L. M. (1978). Interjudge agreement of identifying stuttered words. *Perceptual Motor Skills*, 47:360-62.

HUTCHINSON, J. M. (1976). A review of rhythmic pacing as a treatment strategy for stuttering. *Rehabilitation Literature*, 37:297-303.

HUTCHINSON, J., & BURKE, K. (1973). An investigation of the effects of temporal alterations in the auditory feedback upon stutterers and clutterers. *Journal of Communication Disorders*, 6:193-205.

HUTCHINSON, J. M., & NAVARRE, B. M. (1977). The effect of metronome pacing on selected aerodynamic patterns of stuttered speech. *Journal of Fluency Disorders*, 2:189-204.

HUTCHINSON, J. M., & NORRIS, G. M. (1977). The differential effect of three auditory stimuli on the frequency of stuttering behavior. *Journal of Fluency Disorders*, 2:283-93.

HUTCHINSON, J. M., & WATSON, K. L. (1976). Jaw mechanics during release of the stuttering moment: Some initial observations and interpretations. *Journal of Communication Disorders*, 9:269-79.

INGHAM, R. J. (1975a). Operant methodology in stuttering therapy. J. Eisenson (ed.). *Stuttering, a Second Symposium.* New York: Harper & Row.

INGHAM, R. J. (1975b). A comparison of covert and overt assessment procedures in stuttering therapy outcome evaluation. *Journal of Speech and Hearing Research*, 18:346-54.

INGHAM, R. J. (1979). Comment on "Stuttering therapy: The relation between attitude change and long-term outcome." *Journal of Speech and Hearing Disorders*, 44:397-403.

INGHAM, R. J. (1981). Some effects of the Edinburgh Masker on stuttering during oral reading and spontaneous speech. *Journal of Fluency Disorders*, 6:135-54.

INGHAM, R. J. (1982). The effects of self-evaluation training on maintenance and generalization during stuttering treatment. *Journal of Speech and Hearing Disorders*, 47:271-80.

INGHAM, R. J. (1984). *Stuttering and Behavior Therapy.* San Diego, Calif.: College Hill Press.

INGHAM, R., & ANDREWS, G. (1971). Stuttering: The quality of fluency after treatment. *Journal of Communication Disorders*, 4:279-88.

INGHAM, R., & ANDREWS, G. (1973a). An analysis of a token economy in stuttering therapy. *Journal of Applied Behavioral Analysis*, 6:219-29.

INGHAM, R. J., & ANDREWS, G. (1973b). Behavior therapy and stuttering: A review. *Journal of Speech and Hearing Disorders*, 38:405-41.

INGHAM, R. J., ANDREWS, G., & WINKLER, R. (1972). Stuttering: A comparative evaluation of the short-term effectiveness of four treatment techniques. *Journal of Communication Disorders*, 5:91-117.

INGHAM, R. J., & CARROLL, P. J. (1977). Listener judgement of differences in stutterers' nonstuttered speech during chorus- and non-chorus-reading conditions. *Journal of Speech and Hearing Research*, 20:293-302.

INGHAM, R. J., & PACKMAN, A. C. (1978). Perceptual assessment of normalcy of speech following stuttering therapy. *Journal of Speech and Hearing Research*, 21:63-73.

IRWIN, A. (1972). The treatment and results of "easy stammering." *British Journal of Disorders of Communication*, 7:151-56.

IRWIN, A. (1980). *Successful Treatment of Stuttering*. New York: Walker and Co.

JACOBSON, E. (1938). *Progressive Relaxation*. Chicago: University of Chicago Press.

JAMES, J. E. (1983). Parameters of the influence of self-initiated time-out from speaking on stuttering. *Journal of Communication Disorders*, 16:123-32.

JAMES, J. E., & INGHAM, R. J. (1974). The influence of stutterers' expectancies of improvement to time-out. *Journal of Speech and Hearing Research*, 17:86-93.

JANSSEN, P., WIENEKE, G., & VAANE, E. (1983). Variation in the initiation of articulatory movements in the speech of stutterers and normal speakers. *Journal of Fluency Disorders*, 8:341-58.

JOHNSON, L. (1980). Response to Azrin. *Journal of Speech and Hearing Disorders*, 45:426-27.

JOHNSON, W. (1946). *People in Quandaries*. New York: Harper & Row.

JOHNSON, W. (1955). *Stuttering in Children and Adults*. Minneapolis: University of Minnesota Press.

JOHNSON, W. (1961a). Measurements of oral reading and speaking rate and disfluency of adult male and female stutterers and nonstutterers. *Journal of Speech and Hearing Disorders*, Monograph Supplement, 7:1-20.

JOHNSON, W. (1961b). *Stuttering and What You Can Do About It*. Danville, Ill.: The Interstate Printers and Publishers.

JOHNSON, W., DARLEY, F. L., & SPRIESTERSBACH, D. C. (1963). *Diagnostic Methods in Speech Pathology*. New York: Harper & Row.

JOHNSON, W., & KNOTT, J. R. (1937). Studies in the psychology of stuttering: I. The distribution of moments of stuttering in successive readings of the same material. *Journal of Speech Disorders*, 2:17-19.

JOHNSON, W., & ROSEN, L. (1937). Studies in the psychology of stuttering: VII: Effect of certain changes in speech patterns upon frequency of stuttering. *Journal of Speech Disorders*, 2:105-9.

JONAS, G. (1977). *Stuttering, the Disorder of Many Theories*. New York: Farrar, Strauss, and Giroux.

JONES, H. G. (1969). Behavior therapy and stuttering: The need for a multifarious approach to a multiplex problem. B. B. Gray & G. England (eds.). *Stuttering and the Conditioning Therapies*. Monterey, Calif.: The Monterey Institute for Speech and Hearing.

JONES, R. J., & AZRIN, N. H. (1969). Behavioral engineering: Stuttering as a function of stimulus duration during speech synchronization. *Journal of Applied Behavioral Analysis*, 2:223-29.

JUDD, D. (1983). *King George VI, 1895–1952*. New York: Frankling Watts.

KAASIN, K., & BJERKAN, B. (1982). Critical words and the locus of stuttering in speech. *Journal of Fluency Disorders*, 7:433-46.

KASPRISIN-BURELLI, A. T., EGOLF, D. B., & SHAMES, G. H. (1972). A comparison of parental verbal behavior with stuttering and nonstuttering children. *Journal of Communicative Disorders*, 5:335-46.

KASTEIN, S. (1947). The chewing method of treatment of stuttering. *Journal of Communication Disorders*, 12:195-98.

KATZ, M. (1977). Survey of patented anti-stuttering devices. *Journal of Communication Disorders*, 10:181-206.

KELHAM, R., & MCHALE, A. (1966). The application of learning theory to the treatment of stammering. *British Journal of Disorders of Communication*, 1:114-18.

KELLY, T. L., & STEER, M. D. (1949). Revised concept of rate. *Journal of Speech and Hearing Disorders*, 14:222-26.

KENNEDY, J. G., & ABBS, J. H. (1982). Basic neurophysiological mechanisms underlying oral communication. N. J. Lass, L. V. McReynolds, J. L. Northern, & D. E. Yoder (eds.). *Speech, Language, and Hearing*, Vol. I. Philadelphia: W. B. Saunders.

KENT, L. R. (1961). Carbon dioxide therapy as medical treatment for stuttering. *Journal of Speech and Hearing Disorders*, 26:268-72.

KENT, R. D. (1983). Facts about stuttering: Neurophysiologic perspectives. *Journal of Speech and Hearing Disorders*, 48:249-55.

KIDD, K. K., HEIMBUCH, R. C., RECORDS, M. A., OEHLERT, G., & WEBSTER, R. L. (1980). Familial stuttering patterns are not related to one measure of severity. *Journal of Speech and Hearing Research*, 23:539-45.

KINSTLER, D. B. (1961). Covert and overt maternal rejection in stuttering. *Journal of Speech and Hearing Disorders*, 26:145-56.

KLINGBEIL, G. M. (1972). The historical background of the modern speech clinic, 1939. L. L. Emerick & C. E. Hamre (eds.). *An Analysis of Stuttering, Selected Readings.* Danville, Ill.: Interstate Printers and Publishers.

KNOTT, J. R., JOHNSON, W., & WEBSTER, M. J. (1937). Studies in the psychology of stuttering: II. A quantitative evaluation of expectation of stuttering in relation to occurrence of stuttering. *Journal of Speech Disorders,* 2:20-22.

KONDAS, O. (1967). The treatment of stammering in children by the shadowing method. *Behavior Research and Therapy,* 5:325-29.

KONDAS, O. (1968). Experiment of the shadowing methods with children stammerers. *Psychologica,* 19:109-16.

KORCHIN, S. J. (1976). *Modern Clinical Psychology.* New York: Basic Books.

LADOUCEUR, R., COTE, C., LEBLOND, G., & BOUCHARD, L. (1982). Evaluation of regulated breathing method and awareness training in the treatment of stuttering. *Journal of Speech and Hearing Disorders,* 47:422-26.

LAFOLLETTE, A. C. (1956). Parental environment of stuttering children. *Journal of Speech and Hearing Disorders,* 21:202-8.

LAMENDELLA, J. T. (1977). The limbic system in human communication. H. Whitaker & H. A. Whitaker (eds.). *Studies in Neurolinguistics,* Vol. III. New York: Academic Press.

LANGOVA, J., & MORAVEK, M. (1964). Some results of experimental examinations among stutterers and clutterers. *Folia Phoniatrica,* 16:290-96.

LANYON, R. I. (1965). The relationship of adaptation and consistency to improvement in stuttering therapy. *Journal of Speech and Hearing Research,* 8:263-70.

LANYON, R. I. (1967). The measurement of stuttering severity. *Journal of Speech and Hearing Research,* 10:836-43.

LANYON, R. I. (1968). Some characteristics of nonfluency in normal speakers and stutterers. *Journal of Abnormal Psychology,* 73:550-55.

LANYON, R. I. (1969). Behavior change in stuttering through systematic desensitization. *Journal of Speech and Hearing Disorders,* 34:253-60.

LARSON, C. R., & PFINGST, B. E. (1982). Neuroanatomic basis of hearing and speech. N. J. Lass, L. V. McReynolds, J. L. Northern & D. E. Yoder (eds.). *Speech, Language, and Hearing, Vol. I.* Philadelphia: W. B. Saunders.

LAY, T. (1982). Nonspecific elements in therapy with stutterers. *Journal of Fluency Disorders,* 7:479-86.

LECHNER, B. (1979). The effects of delayed auditory feedback and masking on the fundamental frequency of stutterers and nonstutterers. *Journal of Speech and Hearing Research,* 22:343-53.

LEE, B. S. (1950a). Effects of delayed speech feedback. *Journal of the American Speech Association,* 22:824-26.

LEE, B. S. (1950b). Some effects of sidetone delay. *Journal of the American Speech Association,* 22:639-40.

LEE, B. S. (1951). Artificial stutter. *Journal of Speech and Hearing Disorders,* 16:53-55.

LEE, J. (1976). Application of Martin Schwartz's airflow technique in the treatment of stuttering. *Journal of Speech and Hearing Disorders,* 41:133-34.

LEITH, W. R. (1971). Clinical training in stuttering therapy: A survey. *Journal of the American Speech and Hearing Association,* 13:6-8.

LEITH, W. R., & CHMIEL, C. C. (1980). Delayed auditory feedback and stuttering: Theoretical and clinical implications. N. J. Lass (ed.). *Speech and Language, Advances in Basic Research and Practice.* New York: Academic Press.

LEMERT, E., & VAN RIPER, C. (1958). The use of psychodrama in the treatment of speech defects. C. F. Diehl (ed.). *A Compendium of Research and Theory on Stuttering.* Springfield, Ill.: Charles C Thomas.

LENNON, E. J. (1963). Le begaiment: Therapeutiques moderne (Stuttering: Modern therapies). Paris: G. Doint & Cie, 1962. In *dsh Abstracts,* No. 1581, 3:355-56.

LERMAN, J. W., & SHAMES, G. H. (1965). The effect of situational difficulty on stuttering. *Journal of Speech and Hearing Research,* 8:271-80.

LEWIS, D., & SHERMAN, D. (1951). Measuring the severity of stuttering. *Journal of Speech and Hearing Disorders,* 16:320-26.

LIEBETRAU, R. M., & DALY, D. A. (1981). Auditory processing and perceptual abilities of "organic" and "functional" stutterers. *Journal of Fluency Disorders,* 6:219-31.

LOCKHART, M. S., & ROBERTSON, A. W. (1977). Hypnosis and speech therapy as a combined therapeutic approach to the problem of stammering. *British Journal of Disorders of Communication,* 12:97-108.

LOTZMANN, V. G. (1961). The effect of various auditory delay times on stutterers. *Folia Phoniatrica,* 13:276-312.

LOZANO, R. A., & DREYER, D. E. (1978). Some effects of delayed auditory feedback. *Journal of Communication Disorders,* 11:407-15.

LUPER, H. L., & MULDER, R. L. (1964). *Stuttering Therapy for Children.* Englewood Cliffs, N.J.: Prentice-Hall.

McCABE, R. B., & McCOLLUM, J. D. (1972). The personal reactions of a stutterer to delayed auditory feedback. *Journal of Speech and Hearing Disorders,* 37:536-41.

McCLELLAND, J. K., & COOPER, E. B. (1978). Fluency-related behaviors and attitudes of 178 young stutterers. *Journal of Fluency Disorders,* 3:253-63.

McCormick, B. (1975). Therapeutic and diagnostic implications of delayed auditory feedback. *British Journal of Disorders of Communication*, 10:98-110.

MacCulloch, M. J., Eaton, R., & Long, E. (1970). The long-term effect of auditory masking on young stutterers. *British Journal of Disorders of Communication*, 5:165-73.

McDonald, E., & Frick, J. (1954). Store clerks' reactions to stuttering. *Journal of Speech and Hearing Disorders*, 19:306-11.

McFarlane, S. C., & Prins, D. (1978). Neural response time of stutterers and nonstutterers in selected oral motor tasks. *Journal of Speech and Hearing Research*, 21:768-78.

McFarlane, S. C., & Shipley, K. G. (1981). Latency of vocalization onset for stutterers and nonstutterers under conditions of auditory and visual cueing. *Journal of Speech and Hearing Disorders*, 46:307-11.

McGee, S. R., Hutchinson, J. M., & Deputy, P. N. (1981). The influence of the onset of phonation on the frequency of disfluency among children who stutter. *Journal of Speech and Hearing Research*, 24:269-72.

Mackay, D. G. (1968). Metamorphosis of a critical interval: Age-linked changes in the delay in auditory feedback that produces maximum disruption of speech. *Journal of the Acoustical Society of America*, 43:811-21.

McLean, A. E., & Cooper, E. B. (1978). Electromyographic indications of laryngeal-area activity during stuttering expectancy. *Journal of Fluency Disorders*, 3:205-19.

Mallard, A. R., & Meyer, L. A. (1979). Listener preferences for stuttered and syllable-timed speech production. *Journal of Fluency Disorders*, 4:117-21.

Manning, W. H., & Coufal, K. J. (1976). The frequency of disfluencies during phonatory transitions in stuttered and nonstuttered speech. *Journal of Communication Disorders*, 9:75-81.

Manning, W. H., & Jamieson, W. J. (1974). Listener judgements of fluency: The effect of part-word CV repetition and neutral vowel substitutions. *Journal of Fluency Disorders*, 1:18-22.

Marland, P. M. (1957). "Shadowing"—a contribution to the treatment of stammering. *Folia Phoniatrica*, 9:242-45.

Martin, R. (1965). Direct magnitude-estimation judgements of stuttering severity using audible and visible and audible-visible speech samples. *Speech Monographs*, 32:169-77.

Martin, R. R., & Haroldson, S. K. (1967). The relationship between anticipation and consistency of stuttered words. *Journal of Speech and Hearing Research*, 10:323-27.

Martin, R. R., & Haroldson, S. K. (1979). Effects of five experimental treatments on stuttering. *Journal of Speech and Hearing Research*, 22:132-46.

Martin, R. R., Haroldson, S. K., & Kuhl, P. (1972a). Disfluencies of young children in two speaking situations. *Journal of Speech and Hearing Research*, 15:831-36.

Martin, R. R., Kuhl, P., & Haroldson, S. (1972b). An experimental treatment with two preschool stuttering children. *Journal of Speech and Hearing Research*, 15:743-52.

Maxwell, D. L. (1982). Cognitive and behavioral self-control strategies: Applications for the clinical management of adult stutterers. *Journal of Fluency Disorders*, 7:403-32.

Messbarger, P. (1982). *Criteria for stuttering therapy techniques in the public schools.* Unpublished paper. Athens: Ohio University.

Metraux, R. W. (1950). Speech profiles of the pre-school child 18 to 54 months. *Journal of Speech and Hearing Disorders*, 15:37-53.

Metz, D. E., Conture, E. G., & Caruso, A. (1979). Voice onset time, frication, and aspiration during stutterers' fluent speech. *Journal of Speech and Hearing Research*, 22:649-56.

Meyer, V., & Comley, J. (1969). A preliminary report on the treatment of stammer by the use of rhythmic stimulation. B. B. Gray & G. England (eds.). *Stuttering and the Conditioning Therapies.* Monterey, Calif.: The Monterey Institute for Speech and Hearing.

Meyer, V., & Mair, J. M. M. (1963). A new technique to control stammering. *Behavioral Research Therapy*, 1:751-54.

Miller, S. (1982). Airflow therapy programs: Facts and/or fancy. *Journal of Fluency Disorders*, 7:187-202.

Modigliani, A. (1971). Embarrassment, facework, and eye contact: Testing a theory of embarrassment. *Journal of Personal and Social Psychology*, 17:15-24.

Moleski, R., & Tosi, D. J. (1976). Comparative psychotherapy: Rational-emotive therapy versus systematic desensitization in the treatment of stuttering. *Journal of Consulting Clinical Psychology*, 44:309-11.

Moncur, J., & Brackett, L. (1974). *Modifying Vocal Behavior.* New York: Harper & Row.

Montgomery, A. A., & Cooke, P. A. (1976). Perceptual and acoustic analysis of repetitions in stuttered speech. *Journal of Communication Disorders*, 9:317-30.

Moore, G. P. (1971). *Organic Voice Disorders.* Englewood Cliffs, N.J.: Prentice-Hall.

Moore, W. E. (1954). Relation of stuttering in spontaneous speech to speech content and to adaptation. *Journal of Speech and Hearing Disorders*, 19:208-16.

Moss, S. E. (1976). The influence of varying degrees of voicing on the adaptation effect in the repeated oral readings of stutterers. *Australian Journal of Human Communication Disorders*, 4:127-37.

Mowrer, D. E. (1979). *Fluent Speech.* Columbus, Ohio: Charles E. Merrill.

Mowrer, D. E., & Case, J. L. (1982). *Clinical Management of Speech Disorders.* Rockville, Md.: Aspen Systems.

Muckenhoff, E. (1974). Zum ubungsfaktor in fer stotterntherapie (The exercise factor in the treatment of stutterers). *Rehab.* 15:21-27. In *dsh Abstracts*, No. 517, (1976) 17:104.

MUIRDEN, R. (1968). *Stammering, Its Correction Through The Re-education of the Speech Function.* Springfield, Ill.: Charles C Thomas.

MULDER, R. L. (1961). The student of stuttering as a stutterer, *Journal of Speech and Hearing Disorders,* 26:178-79.

MURPHY, A. T. (1964). *Functional Voice Disorders.* Englewood Cliffs, N.J.: Prentice-Hall.

MURPHY, A. T., & FITZSIMMONS, R. (1960). *Stuttering and Personality Dynamics.* New York: Ronald Press.

MURPHY, M., & BAUMGARTNER, J. M. (1981). Voice initiation and termination times in stuttering and nonstuttering children. *Journal of Fluency Disorders,* 6:257-64.

MURRAY, E. (1932). Dysintegration of breathing and eye movements in stuttering during silent reading and reasoning. *Psychological Monographs,* 43:218-75.

MURRAY, F. P., with EDWARDS, J. G. (1980). *A Stutterer's Story.* Danville, Ill.: The Interstate Printers and Publishers.

MYERS, F. L., & WALL, M. J. (1982). Toward an integrated approach to early childhood stuttering. *Journal of Fluency Disorders,* 7:47-54.

NAYLOR, R. V. (1953). A comparative study of methods of estimating the severity of stuttering. *Journal of Speech and Hearing Disorders,* 18:30-37.

NEAVES, A. (1966). Prognosis in stammering. *Speech Pathology Diagnosis: Theory and Practice.* Report of the National Conference of the College of Speech Therapists. Edinburgh: E & S Livingstone.

NEAVES, A. (1970). To establish a basis for prognosis of stammering. *British Journal of Disorders of Communication,* 5:46-58.

NEELLEY, J. N. (1961). A study of the speech behavior of stutterers and nonstutterers under normal and delayed auditory feedback. *Journal of Speech and Hearing Disorders,* Mongr. Suppl. 7:63-82.

NEILSON, P. D., ANDREWS, G., GUITAR, B. E., & QUINN, P. T. (1979). Tonic stretch reflexes in lip, tongue and jaw muscles. *Brain Research,* 178:311-27.

NEWMAN, P. W. (1954). A study of adaptation and recovery of the stuttering response in self-formulated speech. *Journal of Speech and Hearing Disorders,* 19:450-58.

NUTTALL, E. C., & SCHEIDEL, T. M. (1965). Stutterers' estimates of normal apprehensiveness toward speaking. *Speech Monographs,* 32:455-57.

O'KEEFE, B. M., & KROLL, R. M. (1980). Clinicians' molar and molecular stuttering analyses of expanded and nonexpanded speech. *Journal of Fluency Disorders,* 5:43-54.

OST, L-G., GOTESTAN, G., & LENNERT, M. (1976). A controlled study of two behavioral methods in the treatment of stuttering. *Behavior Therapy,* 7:587-92.

OVERSTAKE, C. P. (1979). *Stuttering: A New Look at an Old Problem Based on Neurophysiological Aspects.* Springfield, Ill.: Charles C Thomas.

OWEN, N. (1980). Facilitating maintenance of behavior change. Boberg, E. (ed.), *Maintenance of Fluency: Proceedings of the Banff Conference.* New York: Elsevier.

PATTIE, F. A., & KNIGHT, B. B. (1944). Why does the speech of stutterers improve in choral readings? *Journal of Abnormal and Social Psychology,* 39:362-67.

PEINS, M. (1961). Adaptation effect and spontaneous recovery in stuttering expectancy. *Journal of Speech and Hearing Research,* 4:91-99.

PEINS, M., LEE, B. S., & McGOUGH, W. E. (1970). A tape-recorded therapy method for stutterers: A case report. *Journal of Speech and Hearing Disorders,* 35:188-93.

PEINS, M., McGOUGH, W. E., & LEE, B. S. (1972). Tape recorder therapy for the rehabilitation of the stuttering handicapped. *Language, Speech and Hearing Services in the Schools,* 3:30-35.

PELLMAN, C. (1947). *Overcoming Stammering.* New York: Beachhurst Press.

PERKINS, W. H. (1973a). Replacement of stuttering with normal speech: I. Rationale. *Journal of Speech and Hearing Disorders,* 38:283-94.

PERKINS, W. H. (1973b). Replacement of stuttering with normal speech: II. Clinical procedures. *Journal of Speech and Hearing Disorders,* 38:295-303.

PERKINS, W. H. (1975). Articulatory rate in the evaluation of stuttering treatments. *Journal of Speech and Hearing Disorders,* 20:277-78.

PERKINS, W. H. (1978). *Human Perspectives in Speech and Language Disorders.* St. Louis, Mo.: C. V. Mosby.

PERKINS, W. H. (1980). Disorders of speech flow. T. J. Hixon, L. D. Shriberg, & J. H. Saxman (eds.). *Introduction to Communication Disorders.* Englewood Cliffs, N.J.: Prentice-Hall.

PERKINS, W. H. (1983). Learning from the negative outcomes in stuttering therapy: II. An epiphany of failures. *Journal of Fluency Disorders,* 8:155-60.

PERKINS, W. H., BELL, J., JOHNSON, L., & STOCKS, J. (1979). Phone rate and the effective planning-time hypothesis of stuttering. *Journal of Speech and Hearing Research,* 22:747-55.

PERKINS, W. H., & CURLEE, R. F. (1969). Clinical impressions of portable masking unit effects in stuttering. *Journal of Speech and Hearing Disorders,* 34:360-62.

PERKINS, W. H., RUDAS, J., JOHNSON, L., & BELL, J. (1976). Stuttering: Discoordination of phonation with articulation and respiration. *Journal of Speech and Hearing Disorders,* 19:509-22.

PERKINS, W. H., RUDAS, J., JOHNSON, L., MICHAEL, W. B., & CURLEE, R. F. (1971). Replacement of stuttering with normal speech: III. Clinical effectiveness. *Journal of Speech and Hearing Disorders,* 36:264-80.

PETERSON, H. A. (1969). Affective meaning of words as rated by stuttering and nonstuttering readers. *Journal of Speech and Hearing Research*, 12:337-43.

PHYSICIAN'S DESK REFERENCE, 36th ed. (1982). Oradell, N.J.: C. E. Baker, Medical Economics Co.

PLOMLEY, A., INGHAM, R., & ANDREWS, G. (1971). The modification of stuttering and the token reinforcement system. *Journal of the Australian College of Speech Therapists*, 21:14-18.

POLLACZEK, P. P., & HOMEFIELD, H. D. (1954). The use of masks as an adjunct to role playing. *Mental Hygiene*, 38:299-304.

POPPEN, R., NUNN, R. G., & HOOK, S. (1977). Effects of several therapies on stuttering in a single case. *Journal of Fluency Disorders*, 2:35-44.

PORFERT, A., & ROSENFIELD, D. (1978). Prevalence of stuttering. *Journal of Neurology, Neurosurgery, and Psychiatry*, 41:954-56.

PRINS, D. (1970). Improvement and regression in stutterers following short-term intensive therapy. *Journal of Speech and Hearing Disorders*, 35:123-34.

PRINS, D. (1972). Personality, stuttering severity, and age. *Journal of Speech and Hearing Research*, 15:148-54.

PRINS, D., & LOHR, F. (1972). Behavioral dimensions of stuttered speech. *Journal of Speech and Hearing Research*, 15:61-71.

QUARRINGTON, B. (1959). Measures of stuttering adaptation. *Journal of Speech and Hearing Research*, 2:105-12.

QUARRINGTON, B. (1965). Stuttering as a function of the information value and sentence position of words. *Journal of Abnormal Psychology*, 70:221-24.

QUARRINGTON, B., & DOUGLASS, E. (1960). Audibility avoidance in nonvocalized stutterers. *Journal of Speech and Hearing Disorders*, 25:358-65.

QUINN, P. T. (1971). Suttering: Some observations on speaking when alone. *Journal of the Australian College of Speech Therapists*, 21:92-94.

RAGSDALE, J. D. (1976). Relationship between hesitation phenomena, anxiety, and self-control in normal communication situations. *Language and Speech*, 19:257-65.

RAMIG, R., & ADAMS, M. R. (1980). Rate reduction strategies used by stutterers and nonstutterers during high- and low-pitched speech. *Journal of Fluency Disorders*, 5:27-41.

RAMIG, R., & ADAMS, M. R. (1981). Vocal changes in stutterers and nonstutterers during high- and low-pitched speech. *Journal of Fluency Disorders*, 6:15-33.

RECORDS, M. A., HEIMBUCH, R. C., & KIDD, K. K. (1977). Handedness and stuttering: A dead horse? *Journal of Fluency Disorders*, 2:271-82.

REICH, A., TIU, J., & GOLDSMITH, H. (1981). Laryngeal and manual reaction time of stuttering and nonstuttering adults. *Journal of Speech and Hearing Research*, 24:192-96.

REVDI, L. (1976). Hypertensive manifestations and consecutive laryngeal alterations in stutterers. *Fül Orr-Gégegyógy*, 22:226-30. In *dsh Abstracts*, No. 560 (1979) 19:112.

RICHTER, E. (1976). Der stellenert der Atmungstherapie in der Ubungsbehandlung des Stotterns (The value of breathing exercises in the treatment of stuttering). *Sprachheilarbeit*, 21:70-77. In *dsh Abstracts*, No. 520 (1977) 17:105.

RIEBER, R. W. (1977). *The Problem of Stuttering: Theory and Therapy*. New York: Elsevier.

RIEBER, R. W., BRESKIN, S., & JAFFE, J. (1972). Pause time and phonation time in stuttering and cluttering. *Journal of Psycholinguistic Research*, 1:149-54.

RILEY, G. D. (1972). A stuttering severity instrument for children and adults. *Journal of Speech and Hearing Disorders*, 37:314-22.

RILEY, G. D., & RILEY, J. (1979). A component model for diagnosing and treating children who stutter. *Journal of Fluency Disorders*, 4:279-93.

RILEY, G. D., & RILEY, J. (1980). Motoric and linguistic variables among children who stutter. *Journal of Speech and Hearing Disorders*, 45:504.

ROBBINS, S. D. (1931). Breath control in stammering. *Proceedings of the American Speech Correction Association*, 1:57-64.

ROBBINS, S. D. (1935). The role of rhythm in the correction of stammering. *Quarterly Journal of Speech*, 21:331-43.

RONSON, I. (1976). Word frequency and stuttering: The relationship to sentence structure. *Journal of Speech and Hearing Research*, 19:813-19.

ROSENFIELD, D. B., & FREEMAN, F. J. (1983). Clinical notes: Stuttering onset after laryngectomy. *Journal of Fluency Disorders*, 8:265-68.

ROSSO, L. J., & ADAMS, M. R. (1969). A study of the relationship between the latency and consistency of stuttering. *Journal of Speech and Hearing Research*, 12:389-93.

ROTHMAN, I. (1969). Practical rhythm desensitization for stuttering, with description of a new electronic pacer used for stuttering, insomnia, and anxiety. *Journal of the American Osteopathic Association*, 68:573-77.

RUBIN, Z., & MCNEIL, E. B. (1981). *The Psychology of Being Human*, 3rd. ed. New York: Harper & Row.

RUDOLF, S. R., MANNING, W. H., & SEWELL, W. R. (1983). The use of self-efficacy scaling in training student clinicians: Implications for working with stutterers. *Journal of Fluency Disorders*, 8:55-76.

RUNYAN, C. M., & ADAMS, M. R. (1979). Unsophisticated judges' perceptual evaluations of the speech of "successfully treated" stutterers. *Journal of Fluency Disorders*, 4:29-38.

RUNYAN, C. M., & BONIFANT, D. C. (1981). A perceptual comparison: All-voiced versus typical reading passage read by children. *Journal of Fluency Disorders*, 6:247-55.

RUSTIN, C. M. (1978). An intensive group programme for adolescent stammerers. *British Journal of Disorders of Communication*, 13:85-92.

RYAN, B. P. (1971). Operant procedures applied to stuttering therapy for children. *Journal of Speech and Hearing Disorders*, 36:264-280.

RYAN, B. P. (1974). *Programmed Therapy for Stuttering in Children and Adults*. Springfield, Ill.: Charles C Thomas.

RYAN, B. P. (1978). An illustration for operant conditioning therapy for stuttering. *Conditioning and Stuttering Therapy*. Memphis, Tenn.: Speech Foundation of America, No. 7.

RYAN, B. P. (1979). Stuttering therapy in a framework of operant conditioning and programmed learning. H. Gregory (ed.). *Controversies About Stuttering Therapy*. Baltimore: University Park Press.

RYAN, B. P., & VAN KIRK, B. (1971). *Programmed Conditioning for Fluency*. Monterey, Calif.: Behavioral Sciences Institute.

RYAN, B. P., & VAN KIRK, B. (1974). The establishment, transfer and maintenance of fluent speech in 50 stutterers using delayed auditory feedback and operant procedures. *Journal of Speech and Hearing Disorders*, 39:3-10.

SAINT LOUIS, K. O. (1979). Linguistic and motor aspects of stuttering. N. J. Lass (ed.). *Speech and Language Advances in Basic Research and Practice*. New York: Academic Press.

ST. ONGE, K. R. (1963). The stuttering syndrome. *Journal of Speech and Hearing Research*, 6:195-97.

SAKATA, R., & ADAMS, M. R. (1972). Comparisons among various forms of individual stutterers disfluency. *Journal of Communication Disorders*, 5:232-39.

SANTOSTEFANO, S. (1960). Anxiety and hostility in stuttering. *Journal of Speech and Hearing Research*, 3:337-47.

SCHAEF, R., & MATTHEWS, J. (1954). A first step in the evaluation of stuttering therapy. *Journal of Speech and Hearing Disorders*, 19:467-73.

SCHILLING, VON, A. (1960). X-ray kymographic investigation of the diaphragmatic action of stutterers. *Folia Phoniatrica*, 12:145-53.

SCHISSEL, R. J., & FLOURNOY, J. E. (1975). An investigation of the variability of experienced and inexperienced listeners in their use of a screening test of articulation. *Journal of Communication Disorders*, 11:459-68.

SCHLESINGER, I. M., FORTE, M., FRIED, B., & MELKMAN, R. (1965). Stuttering, information load, and response strength. *Journal of Speech and Hearing Disorders*, 30:32-36.

SCHWARTZ, D., & WEBSTER, L. M. (1977). A clinical adaptation of the Hollins precision fluency shaping program through deintensification. *Journal of Fluency Disorders*, 2:3-10.

SCHWARTZ, M. F. (1967). Syllable duration in oral and whispered reading. *Journal of the American Speech and Hearing Association*, 41:1,367-69.

SCHWARTZ, M. F. (1974). The core of the stuttering block. *Journal of Speech and Hearing Disorders*, 39:169-77.

SCHWARTZ, M. F. (1976). *Stuttering Solved*. New York: McGraw-Hill.

SERGEANT, R. L. (1961). Concurrent repetition of a continuous flow of words. *Journal of Speech and Hearing Research*, 4:373-80.

SHAMES, G. H. (1953). A utilization of adaptation phenomena in therapy for stuttering. *Journal of Speech and Hearing Disorders*, 18:256-57.

SHAMES, G. H. (1975). Operant conditioning and stuttering. J. Eisenson (ed.). *Stuttering, a Second Symposium*. New York, Harper & Row.

SHAMES, G. H. (1978). Operant conditioning and therapy for stuttering. *Conditioning in Stuttering Therapy*. Memphis, Tenn.: Speech Foundation of America.

SHAMES, G. H., & EGOLF, D. B. (1976). *Operant Conditioning and the Management of Stuttering*. Englewood Cliffs, N.J.: Prentice-Hall.

SHAMES, G. H., EGOLF, D. B., & RHODES, R. C. (1969). Experimental programs in stuttering therapy. *Journal of Speech and Hearing Disorders*, 34:30-47.

SHAMES, G. H., & FLORANCE, C. L. (1980). *Stutter-Free Speech, A Goal for Therapy*. Columbus, Ohio: Charles E. Merrill.

SHAMES, G. H., & WIIG, E. H. (1982). *Human Communication Disorders*. Columbus, Ohio: Charles E. Merrill.

SHANE, M. L. S. (1955). Effect on stuttering of alteration in auditory feedback. W. Johnson (ed.). *Stuttering in Children and Adults*. Minneapolis: University of Minnesota Press.

SHAPIRO, A. I., & DECICCO, B. A. (1982). The relationship between normal disfluency and stuttering: An old question revisited. *Journal of Fluency Disorders*, 7:109-21.

SHEARER, W. M. (1966). Speech: Behavior of middle ear muscles during stuttering. *Science*, 152:1,280.

SHEEHAN, J. G. (1968). Reflections on the behavioral modification of stuttering. *Conditioning in Stuttering Therapy*. Memphis, Tenn.: Speech Foundation of America.

SHEEHAN, J. G. (1969). Cyclic variations in stuttering: A comment on Taylor and Taylor's Test of Prediction from the conflict hypothesis of stuttering. *Journal of Abnormal Psychology*, 74:452-53.

SHEEHAN, J. G. (1970). *Stuttering Research and Therapy*. New York: Harper & Row.

SHEEHAN, J. G. (1974). Stuttering behavior: A phonetic analysis. *Journal of Communication Disorders*, 7:193-212.

SHEEHAN, J. G. (1975). Conflict theory and avoidance-reduction therapy. J. Eisenson (ed.). *Stuttering, a Second Symposium*. New York: Harper & Row.

SHEEHAN, J. G. (1980). Problems in the evaluations of progress and outcome. W. H. Perkins (ed.). *Strategies in Stuttering Therapy*. J. L. Northern (ed.). *Seminars in Speech, Language, and Hearing*. New York: Thieme-Stratton.

SHEEHAN, J. G. (No. 9). Message to a stutterer. M. Fraser (dir.). *To the Stutterer*. Memphis, Tenn.: Speech Foundation of America.

SHEEHAN, J. G., HADLEY, P. A., & HADLEY, R. G. (1962). Guilt, shame and tension in graphic projections of stuttering. *Journal of Speech and Hearing Disorders*, 27:129-39.

SHEEHAN, J. G., & MARTYN, M. M. (1970). Stuttering and its disappearance. *Journal of Speech and Hearing Research*, 13:279-89.

SHERMAN, D. (1952). Clinical and experimental use of the Iowa Scale of Severity of Stuttering. *Journal of Speech and Hearing Disorders*, 17:316-20.

SHERRARD, C. A. (1975). Stuttering as "false alarm" responding. *British Journal of Disorders of Communication*, 10:83-91.

SHINE, R. E. (1980). Direct management of the beginning stutterer. W. H. Perkins (ed.). *Strategies in Stuttering Therapy*. J. L. Northern (ed.). *Seminars in Speech, Hearing and Language*. New York: Thieme-Stratton.

SHULMAN, E. (1955). Factors influencing the variability of stuttering. W. Johnson (ed.). *Stuttering in Children and Adults*. Minneapolis: University of Minnesota Press.

SHUMAK, I. C. (1955). A speech situation rating sheet for stutterers. W. Johnson (ed.). *Stuttering in Children and Adults*. Minneapolis: University of Minnesota Press.

SIEGEL, G. M., FEHST, C. A., GARBER, S. R., & PICK, H. L. (1980). Delayed auditory feedback with children. *Journal of Speech and Hearing Disorders*, 23:802-13.

SIEGEL, G. M., & HAUGEN, D. (1964). Audience size and variations in stuttering behavior. *Journal of Speech and Hearing Research*, 7:381-88.

SILVERMAN, E. M. (1978). Adults' speech disfluency: Single-syllable repetition. *Perceptual and Motor Skills*, 46:970.

SILVERMAN, E. M. (1980). Communication attitudes of women who stutter. *Journal of Speech and Hearing Disorders*, 45:533-39.

SILVERMAN, E. M. (1982). Speech-language clinicians' and university students' impressions of women and girls who stutter. *Journal of Fluency Disorders*, 7:469-78.

SILVERMAN, F. H. (1970). A note on the degree of adaptation by stutterers and nonstutterers during oral reading. *Journal of Speech and Hearing Research*, 13:173-77.

SILVERMAN, F. H. (1971a). The effect of rhythmic auditory stimulation on the disfluency of nonstutterers. *Journal of Speech and Hearing Research*, 14:350-55.

SILVERMAN, F. H. (1971b). A rationale for the use of the hearing aid metronome in a program of therapy for stuttering. *Perceptual and Motor Skills*, 32:34.

SILVERMAN, F. H. (1972). Disfluency and word length. *Journal of Speech and Hearing Research*, 15:788-91.

SILVERMAN, F. H. (1976). Long-term impact of a miniature metronome on stuttering: An interim report. *Perceptual and Motor Skills*, 42:1,322.

SILVERMAN, F. H. (1980). Dimensions of improvement in stuttering. *Journal of Speech and Hearing Research*, 23:137-51.

SILVERMAN, F. H., & TROTTER, W. D. (1973). Impact of pacing speech with a miniature electronic metronome upon the manner in which a stutterer is perceived. *Behavior Therapies*, 4:414-19.

SILVERMAN, F. H., & WILLIAMS, D. E. (1972). Prediction of stuttering by school-age stutterers. *Journal of Speech and Hearing Research*, 15:189-93.

SLORACH, N. (1971). Twenty years of stuttering therapy. *Journal of the Australian College of Speech Therapists*, 21:19-23.

SMITH, K. U., & TIERNEY, D. (1971). Delayed speech feedback and age. *Journal of Speech and Hearing Research*, 14:214-19.

SODERBERG, G. (1962a). Phonetic influences upon stuttering. *Journal of Speech and Hearing Research*, 5:315-20.

SODERBERG, G. (1962b). What is "average" in stuttering? *Journal of Speech and Hearing Disorders*, 27:85-86.

SODERBERG, G. (1967). Linguistic factors in stuttering. *Journal of Speech and Hearing Research*, 10:801-10.

SODERBERG, G. (1969a). A comparison of adaptation trends in the oral reading of stutterers, inferior speakers, and superior speakers. *Journal of Communication Disorders*, 2:99-108.

SODERBERG, G. A. (1969b). DAF and the speech of stutterers: A review of studies. *Journal of Speech and Hearing Disorders*, 34:20-29.

SODERBERG, G. (1971). Relations of word information and word length to stuttering disfluencies. *Journal of Communication Disorders*, 4:9-14.

SOMMERS, R. K., BOBKOFF-LEVENTHAL, K., APPLEGATE, J. A., & SQUARE, P. A. (1979). A critical review of a recent decade of stuttering research. *Journal of Fluency Disorders*, 4:223-37.

SPEECH FOUNDATION OF AMERICA. (No. 5). *Stuttering: Training the Therapist*. M. S. Fraser (dir.). Memphis, Tenn.

SPEECH FOUNDATION OF AMERICA. (No. 9). *To the Stutterer*. M. Fraser (dir.). Memphis, Tenn.
SPEECH FOUNDATION OF AMERICA. (No. 12). *Self-Therapy for the Stutterer*, 3rd. ed. M. Fraser (dir.). Memphis, Tenn.
SPIELBERGER, C. D. (1966). Theory and research on anxiety. C. D. Spielberger (ed.). *Anxiety and Behavior*. New York: Academic Press.
SPIELBERGER, C. D. (1972). Conceptual and methodological issues in anxiety research. C. D. Spielberger (ed.). *Anxiety: Current Trends in Theory and Research*, Vol. III. New York: Academic Press.
SPIELBERGER, C. D., GORSUCH, R. L., & LUSHENE, R. E. (1970). *STAI Manual*. Palo Alto, Calif.: Consulting Psychologists Press.
SPILKA, B. (1954). Relationship between certain aspects of personality and some vocal effects of DAF. *Journal of Speech and Hearing Disorders*, 19:491-503.
STAMPFL, T. G., & LEVIS, D. J. (1967). Essentials of implosive therapy: A learning-theory based on psychodynamic behavioral therapy. *Journal of Abnormal Psychology*, 72:496-503.
STARBUCK, H. B., & STEER, M. D. (1954). Adaptation effect and its relation to thoracic breathing in stutterers and nonstutterers. *Journal of Speech and Hearing Disorders*, 19:440-49.
STARK, R. E., & PIERCE, B. R. (1970). The effects of delayed auditory feedback on a speech-related task in stutterers. *Journal of Speech and Hearing Research*, 13:245-53.
STARKWEATHER, C. W. (1980). A multiprocess behavioral approach to stuttering therapy. W. H. Perkins (ed.). *Strategies in Stuttering Therapy*. J. L Northern (ed.). *Seminars in Speech, Language, and Hearing*. New York: Thieme-Stratton.
STARKWEATHER, C. W. (1982). Stuttering and laryngeal behavior: A review. *ASHA Monographs No. 21*. Rockville, Md.: American Speech, Language, and Hearing Association.
STARKWEATHER, C. W., HIRSCHMAN, P., & TANNENBAUM, R. S. (1976). Latency of vocalization onset: Stutterers versus nonstutterers. *Journal of Speech and Hearing Research*, 19:481-92.
STEIN, J. (1967). (ed.). *The Random House Dictionary of the English Language*. New York: Random House.
STILL, A. W., & GRIGGS, S. (1979). Changes in the probability of stuttering following a stutter: A test of some recent models. *Journal of Speech and Hearing Research*, 22:565-71.
STROTHER, C. R., & KRIEGMAN, L. S. (1944). Rhythmokinesis in stutterers and non-stutterers. *Journal of Speech Disorders*, 9:239-244.
SUE, D., SUE, D. W., & SUE, S. (1981). *Understanding Abnormal Behavior*. Boston: Houghton Mifflin.
SUTTON, S. A., & CHASE, A. (1961). White noise and stuttering. *Journal of Speech and Hearing Research*, 4:72.
ŠVÁB, L., GROSS, J., & LANGOVÁ, J. (1972). Stuttering and social isolation. *Journal of Nervous and Mental Diseases*, 155:1-5.
TATE, M. W., CULLINAN, W. L., & AHLSTRAND, A. (1961). Measurement of adaptation in stuttering. *Journal of Speech and Hearing Research*, 4:321-39.
TIFFANY, W. R., & HANLEY, C. N. (1954). An investigation into the use of electromechanically delayed auditory side tone in training. *Journal of Speech and Hearing Disorders*, 19:367-73.
TIMMONS, B. A., & BOUDREAU, J. P. (1972). Auditory feedback as a major factor in stuttering. *Journal of Speech and Hearing Disorders*, 37:476-84.
TORNICK, G. B., & BLOODSTEIN, O. (1976). Stuttering and sentence length. *Journal of Speech and Hearing Research*, 19:651-54.
TRAVIS, L. E. (1978). The cerebral dominance theory of stuttering: 1931-1978. *Journal of Speech and Hearing Disorders*, 43:278-81.
TREON, M., & TAMAYO, F. M. V. (1974). The separate and combined effects of GSR biofeedback and delayed auditory feedback on stuttering: A preliminary study. *Journal of Fluency Disorders*, 1:3-9.
TROJAN, F. A. (1965). A new method in the treatment of stuttering: The kinetic discharge therapy. *Folia Phoniatrica*, 17:195-201.
TROTTER, W. (1956). Relationship between severity of stuttering and word conspicuousness. *Journal of Speech and Hearing Disorders*, 21:198-201.
TROTTER, W. D., & LESCH, M. M. (1967). Personal experience with a stutter-aid. *Journal of Speech and Hearing Disorders*, 32:270-72.
TROTTER, W. D., & SILVERMAN, F. H. (1973). Experiments with a stutter-aid. *Perceptual and Motor Skills*, 36:1,124-30.
TROTTER, W. D., & SILVERMAN, F. H. (1974). Does the effect of pacing speech with a miniature metronome on stuttering wear off? *Perceptual and Motor Skills*, 39:429-30.
TROTTER, W. D., & SILVERMAN, F. H. (1976). The stutterer as a character in contemporary literature. *Journal of Speech and Hearing Disorders*, 41:553-54.
TURNBAUGH, K. R., GUITAR, B. E., & HOFFMAN, P. R. (1979). Speech clinicians' attribution of personality traits as a function of stuttering severity. *Journal of Speech and Hearing Research*, 22:37-45.
TURNBAUGH, K. R., GUITAR, B. E., & HOFFMAN, P. R. (1981). The attribution of personality traits: The stutterers and nonstutterers. *Journal of Speech and Hearing Research*, 24:288-91.
ULLIANA, L., & INGHAM, R. J. (1984). Behavioral and nonbehavioral variables in the measurement of stutterers' communication attitudes. *Journal of Speech and Hearing Disorders*, 49:83-93.
UNIVERSITY OF EDINBURGH BULLETIN (Feb. 28, 1979). *The Edinburgh Masker*, 15.
VAN DANTZIG, C. (1940). Syllable-tapping: A new method for the help of stammerers. *Journal of Speech Disorders*, 5:127-32.

VAN RIPER, C. (1937). Effect of devices for minimizing stuttering on the creation of symptoms. *Journal of Abnormal and Social Psychology*, 32:185-92.
VAN RIPER, C. (1938). A study of the stutterer's ability to interrupt stuttering spasms. *Journal of Speech Disorders*, 3:117-19.
VAN RIPER, C. (1947). *Speech Correction Principles and Methods*. Englewood Cliffs, N.J.: Prentice-Hall.
VAN RIPER, C. (1949). To the stutterer as he begins his speech therapy. *Journal of Speech Disorders*, 14:303-6.
VAN RIPER, C. (1954). *Speech Correction Principles and Methods*. Englewood Cliffs, N.J.: Prentice-Hall.
VAN RIPER, C. (1958). Experiments in stuttering therapy. J. Eisenson (ed.). *Stuttering, a Symposium*. New York: Harper & Row.
VAN RIPER, C. (1959). Binaural speech therapy. *Journal of Speech and Hearing Disorders*, 24:62-63.
VAN RIPER, C. (1965). Clinical use of intermittent masking noise in stuttering therapy. *Journal of the American Speech and Hearing Association*, 7:381.
VAN RIPER, C. (1970). The use of DAF in stuttering therapy. *British Journal of Disorders of Communication*, 4:40-45.
VAN RIPER, C. (1971). Symptomatic therapy for stuttering. L. E. Travis (ed.). *Handbook for Speech Pathology and Audiology*. New York: Appleton-Century-Crofts, Educ. Div., Meredith Corp.
VAN RIPER, C. (1973). *The Treatment of Stuttering*. Englewood Cliffs, N.J.: Prentice-Hall.
VAN RIPER, C. (No. 9). Putting it together. M. Fraser (dir.). *To the Stutterer*. Memphis, Tenn.: Speech Foundation of America.
VAN RIPER, C. (1974a). Modifying the stuttering. *Therapy for Stutterers*. Memphis, Tenn.: Speech Foundation of America, No. 10.
VAN RIPER, C. (1974b). The *ablauf* problem in stuttering. *Journal of Fluency Disorders*, 1:2-9.
VAN RIPER, C. (1974c). Stuttering: Where and whither? *Journal of the American Speech, Language and Hearing Association*, 16:483-87.
VAN RIPER, C. (1978). *Speech Correction Principles and Methods*. Englewood Cliffs, N.J.: Prentice-Hall.
VAN RIPER, C. (1982). *The Nature of Stuttering*. Englewood Cliffs, N.J.: Prentice-Hall.
VAN RIPER, C., & EMERICK, L. (1984). *Speech Correction Principles and Methods*. Englewood Cliffs, N.J.: Prentice-Hall.
VAN RIPER, C., & GRUBER, L. (1957). *A Casebook in Stuttering*. New York: Harper & Row.
VENKATAGIRI, H. S. (1980). The relevance of DAF-induced speech disruption to the understanding of stuttering. *Journal of Fluency Disorders*, 5:87-98.
VENKATAGIRI, H. S. (1981). Reaction time for voiced and whispered /a/ in stutterers and nonstutterers. *Journal of Fluency Disorders*, 6:265-71.
VENKATAGIRI, H. S. (1982a). A comparison of DAF-induced disfluencies with stuttering. *Journal of Communication Disorders*, 15:385-94.
VENKATAGIRI, H. S. (1982b). Reaction time for /s/ and /z/ in stutterers and nonstutterers: A test of the discoordination hypothesis. *Journal of Communication Disorders*, 15:55-68.
VLASOVA, N. A. (1962). Prevence a leceni koktavosti v detskem veku v USSR (Prevention and treatment of children's stuttering in the USSR). *Caskossslovenska Otolaryngol*, 4:30-32. In *dsh Abstracts*, No. 1046 (1962), 2:266.
VOLZ, H. B., KLEVANS, D. R., NORTON, S. J., & PUTENS, D. L. (1978). Interpersonal communication skills of speech-language pathology undergraduates: The effects of training. *Journal of Speech and Hearing Disorders*, 43:524-42.
WALL, M. J. & MYERS, F. J. (1982). A review of linguistic factors associated with early childhood stuttering. *Journal of Communication Disorders*, 15:441-50.
WALL, M. J., STARKWEATHER, C. W., & HARRIS, K. S., (1981). The influence of voicing adjustments on the location of stuttering in the spontaneous speech of young child stutterers. *Journal of Fluency Disorders*, 6:299-310.
WALLE, E. L. (1980). Masking devices and the Edinburgh Masker—clinical applications within a prison setting. *Journal of Fluency Disorders*, 5:69-74.
WALNUT, F. (1954). A personality inventory item analysis of individuals who stutter and who have other handicaps. *Journal of Speech and Hearing Disorders*, 19:220-27.
WALTON, D., & MATHER, M. D. (1963). The relevance of generalization techniques to the treatment of stammering and phobic systems. *Behavior Research and Therapy*, 1:121-25.
WATSON, B. C., & ALFONSO, P. J. (1982). A comparison of LRT and VOT values between stutterers and nonstutterers. *Journal of Fluency Disorders*, 7:219-42.
WATSON, B. C., & ALFONSO, P. J. (1983). Foreperiod and stuttering severity effects on acoustic laryngeal reaction time. *Journal of Fluency Disorders*, 8:183-205.
WATTS, F. (1971). The treatment of stammering by intensive practice of fluent speech. *British Journal of Communication Disorders*, 6:144-47.
WATTS, F. (1973). Mechanisms of fluency control in stutterers. *British Journal of Disorders of Communication*, 8:131-38.
WEBSTER, L. M. (1970). A clinical report on the measured effectiveness of certain desensitization techniques with stutterers. *Journal of Speech and Hearing Disorders*, 35:369-76.
WEBSTER, R. L. (1972). *An operant response shaping program for the establishment of fluency in stutterers: Final report*, Roanoke, Va.: Hollins College, 80.

WEBSTER, R. L. (1974). Behavioral analysis of stuttering: Treatment and theory. M. Calhoun (ed.). *Innovative Treatment Methods in Psychopathology*. New York: John Wiley.

WEBSTER, R. L. (1977). Concept and theory in stuttering: An insufficiency of empiricism. *Journal of Communication Disorders*, 10:65-71.

WEBSTER, R. L. (1978). Empirical considerations regarding stuttering therapy. H. Gregory (ed.). *Controversies About Stuttering Therapy*. Baltimore: University Park Press.

WEBSTER, R. L. & LUBKER B., (1968). Masking of auditory feedback in stutterers' speech. *Journal of Speech and Hearing Disorders*, 11:219-23.

WEBSTER, R. L., SCHUMACHER, S., & LUBKER, B. (1970). Changes in stuttering frequency as a function of various intervals of DAF. *Journal of Abnormal Psychology*, 75:45-49.

WEINER, A. E. (1978). Vocal control therapy for stutterers: A trial program. *Journal of Fluency Disorders*, 3:115-26.

WELLER, H. C. (1941). Vegetative rhythm determinative of speech patterns. *Journal of Speech Disorders*, 6:161-71.

WELLS, G. B. (1983). A feature analysis of stuttered phonemes. *Journal of Fluency Disorders*, 8:119-24.

WENDAHL, R. W., & COLE, J. (1961). Identification of stuttering during relatively fluent speech. *Journal of Speech and Hearing Research*, 4:281-86.

WERTHEIM, E. S. (1974). Key features of the bio-adaptive theory of stuttering and its clinical implications. *Australian Journal of Human Communication Disorders*, 2:86-94.

WEST, R. (1942). The pathology of stuttering. *The Nervous Child*, 2:96-106.

WHITTEN, I. F. (1938). Therapies used for stuttering: A report of the author's own case. *Quarterly Journal of Speech*, 24:227-33.

WILLIAMS, D. E. (1982). Stuttering therapy: Where are we going—and why? *Journal of Fluency Disorders*, 7:159-70.

WILLIAMS, D. E., & KENT, L. R. (1958). Listener evaluations of speech interruptions. *Journal of Speech and Hearing Research*, 1:124-31.

WILLIAMS, J. D., Comments on the use of the "Edinburgh Masker" device, Northern Illinois University, Dekalb, Ill.: Undated, received 1984.

WINGATE, M. E. (1962). Evaluation and stuttering, Part III: Identification of stuttering and the use of a label. *Journal of Speech and Hearing Disorders*, 27:368-77.

WINGATE, M. E. (1964). Recovery from stuttering. *Journal of Speech and Hearing Disorders*, 29:312-21.

WINGATE, M. E. (1966). Stuttering adaptation and learning: I. The relevance of adaptation studies to stuttering as "learned behavior." *Journal of Speech and Hearing Disorders*, 31:147-56.

WINGATE, M. E. (1967). Slurvian skill of stutterers. *Journal of Speech and Hearing Research*, 10:844-48.

WINGATE, M. E. (1969). Sound and pattern in "artificial" fluency. *Journal of Speech and Hearing Research*, 12:677-86.

WINGATE, M. E. (1973). A reply to Conture's "Comments on 'Effect on stuttering of changes in audition.'" *Journal of Speech and Hearing Research*, 13:861-73.

WINGATE, M. E. (1971a). The fear of stuttering. *Journal of American Speech and Hearing Association*, 13:3-5.

WINGATE, M. E. (1971b). Phonetic ability in stuttering. *Journal of Speech and Hearing Research*, 14:189-94.

WINGATE, M. E. (1976). *Stuttering Theory and Treatment*. New York: Irvington Publishers, John Wiley.

WINGATE, M. E. (1979a). The first three words. *Journal of Speech and Hearing Research*, 22:604-12.

WINGATE, M. E. (1979b). The loci of stuttering: Grammar or prosody? *Journal of Communication Disorders*, 12:283-90.

WINGATE, M. E. (1981). Sound and pattern in artificial fluency: Spectrographic evidence. *Journal of Fluency Disorders*, 6:95-118.

WINGATE, M. E. (1982). Early position and stuttering occurrence. *Journal of Fluency Disorders*, 7:243-58.

WINGATE, M. E. (1983). Speaking unassisted: Comments on a paper by Andrews, et al. *Journal of Speech and Hearing Disorders*, 48:255-63.

WOHL, M. T. (1966). Reciprocal inhibition—a process of continuous diagnosis. *Speech Pathology Diagnosis: Theory and Practice*. Report of the National Conference of the College of Speech Therapists. Edinburgh: E. & S. Livingston.

WOHL, M. T. (1968). The electronic metronome—an evaluative study. *British Journal of Disorders of Communication*, 3:89-98.

WOHL, M. T. (1970). The treatment of non-fluent utterance—a behavioral approach. *British Journal of Disorders of Communication*, 5:66-76.

WOLF, A. A., & WOLF, E. G. (1959). Feedback processes in the theory of certain speech disorders. *Speech Pathology and Therapy*, 2:48-55.

WOLK, L. (1981). Vocal tract dynamics in an adult stutterer. *South African Journal of Communication Disorders*, 28:38-52.

WOLPE, J. (1958). *Psychotherapy by Reciprocal Inhibition*. Stanford, Calif.: Stanford University Press.

WOLPE, J. (1973). *The Practice of Behavior Therapy*. New York: Pergamon Press.

WOODS, C. L. (1976). Stigma of a disorder. *Australian Journal of Human Disorders of Communication*, 4:133-39.

WOODS, C. L. (1977). Dimensions of the stutterer stereotype. *Australian Journal of Human Disorders of Communication*, 5:119-25.

Woods, C. L., & Williams, D. E. (1976). Traits attributed to stuttering and normally fluent males. *Journal of Speech and Hearing Research*, 19:267-78.

Wyke, B. (1974). Phonatory reflex mechanisms and stammering. *Folia Phoniatrica*, 26:321-28.

Wynne, M. K., & Boehmler, R. M. (1982). Central auditory function in fluent and disfluent normal speakers. *Journal of Speech and Hearing Research*, 25:54-57.

Yairi, E. (1972). Disfluency rate and patterns of stutterers and nonstutterers. *Journal of Communication Disorders*, 5:225-31.

Yairi, E., & Lewis, B. (1984). Disfluencies at the onset of stuttering. *Journal of Speech and Hearing Research*, 27:154-59.

Yates, A. J. (1963). Recent empirical and theoretical approaches to the experimental manipulation of speech in normal subjects and in stammerers. *Behavioral Research and Therapy*, 1:95-119.

Yonovitz, A., & Shepherd, W. J. (1977). Electrophysical measurement during a time-out procedure in stuttering and normal speakers. *Journal of Fluency Disorders*, 2:129-39.

Yonovitz, A., Shepherd, W. F. & Garrett, S. (1977). Hierarchial stimulation: Two cases of stuttering modification using systematic desensitization. *Journal of Fluency Disorders*, 2:21-28.

Young, M. A. (1964). Identification of stutterers from recorded samples of their fluent speech. *Journal of Speech and Hearing Research*, 7:302-3.

Young, M. (1965). Audience size, perceived situational difficulty, and stuttering frequency. *Journal of Speech and Hearing Research*, 8:401-7.

Young, M. A. (1975a). Observer agreement for marking moments of stuttering. *Journal of Speech and Hearing Research*, 18:530-40.

Young, M. A. (1975b). Onset, prevalence, and recovery from stuttering. *Journal of Speech and Hearing Disorders*, 40:49-58.

Young, M. A. (1980). Comparison of stuttering frequencies during reading and speaking. *Journal of Speech and Hearing Research*, 23:210-22.

Young, M. A., & Prather, E. M. (1962). Measuring severity of stuttering using short segments of speech. *Journal of Speech and Hearing Research*, 5:256-62.

Yovetich, W. S., Booth, J. C., & Tyler, R. S. (1977). The efects of dysfluencies on attention in stutterers and non-stutterers. *Human Communication*, 1:29-39.

Zalosh, S. & Salzman, L. F. (1965). After effects of delayed auditory feedback. *Perceptual and Motor Skills*, 20:817-23.

Zemlin, W. R. (1980). *Speech and Hearing Science, Anatomy, and Physiology*, Englewood Cliffs, N.J.: Prentice-Hall.

Zimmerman, G. (1980a). Articulation behaviors associated with stuttering: A cinefluorographic analysis. *Journal of Speech and Hearing Research*, 23:108-21.

Zimmerman, G. (1980b). Articulatory dynamics of fluent utterances of stutterers ad nonstutterers. *Journal of Speech and Hearing Research*, 23:95-107.

Zimmerman, G. (1980c). Stuttering: A disorder of movement. *Journal of Speech and Hearing Research*, 23:122-36.

Zsilavecz, U. (1981). Cybernetic functioning in stuttering. *South African Journal of Communication Disorders*, 28:60-66.

INDEX